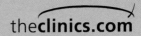

ULTRASOUND CLINICS

Genitourinary Ultrasound

Guest Editor

VIKRAM S. DOGRA, MD

Vascular Ultrasound

Guest Editor

DEBORAH J. RUBENS, MD

January 2006 • Volume 1 • Number 1

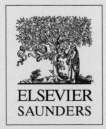

ELSEVIER
SAUNDERS

An imprint of Elsevier, Inc
PHILADELPHIA LONDON TORONTO MONTREAL SYDNEY TOKYO

W.B. SAUNDERS COMPANY
A Division of Elsevier Inc.

1600 John F. Kennedy Boulevard • Suite 1800 • Philadelphia, Pennsylvania 19103-2899

http://www.theclinics.com

ULTRASOUND CLINICS Volume 1, Number 1
January 2006 ISSN 1556-858X, ISBN 1-4160-3469-2

Editor: Barton Dudlick

Ultrasound Clinics (ISSN 1556-858X) is published bimonthly by W.B. Saunders Company. Corporate and editorial offices: 1600 John F. Kennedy Boulevard, Suite 1800, Philadelphia, Pennsylvania 19103-2899. Accounting and circulation offices: 6277 Sea Harbor Drive, Orlando, FL 32887-4800. Periodicals postage paid at Orlando, FL 32862, and additional mailing offices. Subscription prices are USD 150 per year for US individuals, USD 210 per year for US institutions, USD 75 per year for US students and residents, USD 170 per year for Canadian individuals, USD 200 per year for Canadian institutions, USD 170 per year for international individuals, USD 230 per year for international institutions and USD 85 per year for Canadian and foreign students/residents. To receive student and resident rate, orders must be accompanied by name of affiliated institution, date of term, and the signature of program/residency coordinator on institution letterhead. Orders will be billed at individual rate until proof of status is received. Foreign air speed delivery is included in all Clinics subscription prices. All prices are subject to change without notice. POSTMASTER: Send address changes to *Ultrasound Clinics*, W.B. Saunders Company, Periodicals Fulfillment, Orlando, FL 32887-4800. **Customer Service: 1-800-654-2452 (US). From outside of the US, call (+1) 407-345-4000.**

Printed in the United States of America.

GENITOURINARY ULTRASOUND
VASCULAR ULTRASOUND

PATRICK FULTZ, MD
Department of Radiology, University of Rochester School of Medicine and Dentistry, Rochester, New York

MARK KLIEWER, MD
Professor, Diagnostic Radiology, University of Wisconsin Medical School, Madison, Wisconsin

FELIX L. LIN, MD
Chief Resident, Diagnostic Radiology, Yale University School of Medicine, New Haven, Connecticut

MARK E. LOCKHART, MD, MPH
Associate Professor of Radiology, University of Alabama at Birmingham Hospital, Birmingham, Alabama

SARAH E. McACHRAN, MD
Resident, Department of Urology, Case School of Medicine, Cleveland, Ohio

SHANNON NEDELKA, MD
Adjunct Assistant Professor, Department of Radiology, University of Rochester Medical Center, Rochester, New York

RAJ MOHAN PASPULATI, MD
Assistant Professor, Department of Radiology, University Hospitals of Cleveland, Case Western Reserve University, Cleveland, Ohio

MARTIN I. RESNICK, MD
Lester Persky Professor and Chairman, Department of Urology, Case School of Medicine, Cleveland, Ohio

MICHELLE L. ROBBIN, MD
Professor of Radiology, Chief of Ultrasound, University of Alabama at Birmingham Hospital, Birmingham, Alabama

DEBORAH J. RUBENS, MD
Professor and Associate Chair, Department of Radiology and Surgery, University of Rochester School of Medicine and Dentistry, Rochester, New York

NAEL E.A. SAAD, MB, Bch
Diagnostic Radiology Resident, Vascular and Interventional Radiology Tract, Department of Radiology, University of Rochester Medical Center, Rochester, New York

WAEL E.A. SAAD, MB, Bch
Assistant Professor of Radiology, Department of Radiology, University of Rochester Medical Center, Rochester, New York

LESLIE M. SCOUTT
Professor, Diagnostic Radiology, Chief Section of Ultrasound, Yale University School of Medicine, New Haven, Connecticut

CARLOS J. SIVIT, MD
Professor of Radiology and Pediatrics, Case School of Medicine; Director of Pediatric Radiology, Rainbow Babies and Children's Hospital, Cleveland, Ohio

SUSAN L. VOCI, MD
Associate Professor of Radiology, Department of Radiology, University of Rochester Medical Center, Rochester, New York

SRINIVAS VOURGANTI, MD
University Hospitals of Cleveland; Professor, Department of Urology, Case Western Reserve School of Medicine, Cleveland, Ohio

THERESE M. WEBER, MD
Associate Professor, Department of Radiology, Wake Forest University School of Medicine, Winston-Salem, North Carolina

GENITOURINARY ULTRASOUND
VASCULAR ULTRASOUND

Volume 1 • Number 1 • January 2006

Contents

provocative maneuvers also can help to distinguish accurately between the internal carotid artery and external carotid artery and to identify a subclavian stenosis by converting a presteal to a complete vertebral steal. Certain iatrogenic conditions can be recognized by their Doppler waveforms and gray-scale features. It is important to recognize the effect of such conditions on the Doppler waveform to avoid pitfalls in grading carotid stenosis.

FORTHCOMING ISSUES

ULTRASOUND CLINICS JANUARY 2006

GOAL STATEMENT

The goal of the *Ultrasound Clinics* is to keep practicing radiologists and radiology residents up to date with current clinical practice in ultrasound by providing timely articles reviewing the state-of-the-art in patient care.

ACCREDITATION

The *Ultrasound Clinics* is planned and implemented in accordance with the Essential Areas and Policies of the Accreditation Council for Continuing Medical Education (ACCME) through the joint sponsorship of the University of Virginia School of Medicine and Elsevier. The University of Virginia School of Medicine is accredited by the ACCME to provide continuing medical education for physicians.

The University of Virginia School of Medicine designates this educational activity for a maximum of 60 category 1 credits per year, 15 category 1 credits per issue, toward the AMA Physician's Recognition Award. Each physician should claim only those credits that he/she actually spent in the activity.

The American Medical Association has determined that physicians not licensed in the US who participate in this CME activity are eligible for AMA PRA category 1 credit.

Category 1 credit can be earned by reading the text material, taking the CME examination online at http://www.theclinics.com/home/cme, and completing the evaluation. After taking the test, you will be required to review any and all incorrect answers. Following completion of the test and evaluation, your credit will be awarded and you may print your certificate.

FACULTY DISCLOSURE/CONFLICT OF INTEREST

The University of Virginia School of Medicine, as an ACCME accredited provider, endorses and strives to comply with the Accreditation Council for Continuing Medical Education (ACCME) Standards of Commercial Support, Commonwealth of Virginia statutes, University of Virginia policies and procedures, and associated federal and private regulations and guidelines on the need for disclosure and monitoring of proprietary and financial interests that may affect the scientific integrity and balance of content delivered in continuing medical education activities under our auspices.

The University of Virginia School of Medicine requires that all CME activities accredited through this institution be developed independently and be scientifically rigorous, balanced and objective in the presentation/discussion of its content, theories and practices.

All authors/editors participating in an accredited CME activity are expected to disclose to the readers relevant financial relationships with commercial entities occurring within the past 12 months (such as grants or research support, employee, consultant, stock holder, member of speakers bureau, etc.). The University of Virginia School of Medicine will employ appropriate mechanisms to resolve potential conflicts of interest to maintain the standards of fair and balanced education to the reader. Questions about specific strategies can be directed to the Office of Continuing Medical Education, University of Virginia School of Medicine, Charlottesville, Virginia.

The authors/editors listed below have identified no professional or financial affiliations for themselves or their spouse/partner:
Piyush K. Agarwal, MD; Shweta Bhatt, MD; Nancy Carson, MBA, RDMS, RVT; Jeanne Cullinan, MD; Vikram S. Dogra, MD; Barton Dudlick, Acquisitions Editor; Mark Kliewer , MD; Felix L. Lin, MD; Mark E. Lockhart, MD, MPH; Sarah E. McAchran, MD; Shannon Nedelka, MD; Raj Mohan Paspulati, MD; Martin I. Resnick, MD; Michelle L. Robbin, MD; Deborah J. Rubens, MD; Nael E. A. Saad, MBBCh; Wael E. A. Saad, MBBCh; Leslie M. Scoutt, MD; Carlos J. Sivit, MD; Susan L. Voci, MD; Srinivas Vourganti, MD; and Therese M. Weber, MD.

The authors/editors listed below have identified the following professional or financial affiliations for themselves or their spouse/partner:
David R. Bodner, MD is on the speakers' bureau and has teaching engagements for Merck, Sanofi Aventis, Boehringer Ingelheim, and Novartis. Additionally, he owns stock in Merck and Medtronics.
W. Scott Burgin, MD has research support from Spencer Technologies for TCD research.

Disclosure of Discussion of non-FDA approved uses for pharmaceutical products and/or medical devices:
The University of Virginia School of Medicine, as an ACCME provider, requires that all faculty presenters identify and disclose any "off label" uses for pharmaceutical and medical device products. The University of Virginia School of Medicine recommends that each physician fully review all the available data on new products or procedures prior to instituting them with patients.

TO ENROLL

To enroll in the *Ultrasound Clinics* Continuing Medical Education program, call customer service at 1-800-654-2452 or visit us online at www.theclinics.com/home/cme. The CME program is available to subscribers for an additional fee of $205.00

ULTRASOUND CLINICS

Ultrasound Clin 1 (2006) xi–xii

Preface
Genitourinary Ultrasound

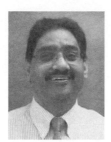

Vikram S. Dogra, MD
Guest Editor

Vikram S. Dogra, MD
Department of Imaging Sciences
University of Rochester Medical Center
601 Elmwood Avenue, Box 648
Rochester NY 14642, USA

E-mail address:
vikram_dogra@urmc.rochester.edu

The rapid advances and refinements of modern imaging systems have provided a wide array of diagnostic tools for practicing radiologists. Ultrasound has enjoyed considerable technical improvement as a result of improved materials, electronics, and computer processing, as has also been the case with CT and MR imaging. These changes have resulted in the availability of high-resolution real-time grayscale imaging, tissue harmonic evaluation, and color and power Doppler analysis. As a consequence of this revival of ultrasound imaging, there has been tremendous growth in the number of ultrasound examinations performed. The increased popularity of ultrasound imaging has therefore encouraged an increased demand for knowledge pertaining to medical ultrasound. There are few ultrasound journals currently available that address all the issues pertaining to sonography in its totality.

There has long been a need for a new medical periodical devoted to medical ultrasound. This new publication, the *Ultrasound Clinics*, is devoted to furthering the knowledge of ultrasound imaging involving every aspect of sonography. This quarterly periodical will have issues dedicated to obstetrics and gynecology, abdominal, vascular, emergency, genitourinary disease, and cardiac imaging. It will also cover topics pertaining to advances in ultrasound technology and new developments.

I am honored to be the Guest Editor of this inaugural issue of the *Ultrasound Clinics* together with Deborah Rubens, who is a very close friend and colleague.

The topics in this issue have been chosen with particular attention to genitourinary and vascular sonography. The review articles have been written by very experienced radiologists who have dedicated their lives to the field of ultrasonography. Most of the articles have a section devoted to the pertinent anatomy and sonographic technique where relevant to aid those readers who are new to the practice of ultrasonography. There is a liberal use of line drawings to explain the ultrasound concepts for easy understanding and reading. Key concepts have been stressed. This issue provides both imaging specialists and clinicians with up-to-date information regarding what is new, exciting, and

doi:10.1016/j.cult.2005.10.001

relevant in the practice of ultrasonography as it pertains to genitourinary and sonography.

I wish to express my sincere thanks to Shweta Bhatt, MD, for her assistance in helping me to complete this issue on schedule. I would also like to thank Bonnie Hami, MA, for her editorial assistance and Joseph Molter for preparation of the illustrations. I am also extremely thankful to Barton Dudlick at Elsevier for his administrative and editorial assistance.

ULTRASOUND
CLINICS

Ultrasound Clin 1 (2006) 1–13

Ultrasonographic Evaluation of Renal Infections

Srinivas Vourganti, MD[a], Piyush K. Agarwal, MD[a],
Donald R. Bodner, MD[a,*], Vikram S. Dogra, MD[b]

Medical ultrasonography dates back to the 1930s when it was adapted from technology used to test the strength of metal hulls of ships and applied to detect brain tumors [1]. Now with ultrasound being performed outside of the radiology suite and in emergency departments, patient clinics, hospital rooms, and doctors' offices, it compromises approximately 25% of all imaging studies performed worldwide [2]. Ultrasonography is non-invasive, rapid, readily available, portable, and offers no exposure to contrast or radiation. Furthermore, it is easily interpretable by physicians of several different disciplines and can result in quick diagnosis and treatment of potentially life-threatening conditions. Some of these conditions include severe kidney infections. This article focuses on reviewing ultrasound characteristics of various renal infections.

Ultrasound principles

Electric waveforms are applied to piezoelectric elements in the transducer causing them to vibrate and emit sound waves. The frequency range of

[a] Department of Urology, Case Western Reserve University School of Medicine and University Hospitals of Cleveland, 11100 Euclid Avenue, Cleveland, OH 44022, USA
[b] Department of Imaging Sciences, University of Rochester School of Medicine, 601 Elmwood Avenue, Box 648, Rochester, NY 14642, USA
* Corresponding author.
E-mail address: Dbodner180@aol.com (D.R. Bodner).

doi:10.1016/j.cult.2005.09.002

the sound waves emitted is above the audible human range of 20 to 20,000 Hz (cycles per second). The sound waves generated range in frequency from 1 to 15 MHz (1,000,000 cycles per second) and are directed by the transducer into the body where they are either reflected, absorbed, or refracted based on the density of the different tissues the waves pass through. Sound passes through soft tissue at an average velocity of 1540 m/s. As the sound passes through tissues of differing densities, a portion of the sound waves is reflected back to the transducer and converted into electrical signals that are then amplified to produce an image. The strength of the returning sound waves or echoes is proportional to the difference in density between the two tissues forming the interface through which the sound waves are traveling [3]. If the sound waves encounter a homogenous fluid medium, such as the fluid in a renal cyst, they are transmitted through without interruption. As a result, no echoes are reflected back to the transducer, which produces an anechoic image [4]. Sound waves that are strongly reflected generate strong echoes and are visualized as bright white lines, creating a hyperechoic image.

In imaging the kidney, the highest frequency that produces adequate tissue penetration with a good resolution is selected. Tissue penetration is inversely related to the frequency of the transducer. Therefore, as the frequency increases, the depth of tissue penetration decreases. Conversely, image resolution is directly related to the frequency of the transducer. Therefore, as the frequency increases, the spatial resolution of the image increases [5]. To balance these two competing factors, a 3.5- or 5-MHz transducer is used to image the kidneys.

Ultrasound technique

Patients are imaged in the supine position and a coupling medium (eg, gel) is applied to the transducer to reduce the interference that may be introduced by air between the transducer and the skin. Generally a 3.5-MHz transducer is used, but a 5-MHz transducer can provide high-quality images in children or thin, adult patients. A breath-hold may be elicited by instructing the patient to hold their breath at maximal inspiration. This action will displace the kidneys inferiorly by approximately 2.5 cm and may provide a better view. The right kidney can be found by placing the transducer along the right lateral subcostal margin in the anterior axillary line during an inspiratory breath-hold. If the kidney cannot be imaged because of overlying bowel gas, then the probe can be moved laterally to the midaxillary line or the posterior axillary line. Imaging the left kidney is often more

challenging as it is located more superiorly, lacks an acoustic window such as the liver, and is covered by overlying gas from the stomach and small bowel. The left kidney can be localized by positioning the patient in the right lateral decubitus position and by placing the probe in the left posterior axillary line or in the left costovertebral angle [6]. The renal examination should include long-axis and transverse views of the upper poles, midportions, and lower poles. The cortex and renal pelvic regions should then be assessed. A maximum measurement of renal length should be recorded for both kidneys. Decubitus, prone, or upright positioning may provide better images of the kidney. When possible, renal echogenicity should be compared with the adjacent liver and spleen. The kidneys and perirenal regions should be assessed for abnormalities. Doppler may be used to differentiate vascular from nonvascular structures [7].

The normal kidney appears elliptical in longitudinal view [**Fig. 1**]. The right kidney varies in length from 8 to 14 cm, whereas the left kidney measures 7 to 12.5 cm. The kidneys are generally within 2 cm of each other in length and are 4 to 5 cm in width [8]. The renal cortex is homogenous and hypoechoic to the liver or spleen. The renal sinus contains the peripelvic fat; lymphatic and renal vessels; and the collecting system, and appears as a dense, central echogenic complex. The medulla can sometimes be differentiated from the cortex by the presence of small and round hypoechoic structures adjacent to the renal sinus [9].

Renal infections

Acute pyelonephritis

A patient who has acute pyelonephritis will classically appear with localized complaints of flank pain and costovertebral angle tenderness accompanied by generalized symptoms of fever, chills, nausea, and vomiting. In addition, these findings may be accompanied by further lower urinary tract symptoms, including dysuria, increased urinary frequency, and voiding urgency [10]. Laboratory abnormalities indicative of the underlying infection can be expected, including neutrophilic leukocytosis on the complete blood count and elevated erythrocyte sedimentation rate and serum C–reactive protein levels. If the infection is severe, it may interfere with renal function and cause an elevation of serum creatinine [11].

Evaluation of the urine will usually demonstrate frank pyuria with urinalysis demonstrating the presence of leukocyte esterase and nitrites and microscopic findings of numerous leukocytes and bacteria [12]. However, sterile urine can be seen despite acute

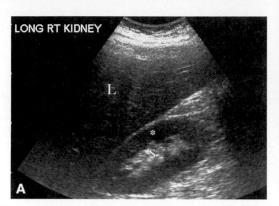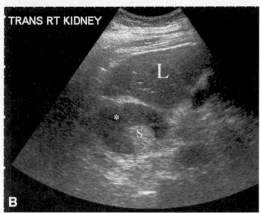

Fig. 1. Normal kidney. Longitudinal (*A*) and transverse (*B*) gray-scale sonogram of the right kidney demonstrates a hypoechoic renal cortex (*asterisk*) as compared with the liver, and a central hyperechoic renal sinus. L, liver; S, renal sinus.

pyelonephritis, especially in the setting of obstruction of the infected kidney [11]. Urine cultures, which should be collected before starting antibiotic therapy, will almost exclusively demonstrate ascending infection from gram-negative bacteria. Eighty percent of infections are caused by *Escherichia coli.* The remainder of cases is mostly caused by other gram-negative organisms, including *Klebsiella, Proteus, Enterobacter, Pseudomonas, Serratia,* and *Citrobacter.* With the exception of *Enterococcus faecalis* and *Staphylococcus epidermidis,* gram-positive bacteria are rarely the cause of acute pyelonephritis [10].

In addition to bacterial nephritis, fungal infections of the kidney are also possible. Infections with fungi are more commonly present in the setting of diabetes, immunosuppression, urinary obstruction, or indwelling urinary catheters [12]. Most commonly, *Candida* sp such as *Candida albicans* and *Candida tropicalis* are the causative organisms. In addition to the Candida, other fungi such as *Torulopsis glabrata, Aspergillus* sp, *Cryptococcus neoformans,* Zygomycetes (ie, *Rhizopus, Rhizomucor, Mucor,* and *Absidia* sp), and *Histoplasma capsulatum* may cause renal infections with less frequency. Clinically, these infections present similarly to bacterial infections. Diagnosis can be accomplished by evaluation of the urine where fungus can be found microscopically or through fungal cultures. These infections can cause the formation of fungal balls, otherwise called bezoars, in the renal pelvis and collecting system, which can contribute to obstruction [13].

Ultrasonographic features of acute pyelonephritis

Imaging is generally not necessary for the diagnosis and treatment of acute pyelonephritis. In un-

complicated cases, ultrasound imaging will usually find a normal-appearing kidney [6]. However, in 20% of cases, generalized renal edema attributed to inflammation and congestion is present, which can be detected by ultrasound evaluation. This edema is formally defined as an overall kidney length in excess of 15 cm or, alternatively, an affected kidney that is at least 1.5 cm longer than the unaffected side [11]. Dilatation of the collecting system in the absence of appreciable obstructive cause may also be detected by ultrasound. A proposed mechanism of this dilatation is that bacterial endotoxins may inhibit normal ureteric peristaltic motion, resulting in hydroureter and hydronephrosis [10]. Parallel lucent streaks in the renal pelvis and ureter, which are most likely caused by mucosal edema, may also be detected on ultrasound. This finding is the equivalent of a striated nephrogram appearance on CT. Additionally, the renal parenchyma may be hypoechoic or attenuated. In cases of fungal infection, collections of air may be seen in the bladder or collecting system as the fungus may be gas-forming. In addition, ultrasonography may demonstrate evidence of fungal debris in the collecting system, such as a bezoar and consequent obstruction [**Fig. 2**] [13].

In relation to other modalities of renal imaging (Tc-99m dimercaptosuccinic acid [DMSA] scintigraphy, spiral CT, and MR), ultrasound has been found to be less sensitive and specific in the diagnosis of acute pyelonephritis [14]. In the pediatric population, where a missed diagnosis can mean irreversible damage, Tc-99m DMSA scintigraphy is still considered the gold standard of imaging [15]. Improvements in ultrasound techniques by way of power Doppler ultrasonography have resulted in better imaging than B-mode ultrasonography alone, but do not improve on the accuracy of Tc-99m DMSA

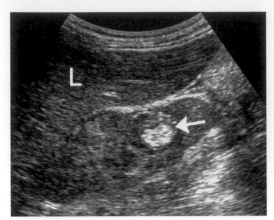

Fig. 2. Fungal ball. Longitudinal gray-scale sonogram of the right kidney in an immunocompromised patient demonstrates an echogenic mass (*arrow*) within a dilated calyx confirmed to be a fungus ball. L, liver.

scintigraphy [16]. Some authors suggest that although power Doppler cannot replace Tc-99m DMSA scintigraphy because of its lack of sensitivity, a positive power Doppler ultrasound finding can obviate the need for further imaging [17]. In addition, when combined with concomitant laboratory findings such as an elevated serum C–reactive protein level, sensitivity and specificity can be improved, and results correlate with those of DMSA findings [18]. However, suggestions that ultrasound can serve as a replacement to other more sensitive modalities in the detection of acute pyelonephritis remain controversial.

Acute focal and multifocal pyelonephritis (acute lobar nephronia)

Acute focal and multifocal pyelonephritis occur when infection is confined to a single lobe or occurs in multiple lobes, respectively, of the kidney. More common in patients who have diabetes and those who are immunosuppressed, these infections will present with clinical features similar to acute pyelonephritis. However, the patient will generally experience more severe symptoms than patients

who have uncomplicated pyelonephritis. In addition, focal pyelonephritis commonly progresses to sepsis [10]. Treatment is similar to other complicated cases of acute pyelonephritis, with 7 days of parenteral antibiotics followed by a 7-day course of oral antibiotics [11].

Ultrasonographic features of acute focal and multifocal pyelonephritis

In imaging acute focal pyelonephritis, it is important to differentiate it from the more severe case of a renal abscess that requires more aggressive management. On ultrasound, the classic description of acute focal pyelonephritis is of a sonolucent mass that is poorly marginated with occasional low-amplitude echoes that disrupt the corticomedullary junction [**Fig. 3**] [6]. The absence of a distinct wall is a defining feature that differentiates focal nephritis from the more serious renal abscess [19]. Farmer and colleagues suggest that an ultrasonographic appearance of increased echogenicity, rather than sonolucent masses, may also be commonly seen in focal nephritis [20]. The ultrasound evaluation should be complemented with a CT evaluation, which is more sensitive in detecting focal pyelonephritis [21]. CT findings demonstrate a lobar distribution of inflammation that appears as a wedge-shaped area of decreased contrast enhancement on delayed images. In more severe disease, a hypodense mass lesion can be seen [19]. The radiologic appearance of multifocal disease is identical to focal disease except that it is seen in more than one lobe.

Renal abscess

Before the advent of antibiotics, most abscesses in the kidney were caused by hematogenous spread (usually of *Staphylococcus* sp) from distant sites. These renal carbuncles would be associated with a history (often remote) of a gram-positive infection elsewhere in the body, such as a carbuncle of the skin [10]. With antibiotic therapy now common, renal carbuncles are now rare, and instances of

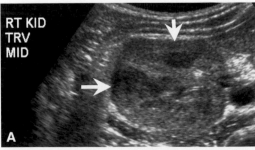

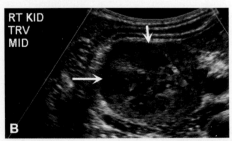

Fig. 3. Pyelonephritis. Transverse gray-scale (*A*) and color flow Doppler (*B*) sonography of the right kidney demonstrate two wedge-shaped areas of decreased echogenicity (*arrows*) in the renal cortex with absence of color flow, consistent with multifocal pyelonephritis.

renal abscess are now primarily caused by ascending infection with enteric, aerobic, gram-negative bacilli, including *Escherichia coli*, *Klebsiella* sp, and *Proteus* sp [19]. Patients are at an increased risk for these abscesses if they have a complicated urinary tract infection (with stasis or obstruction), are diabetic, or are pregnant [10]. Patients will present with fever, chills, and pain in their back and abdomen. In addition, many will have symptoms characteristic of a urinary tract infection, such as dysuria, frequency, urgency, and suprapubic pain. Constitutional symptoms of malaise and weight loss may also be seen [10]. Laboratory studies will demonstrate a leukocytosis. In nearly all renal carbuncles, and up to 30% of gram-negative abscesses, the abscess does not involve the collecting system and urine cultures will be negative [19]. In general, any positive urine culture will match the blood culture in the setting of an ascending gram-negative abscess. In the event of a gram-positive renal carbuncle, the urine culture and blood cultures may isolate different organisms from one another [10].

The management of renal abscesses is generally dictated by their size. Small abscesses (smaller than 3 cm) are treated conservatively with observation and parenteral antibiotics. Similar-sized lesions in patients who are immunocompromised may be treated more aggressively with some form of abscess drainage. Lesions between 3 and 5 cm are often treated with percutaneous drainage. Any abscess larger than 5 cm usually requires surgical drainage.

Ultrasonographic features of renal abscess

Ultrasound is particularly useful in the diagnosis of renal abscess [19]. It usually shows an enlarged kidney with distortion of the normal renal contour [**Fig. 4**]. Acutely, the abscess will appear to have indistinct margins with edema in the surrounding renal parenchyma. However, after convalescence, it will appear as a fluid-filled mass with a distinct wall. This clear margin helps to distinguish this entity from the less severe focal nephritis. Once identified by ultrasound, CT scanning with contrast enhancement can better characterize these lesions. The abscess will be seen as a round or oval pa-

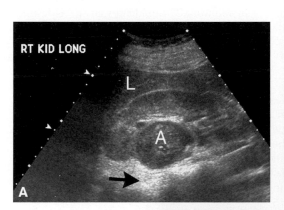

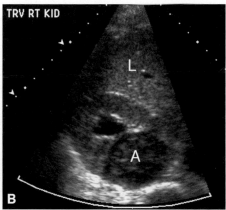

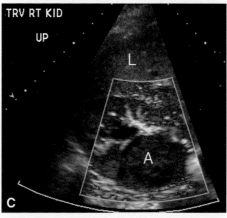

Fig. 4. Renal abscess. Longitudinal (*A*) and transverse (*B*) gray-scale ultrasound of the right kidney reveal presence of a well-defined hypoechoic lesion (A) near the superior pole, with posterior through transmission (*arrow*). Corresponding power Doppler image (*C*) demonstrates an increased peripheral vascularity. L, Liver.

renchymal mass with decreased levels of attenuation. A ring circumscribing the lesion will form with contrast enhancement ("ring sign") because of the increased vascularity of the abscess wall [10]. In many instances, it will be difficult to definitively distinguish a renal abscess from a renal tumor. In these cases, radiologic-guided drainage with analysis of fluid can be helpful in establishing the diagnosis.

Emphysematous pyelonephritis

Emphysematous pyelonephritis is a complication of acute pyelonephritis in which gas-forming organisms infect renal parenchyma. It is usually caused by *E coli* (70% of cases), but *Klebsiella pneumoniae* and *Proteus mirabilis* can cause emphysematous pyelonephritis with less frequency [22]. A necrotizing infection occurs in the renal parenchyma and perirenal tissues in which tissue is used as a substrate with carbon dioxide gas released as a byproduct. Clinically, this infection usually occurs in patients who have diabetes in the setting of urinary tract obstruction. Women are affected more than men. There have been no reported cases in children. Nearly all patients will present with the following triad of symptoms: fever, vomiting, and flank pain. Pneumaturia can be seen when the collecting system is involved. However, focal physical findings are commonly absent [11].

Once discovered, prompt treatment is imperative. Management should begin with supportive care, management of diabetes, and relief of any underlying obstruction. If infection is discovered in one kidney, the contralateral kidney should also be thoroughly investigated, as bilateral involvement is seen in up to 10% of cases. The classic management for emphysematous pyelonephritis is administration of broad-spectrum antibiotics along with emergent nephrectomy [10]. Despite this aggressive therapy, mortality is seen in 30% to 40% of cases.

Ultrasonographic findings of emphysematous pyelonephritis

Emphysematous pyelonephritis is diagnosed by demonstrating gas in the renal parenchyma with or without extension into the perirenal tissue [10]. Ultrasound examination will characteristically show an enlarged kidney containing high-amplitude echoes within the renal parenchyma, often with low-level posterior dirty acoustic shadowing known as reverberation artifacts [**Fig. 5**]. However, the depth of parenchymal involvement may be underestimated during the ultrasound examination. Consequently, multiple renal stones may also manifest as echogenic foci without

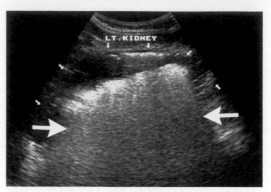

Fig. 5. Emphysematous pyelonephritis. Longitudinal gray-scale sonogram of the left kidney (*small arrows*) demonstrates air within the renal parenchyma with reverberation artifact (*large arrows*).

"clean" posterior shadowing [23,24]. The isolated presence of gas within the collecting system can be seen after many interventional procedures and should not be confused with emphysematous pyelonephritis. In these cases, an evaluation using CT is always warranted and is considered the ideal study to visualize the extent and amount of gas. In addition, CT can identify any local destruction to perirenal tissues. Radiologic studies play an important role in evaluation of the effectiveness of therapy in emphysematous pyelonephritis. As carbon dioxide is rapidly absorbed, any persistence of gas after 10 days of appropriate treatment is indicative of failed therapy [10].

Pyonephrosis

Pyonephrosis is a suppurative infection in the setting of hydronephrosis, which occurs as the result of obstruction. The renal pelvis and calyces become distended with pus [6]. Patients present with fevers, chills, and flank pain. Because of the obstruction, bacteriuria can be absent. It is imperative that this obstruction is relieved through a nephrostomy or ureteral stent. If untreated, pyonephrosis can cause destruction of renal parenchyma and irreversible loss of renal function [10].

Ultrasonographic features of pyonephrosis

Ultrasound findings are useful in early and accurate diagnosis of pyonephrosis. On examination, persistent echoes are seen in a dilated collecting system [**Fig. 6**]. This echogenicity is caused by debris in the collecting system, and is therefore seen in dependent areas of the collecting system. Shifts in this debris can sometimes be appreciated if the patient is asked to change positions during the ultrasound examination. In addition, air can be seen in these infections. In this event, strong echoes with acous-

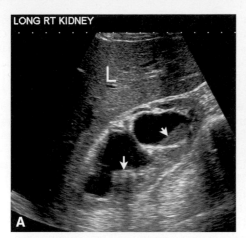
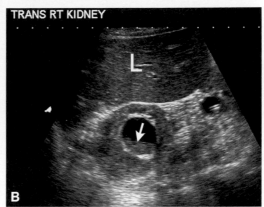

Fig. 6. Pyohydronephrosis. Longitudinal (*A*) and transverse (*B*) gray-scale sonogram of the right kidney demonstrate an enlarged hydronephrotic kidney with a fluid–fluid level (*arrows*) in the dilated calyces secondary to pus appearing as echogenic debris. L, liver.

tic shadowing can be seen behind the affected area of the collecting system [11].

Xanthogranulomatous pyelonephritis

Xanthogranulomatous pyelonephritis (XGP) is a rare inflammatory condition that is seen in the setting of long-term and recurrent obstruction from nephrolithiasis accompanied by infection. It results in the irreversible destruction of renal parenchyma. This damage begins in the renal pelvis and calyces and eventually extends into the renal parenchyma and can occur in either a diffuse or segmental pattern [11]. Though the cause of XGP is unknown, it is thought that the inflammatory process that occurs in response to tissue damage by bacterial infection (usually *Proteus mirabilis* or *E coli*) results in the deposition of lipid-laden histiocytes at the site of infection. These macrophages, or xanthoma cells, along with other inflammatory cells result in the formation of fibrous tissue. This granulomatous process eventually replaces the adjacent normal renal parenchyma and adjacent renal tissue [10].

Clinically, XGP is seen more commonly in women than men. Incidence peaks during the fifth to sixth decade of life. Patients who have diabetes are predisposed to the formation of XGP. Symptoms include those that suggest underlying chronic infection in the setting of obstruction, such as fever, flank pain, persistent bacteriuria, or history of recurrent infected nephrolithiasis. XGP results in the irregular enlargement of the kidney and is often misdiagnosed as a tumor. Even by pathologic examination, XGP can closely resemble malignancy, such as renal cell carcinoma. Definitive diagnosis is often made only after surgical removal, which allows thorough pathologic examination. Treatment of XGP involves surgical removal

of the entire inflammatory process. Limited disease may be amenable to partial nephrectomy; however, more widespread XGP requires total nephrectomy and removal of the involved adjacent tissue [11]. Though classic management suggests that conservative intervention through simple incision and drainage commonly results in further complications, some investigators suggest this course in cases of limited focal disease [25].

Ultrasonographic features of xanthogranulomatous pyelonephritis

Definitive preoperative diagnosis is extremely difficult to establish in XGP. By ultrasound evaluation, multiple hypoechoic round masses can be seen in the affected kidney. These masses can demonstrate internal echoes and can be abscesses (with increased sound through-transmission) or solid granulomatous processes (with decreased sound through-transmission) [11]. Global enlargement with relative preservation of the renal contour can be seen with diffuse disease. However, in focal or segmental XGP a mass-like lesion may be appreciated. In addition, evidence of obstruction and renal calculus is commonly seen (85%) [26]. In general, CT evaluation is considered more informative than ultrasound in describing XGP. A large reniform mass within the renal pelvis tightly surrounding a central calcification is seen on CT imaging [10]. Dilated calyces and abscesses that replace normal renal parenchyma will appear as water-density masses. Calcifications and low attenuation areas attributed to lipid-rich xanthogranulomatous tissue may be seen within the masses [27]. If contrast is used, a blush is seen in the walls of these masses because of their vascularity. This enhancement, which is limited to the mass wall only, will help distinguish XGP from renal tumors and other inflammatory processes that do enhance throughout [11].

Renal malakoplakia

Renal malakoplakia is a rare inflammatory disorder associated with a chronic coliform gram-negative urinary tract infection (usually *E coli*) resulting in the deposition of soft, yellow-brown plaques within the bladder and upper urinary tract. The cause is thought to be abnormal macrophage function that causes incomplete intracellular bacterial lysis. This lysis results in the deposition of histiocytes, called von Hansemann cells, that are filled with these bacteria and bacterial fragments. The bacteria form a nidus for calcium phosphate crystals, which form small basophilic bodies called Michaelis-Gutmann bodies [10].

Clinically, malakoplakia of the urinary tract usually occurs in women. Most patients are older than 50 years. There is often an underlying condition compromising the immune system, such as diabetes, immunosuppression, or the presence of a chronic debilitating disease. Symptoms of a urinary tract infection may be present, such as fever, irritative voiding symptoms, and flank pain. In addition, a palpable mass may be appreciated [11]. If the disease involves the bladder, symptoms of bladder irritability and hematuria may be seen.

Ultrasonographic features of malakoplakia

Imaging findings of malakoplakia are nonspecific and can often mimic other pathology, such as renal tumors [28]. The most common ultrasonographic feature of renal malakoplakia is diffuse enlargement of the affected kidney [29]. Increased echogenicity of the renal parenchyma can be seen because of a confluence of the plaques [10]. In addition, hypoechoic lesions and distortion of parenchymal echoes may be appreciated [29].

Hydatid disease of the kidney (renal echinococcosis)

Echinococcosis is a parasitic infection that is most commonly seen in South Africa, the Mediterranean, Eastern Europe, Australia, and New Zealand. It is caused by the tapeworm *Echinococcus granulosis*. Although the adult form is zoonotic, mostly found in the intestines of dogs, humans may serve as an intermediate host of this parasite while it is in the larval stage [11]. Infection more commonly manifests in the liver and lungs, with only 4% of echinococcosis involving the kidney, because the larvae, which originally invade the body through the gastrointestinal tract, must first escape sequestration in the liver and subsequently the lungs. Only after these two defenses are surpassed are the larvae able to gain widespread access to the systemic circulation, and correspondingly, the kidneys [30].

The offending lesion will most commonly form as a solitary mass in the renal cortex. It is divided into three distinct zones. The outermost adventitial layer consists of host fibroblasts that may become calcified. A middle laminated layer consists of hyaline that surrounds a third inner germinal layer. The germinal layer is composed of nucleated epithelium and is where the echinococcal larvae reproduce. The larvae attach to the surrounding germinal layer and form brood capsules. These brood capsules grow in size and will remain connected to the germinal layer by a pedicle for nutrition. The core of this hydatid cyst contains detached brood capsules (daughter cysts), free larvae, and fluid, a combination known as hydatid sand [10].

Clinically, most patients who have renal echinococcosis are asymptomatic, especially in the beginning stages of the disease process because the cyst starts small and grows at a rate of only 1 cm annually. Because of their focal nature, small hydatid cysts will rarely affect renal function. As the lesion progresses, a mass effect will contribute to symptoms of dull flank pain, hematuria, and a palpable mass on examination [10]. If the cyst ruptures, a strong antigenic immune response ensues with possible urticaria and even anaphylaxis [30]. If a cyst ruptures into the collecting system, the patient will develop symptoms of hydatiduria, including renal colic and passage of urinary debris resembling grape skins [11].

Treatment of echinococcal disease in the kidney is primarily surgical. Medical therapy with antiparasitic agents, such as mebendazole, has been shown to be largely unsuccessful. In removing a cyst, great care must be taken to avoid its rupture. Any release of cyst contents can contribute to anaphylaxis. In addition, the release of the larvae can result in the dissemination of the disease. In the event of rupture, or if resection of the entire cyst is not possible, careful aspiration of the cyst is indicated. After the contents of the cyst are removed, an infusion of an antiparasitic agent (eg, 30% sodium chloride, 0.5% silver nitrate, 2% formalin, or 1% iodine) is reinfused into the cyst [11].

Ultrasonographic features of renal echinococcosis

Ultrasonographic findings of echinococcosis demonstrate different findings based on the age, extent, and complications of the hydatid cyst [30]. These lesions can be classified by the Gharbi ultrasono-

Table 1: Gharbi ultrasonographic classification of hyatid cysts

Type	Pathology	Frequency	Ultrasonographic findings
I	Discrete univesicular mass	22%	Liquid-filled cyst with parietal echo backing
II	Univesicular mass with detached membranes	4%	Liquid-filled cyst with ultrasonographic water lily sign
III	Multivesicular mass	54%	Partitioned cyst with a spoke wheel appearance
IV	Heterogenous mass	12%	Heterogeneous echo structure with mixed solid and liquid components
V	Heterogenous mass with calcifications	8%	Dense reflections with a posterior shade cone caused by calcifications

graphic classification [Table 1] [30]. The Gharbi classification assists in the characterization of renal masses that are caused by hydatid disease. Higher Gharbi type corresponds with further disease progression. Consequently, Gharbi type I cysts are most commonly seen in children. Accordingly, Gharbi types III through V are consistent with more advanced disease and are seen almost exclusively in adults. Most common are the Gharbi type III cysts, which are multivesicular masses that can be de-

tected on ultrasound as a partitioned cyst with a spoke wheel appearance [**Fig. 7**A, B] [31]. Changes in patient position can cause any hydatid sand that is present to be disturbed and will result in the shifting of bright echoes within the mass. This finding has been described as the snowstorm sign [11,32]. Less commonly seen are the univesicular Gharbi type I and type II cysts, which demonstrate less disease progression and are seen more commonly in young adults and children. Type I cysts

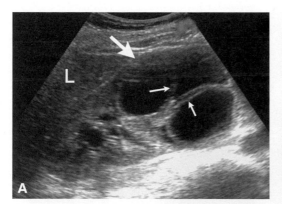
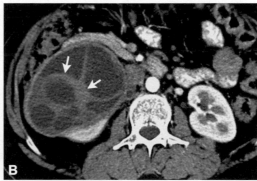
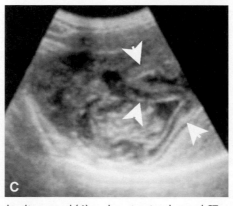

Fig. 7. Renal hydatid cyst. Gray-scale ultrasound (*A*) and contrast-enhanced CT scan (*B*) of the right kidney reveal a well-defined cystic lesion (*large arrow*) with multiple internal septae (*small arrows*) suggestive of a hydatid cyst with multiple daughter cysts. (Courtesy of SA Merchant, India.) (*C*) Gray-scale sonography of the right kidney on a different patient demonstrates the floating membranes (*arrowheads*) of the hydatid cyst following rupture of the cyst, referred to as the water lily sign. (Courtesy of Ercan Kocakoc, Turkey.)

are well-limited liquid cysts that can be differentiated from simple nonhydatid cysts by the presence of a parietal echo. Gharbi type II cysts demonstrate a detached and floating membrane that is pathognomonic for hydatid disease. This detachment of the membranes inside the cyst has been referred to as the ultrasound water lily sign because of its resemblance to the radiographic water lily sign seen in pulmonary cysts [**Fig. 7**C] [33,34]. In contrast, the Gharbi type IV and V cysts demonstrate more advanced disease and are correspondingly seen in older patients. Gharbi type IV hydatid cysts will demonstrate heterogeneity of echo structure with a combination of liquid and solid cyst contents. Gharbi type V hydatid cysts are calcified and will show dense reflections with a posterior shade cone. The varying echogenic aspects of these type IV and V lesions make diagnosis by ultrasound more difficult [30]. In these cases, CT studies can aid in characterization. On CT, the presence of smaller round daughter cysts within the mother cysts can help differentiate hydatid

lesions from other similar appearing pathology, such as simple cysts, abscesses, and necrotic neoplasm [10].

Renal tuberculosis

Tuberculosis is an infection caused by *Mycobacterium tuberculosis*. Typically acquired by inhalation, exposure initially results in a primary infection with a silent bacillemia. This infection will result in systemic dissemination of mycobacteria. Latent foci may result in kidney lesions many years following primary infection, though only 5% of patients who have active tuberculosis will have cavitary lesions in the urinary tract [11].

Clinically, this infection presents in younger patients, with 75% of those affected being younger than 50 years. Renal tuberculosis should be considered in any patient who has a diagnosed history of tuberculosis. Often patients will present asymptomatically, even in cases of advanced disease. If disease involves the bladder, symptoms of urinary

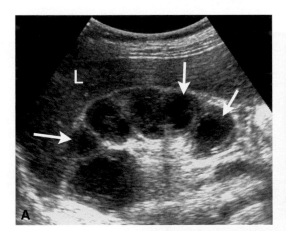
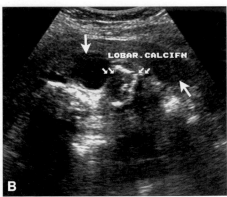
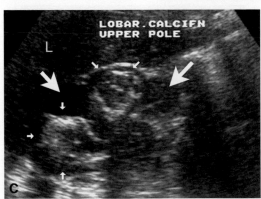

Fig. 8. Renal tuberculosis. (A) Longitudinal gray-scale ultrasound of the right kidney demonstrates hypoechoic areas (*arrows*) in the renal cortex suggestive of lobar caseation in this known case of tuberculosis. Longitudinal gray-scale sonography (*B, C*) of the kidney in another patient who has renal tuberculosis demonstrates hypoechoic areas of caseous necrosis (*large arrows*) with dense peripheral calcification (*small arrows*) with posterior acoustic shadowing. (Panels B, C, Courtesy of SA Merchant, Mumbai, India.)

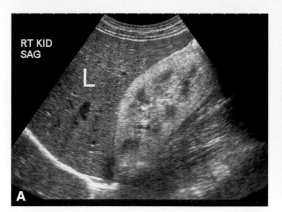 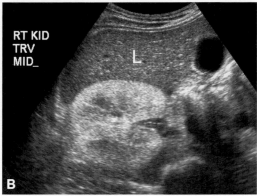

Fig. 9. HIV nephropathy. Longitudinal (*A*) and transverse (*B*) gray-scale sonograms of the right kidney in young man who has no known history of medical disease reveals an enlarged, markedly echogenic kidney (bilateral; left not shown) with loss of corticomedullary differentiation and obliteration of sinus fat suggestive of HIV-nephropathy. Subsequently confirmed by histopathology. L, liver.

frequency may result. One quarter of patients will present with findings of a unilateral poorly functioning kidney. Other suspicious findings include chronic cystitis or epididymitis that is recalcitrant to treatment; firm seminal vesicles on digital rectal examination; or a chronic fistula tract that forms at surgical sites. Diagnosis of urinary tract tuberculosis can be established through a urine culture that demonstrates growth of *M tuberculosis*.

Ultrasonographic features of renal tuberculosis

Early findings of urinary tract tuberculosis are best characterized by intravenous urography. Initially, cavities appear as small irregularities of the minor calyces. These irregular changes are classically described as "feathery" and "moth-eaten." As disease progresses, it extends from the calyces into the underlying renal parenchyma. Calcifications may be appreciated in these areas of caseating necrosis. In addition, tuberculosis involvement of the ureter can result in ureteral strictures, which cause a urographic appearance of a rigid, irregular, "pipe-stem" ureter [11]. Ultrasound findings in the diagnosis of renal tuberculosis have traditionally been described as limited. However, recent reports describe the role of high-resolution ultrasonography in characterizing late and chronic changes in renal tuberculosis [35]. Granulomatous mass lesions in the renal parenchyma can be seen as masses of mixed echogenicity, with or without necrotic areas of caseation and calcifications [**Fig. 8**]. Mucosal thickening and stenosis of the calyces is detectable by ultrasonography. In addition, findings of mucosal thickening of the renal pelvis and ureter, ureteral stricture, and hydronephrosis are seen. Finally, bladder changes such as mucosal thickening and reduced capacity are commonly detectable.

HIV-associated nephropathy

Renal disease is a common complication in patients who have HIV. This complication can result primarily from direct kidney infection with HIV or secondarily from adverse effects of the medications used to treat HIV. HIV-associated nephropathy (HIVAN) accounts for approximately 10% of new end stage renal disease cases in the United States. Patients who have HIVAN are not typically hypertensive.

Ultrasonographic features of HIV-associated nephropathy

Sonography is a critical component in the evaluation of HIVAN. The major sonographic findings include increased cortical echogenicity, decreased corticomedullary definition, and decreased renal sinus fat [**Fig. 9**]. Renal size may be enlarged [36,37]. The increased cortical echogenicity is attributable to prominent interstitial expansion by cellular infiltrate and markedly dilated tubules containing voluminous casts. Histologically, HIVAN demonstrates tubular epithelial cell damage, glomerulosclerosis, and tubulointerstitial scarring [38]. Most patients who have HIVAN have proteinuria secondary to tubular epithelial cell damage. In the presence of marked increased cortical echogenicity in a young patient who has known history of medical renal disease, HIVAN must be considered.

Summary

The growing ubiquity, well-established safety, and cost-effectiveness of ultrasound imaging have cemented its role in the diagnosis of renal infectious diseases. It is imperative that all practitioners of renal medicine understand the ultrasonographic manifestations of these diseases, as early diagnosis and treatment are the cornerstones of avoidance of long-term morbidity and mortality. If the strengths and limitations of ultrasonography are understood properly, a practitioner will be able to achieve the quickest and safest diagnosis with the minimal amount of further invasive imaging. The advent of new ultrasonographic techniques may allow it to serve a more central role in the diagnosis and characterization of renal infections.

References

[1] Newman PG, Rozycki GS. The history of ultrasound. Surg Clin North Am 1998;78(2):179–95.

[2] Harvey CJ, Pilcher JM, Eckersley RJ, et al. Advances in ultrasound. Clin Radiol 2002;57(3):157–77.

[3] McAchran SE, Dogra VS, Resnick MI. Office based ultrasound for urologists. Part I: ultrasound physics, and of the kidney and bladder. AUA Update 2004;23:226–31.

[4] Spirnak JP, Resnick MI. Ultrasound. In: Gillenwater JY, Grayhack JT, Howards SS, et al, editors. Adult & pediatric urology. 4th edition. Philadelphia: Lippincott, Williams & Williams; 2002. p. 165–93.

[5] Smith RS, Fry WR. Ultrasound instrumentation. Surg Clin North Am 2004;84(4):953–71.

[6] Noble VE, Brown DF. Renal ultrasound. Emerg Med Clin North Am 2004;22(3):641–59.

[7] Grant EG, Barr LL, Borgstede J, et al. AIUM standard for the performance of an ultrasound examination of the abdomen or retroperitoneum. American Institute of Ultrasound in Medicine. J Ultrasound Med 2002;21(10):1182–7.

[8] Brandt TD, Neiman HL, Dragowski MJ, et al. Ultrasound assessment of normal renal dimensions. J Ultrasound Med 1982;1(2):49–52.

[9] Horstman W, Watson L. Ultrasound of the genitourinary tract. In: Resnick MI, Older RA, editors. Diagnosis of genitourinary disease. 2nd edition. New York: Thieme; 1997. p. 79–130.

[10] Schaeffer AJ. Infections of the urinary tract. In: Walsh PC, Retik AB, Vaughn ED, et al, editors. Campbell's urology. 8th edition. Philadelphia: Elsevier; 2002. p. 516–602.

[11] Schaeffer AJ. Urinary tract infections. In: Gillenwater JY, Grayhack JT, Howards SS, et al, editors. Adult & pediatric urology. 4th edition. Philadelphia: Lippincott, Williams & Williams; 2002. p. 289–351.

[12] Ramakrishnan K, Scheid DC. Diagnosis and management of acute pyelonephritis in adults. Am Fam Physician 2005;71(5):933–42.

[13] Wise G. Fungal and actinomycotic infections of the genitourinary system. In: Walsh PC, Retik AB, Vaughn ED, et al, editors. Campbell's urology. 8th edition. Philadelphia: Elsevier; 2002. p. 797–827.

[14] Majd M, Nussbaum Blask AR, Markle BM, et al. Acute pyelonephritis: comparison of diagnosis with 99mTc-DMSA, SPECT, spiral CT, MR imaging, and power Doppler US in an experimental pig model. Radiology 2001;218(1):101–8.

[15] Johansen TE. The role of imaging in urinary tract infections. World J Urol 2004;22(5):392–8.

[16] Berro Y, Baratte B, Seryer D, et al. Comparison between scintigraphy, B-mode, and power Doppler sonography in acute pyelonephritis in children. J Radiol 2000;81(5):523–7.

[17] Bykov S, Chervinsky L, Smolkin V, et al. Power Doppler sonography versus Tc-99m DMSA scintigraphy for diagnosing acute pyelonephritis in children: are these two methods comparable? Clin Nucl Med 2003;28(3):198–203.

[18] Wang YT, Chiu NT, Chen MJ, et al. Correlation of renal ultrasonographic findings with inflammatory volume from dimercaptosuccinic acid renal scans in children with acute pyelonephritis. J Urol 2005;173(1):190–4.

[19] Dembry LM, Andriole VT. Renal and perirenal abscesses. Infect Dis Clin North Am 1997;11(3):663–80.

[20] Farmer KD, Gellett LR, Dubbins PA. The sonographic appearance of acute focal pyelonephritis 8 years experience. Clin Radiol 2002;57(6):483–7.

[21] Cheng CH, Tsau YK, Hsu SY, et al. Effective ultrasonographic predictor for the diagnosis of acute lobar nephronia. Pediatr Infect Dis J 2004;23(1):11–4.

[22] Stone SC, Mallon WK, Childs JM, et al. Emphysematous pyelonephritis: clues to rapid diagnosis in the Emergency Department. J Emerg Med 2005;28(3):315–9.

[23] Narlawar RS, Raut AA, Nagar A, et al. Imaging features and guided drainage in emphysematous pyelonephritis: a study of 11 cases. Clin Radiol 2004;59(2):192–7.

[24] Best CD, Terris MK, Tacker JR, et al. linical and radiological findings in patients with gas forming renal abscess treated conservatively. J Urol 1999;162(4):1273–6.

[25] Bingol-Kologlu M, Ciftci AO, Senocak ME, et al. Xanthogranulomatous pyelonephritis in children: diagnostic and therapeutic aspects. Eur J Pediatr Surg 2002;12(1):42–8.

[26] Tiu CM, Chou YH, Chiou HJ, et al. Sonographic features of xanthogranulomatous pyelonephritis. J Clin Ultrasound 2001;29(5):279–85.

[27] Kim JC. US and CT findings of xanthogranulomatous pyelonephritis. Clin Imaging 2001;25(2):118–21.

[28] Evans NL, French J, Rose MB. Renal malacoplakia: an important consideration in the differential diagnosis of renal masses in the presence of Escherichia coli infection. Br J Radiol 1998;71(850):1083–5.

[29] Venkatesh SK, Mehrotra N, Gujral RB. Sonographic findings in renal parenchymal malacoplakia. J Clin Ultrasound 2000;28(7):353–7.

[30] Zmerli S, Ayed M, Horchani A, et al. Hydatid cyst of the kidney: diagnosis and treatment. World J Surg 2001;25(1):68–74.

[31] von Sinner WN. New diagnostic signs in hydatid disease; radiography, ultrasound, CT and MRI correlated to pathology. Eur J Radiol 1991;12(2):150–9.

[32] Marti-Bonmati L, Menor Serrano F. Complications of hepatic hydatid cysts: ultrasound, computed tomography, and magnetic resonance diagnosis. Gastrointest Radiol 1990;15(2):119–25.

[33] Beggs I. The radiology of hydatid disease. AJR Am J Roentgenol 1985;145(3):639–48.

[34] Moguillanski SJ, Gimenez CR, Villavicencio RL. Radiología de la hidatidosis abdominal. In: Stoopen ME, Kimura K, Ros PR, editors. Radiología e imagen diagnóstica y terapeútica: abdomen, Vol. 2. Philadelphia: Lippincott Williams & Wilkins; 1999. p. 47–72.

[35] Vijayaraghavan SB, Kandasamy SV, Arul M, et al. Spectrum of high-resolution sonographic features of urinary tuberculosis. J Ultrasound Med 2004;23(5):585–94.

[36] Di Fiori JL, Rodrigue D, Kaptein EM, et al. Diagnostic sonography of HIV-associated nephropathy: new observations and clinical correlation. AJR Am J Roentgenol 1998;171(3):713–6.

[37] Atta MG, Longenecker JC, Fine DM, et al. Sonography as a predictor of human immunodeficiency virus-associated nephropathy. J Ultrasound Med 2004;23(5):603–10.

[38] Hamper UM, Goldblum LE, Hutchins GM, et al. Renal involvement in AIDS: sonographic-pathologic correlation. AJR Am J Roentgenol 1988;150(6):1321–5.

ULTRASOUND CLINICS

Ultrasound Clin 1 (2006) 15–24

Sonography of Benign Renal Cystic Disease

Therese M. Weber, MD

- Simple cortical cysts
- Complex renal cysts
- Renal sinus cysts
- Medullary cystic disease
- Multiple renal cysts
- Autosomal dominant polycystic kidney disease
- Autosomal recessive polycystic kidney disease
- Von Hippel-Lindau disease
- Tuberous sclerosis
- Acquired cystic kidney disease associated with dialysis
- Multiloculated cystic renal masses
- Multicystic dysplastic kidney
- Multilocular cystic nephroma
- Summary
- Acknowledgments
- References

When evaluating renal masses, differentiating cysts from solid lesions is the primary role of ultrasound (US). US is also helpful and frequently superior to CT, in demonstrating the complex internal architecture of cystic lesions in terms of internal fluid content, septations, tiny nodules, and wall abnormalities, including associated soft tissue masses. Renal cysts are common in the population older than 50 years, occurring in at least 50% of people [1]. Scanning technique is important to the success of demonstrating renal masses with US. The kidneys should be evaluated in multiple patient positions, including supine, lateral decubitus, and occasionally oblique or prone positions. The mass should be scanned with an appropriate focal zone. Simple renal cysts will frequently be better demonstrated with tissue harmonic imaging, which can eliminate low-level internal echoes by reducing background noise [2]. The Bosniak Classification System of renal cysts, shown in Box 1, has become an important tool used by radiologists and urologists to communicate the significance of renal cyst imaging characteristics [3,4]. The primary goal of the radiologist in evaluating cystic renal masses is the differentiation of nonsurgical from surgical lesions [5].

Simple cortical cysts

The sonographic criteria used to diagnose a simple cyst include the following characteristics: internally anechoic, posterior acoustic enhancement, and a sharply defined, imperceptible, smooth far wall. Simple cysts are usually round or ovoid in shape. If all these sonographic criteria are met, further evaluation or follow-up is not required. Maintaining rigid criteria is necessary to ensure the highest possible accuracy with US [6]. The simple renal cyst is a Bosniak category I cyst [**Fig. 1**] [3].

Complex renal cysts

Complex cysts do not meet the strict US criteria of a simple renal cyst. Five to ten percent of all renal cysts are not simple cysts, and 5% to 10% of renal cysts with complex features prove to be tumors [7]. These complex renal cysts may contain complex fluid, septations, calcification, perceptible defined

Department of Radiology, Wake Forest University School of Medicine, Medical Center Boulevard, Winston-Salem, NC 27157-1088, USA
E-mail address: tweber@wfubmc.edu

doi:10.1016/j.cult.2005.09.005

autosomal recessive disorder. There is an association with extrarenal, ophthalmologic abnormalities. The adult form, inherited as an autosomal dominant pattern, tends to present in early adulthood and is not associated with extrarenal abnormalities. US findings include kidneys that are small to normal in size, are hyperechoic, and have small (0.1 to 1.0 cm) cysts in the medulla and at the corticomedullary junction [16,17]. Acquired cystic kidney disease may resemble medullary cystic disease; however, cyst location in the cortex and a history of dialysis supports the diagnosis of acquired cystic kidney disease.

Multiple renal cysts

With increased use of CT, US, and MR, patients who are harboring multiple simple cysts or lesions too small to characterize are being seen with increasing frequency. Multiple renal cysts can be seen in polycystic kidney disease, Von Hippel-Lindau disease (VHL), tuberous sclerosis (TS), acquired cystic kidney disease associated with dialysis (ACKDD), and mulitcystic dysplastic kidney.

Autosomal dominant polycystic kidney disease

Autosomal dominant polycystic kidney disease (ADPKD) is the third most common systemic hereditary condition and accounts for 10% to 15% of all patients on dialysis [18]. Because the disease is characterized by variable expression and occurs with spontaneous mutation, up to 50% of patients will have no family history of the disease [19]. Renal failure develops in 50% of patients and is usually present by 60 years of age. Early signs of the disease include hypertension and flank or back pain with variable progression to ESRD. Nephrolithiasis occurs in 20% to 36% of patients because

of metabolic (lower glomerular filtration rate and urine volume) and anatomic (associated with larger and more numerous renal cysts) factors [20]. Extrarenal manifestations of ADPKD include hepatic, pancreatic, ovarian, splenic, arachnoid, and other cysts, and intracranial berry aneurysms with associated intracranial hemorrhage, abdominal aortic aneurysm, cardiac valve abnormalities, and hernias. The vascular abnormalities and cyst development are related to a basement membrane defect [18]. Eighty percent of people who have ADPKD and ESRD will have colonic diverticulosis. At least two different genes involving chromosomes 4 and 16 have been found to be associated with ADPKD [21].

US, because of high sensitivity and low cost, has become the primary method of diagnosing ADPKD and following the cysts. US screening for ADPKD typically begins between ages 10 and 15 years, but has the problem of false negatives in about 14% of patients younger than 30 years. Bear and colleagues [22] developed criteria that are widely used to diagnose ADPKD. In adults who have a family history of ADPKD, the presence of at least three cysts in both kidneys, with at least one cyst in each kidney, is a positive finding [23]. The cysts tend to involve all portions of the kidney and are of variable size. US typically reveals kidneys that are bilaterally enlarged with compression of the central sinus echo complex [**Fig. 3**]. When the kidneys are markedly enlarged with multiple complex cysts, detection of solid lesions may be difficult, and correlation with MR may be necessary to evaluate for renal cell carcinoma (RCC). When a solid mass is seen it can be confirmed with confidence sonographically [**Fig. 4**]. Nephrolithiasis may be difficult to demonstrate sonographically because of distortion of the collecting system by numerous large cysts. There is no increased risk for RCC in patients who have ADPKD, except for increased risk

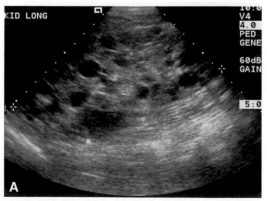 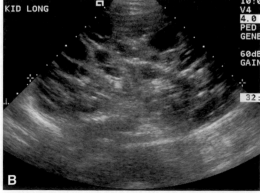

Fig. 3. Bilaterally enlarged kidneys (*A, B*) with multiple cysts of various sizes in adult polycystic kidney disease. The kidneys measure 15.6 cm in length bilaterally.

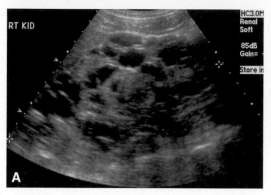 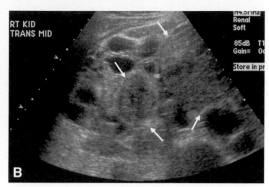

Fig. 4. (*A*) Adult polycystic kidney disease with (*B*) solid renal masses (*white arrows*) in the right kidney confirmed as papillary renal cell carcinoma following nephrectomy.

related to dialysis and the generally increased risk for RCC in men.

Autosomal recessive polycystic kidney disease

Autosomal recessive polycystic kidney disease (ARPKD) is characterized by varying degrees of renal failure and portal hypertension as a result of dilatation of renal collecting tubules, dilatation of biliary radicals, and periportal fibrosis that influences its presentation. The involved gene is located on chromosome 6 [24]. In its severest form, renal disease predominates and ARPKD manifests itself immediately after birth with the early complication of severe pulmonary failure. The diagnosis may be made at fetal or neonatal US. Characteristically, the kidneys are enlarged bilaterally, and oligohydramnios, Potter's facies, and pulmonary complications may be encountered. Children who present later will have some element of renal impairment with the complications of congenital hepatic fibrosis, including portal hypertension, splenomegaly, and bleeding varices [25]. With US, the kidneys maintain a reniform shape, but may be normal to bilaterally enlarged and echogenic [**Fig. 5**].

Von Hippel-Lindau disease

VHL disease is an uncommon condition characterized by multiple lesions, including hemangioblastomas in the central nervous system (CNS) and retina; RCC; pheochromocytomas; pancreatic neuroendocrine tumors; epididymal cystadenomas; endolymphatic sac tumors; carcinoid tumors; and multiple cysts of the kidney, pancreas, and epididymis. The condition is inherited in an autosomal dominant pattern [26]. The VHL tumor suppressor gene is located on chromosome 3 [27]. Inactivation of the VHL suppressor gene gives rise to premalignant renal cysts. Additional genetic alterations are probably required for conversion of these cysts to RCC. Renal involvement in VHL includes multiple, bilateral renal cysts and solid tumors. RCC, one of the major complications of VHL disease, occurs in up to 75% of patients by the age of 60 and occurs 25 years earlier than sporadic RCC [28]. In addition to the development of RCC at a younger age, these tumors tend to be bilateral and multicentric. Cysts, as the most common renal manifestation of the disease, are seen in 75% of patients. Although multiple, these cysts are generally fewer than in patients who have ADPKD. In ADPKD, pancreatic cysts almost

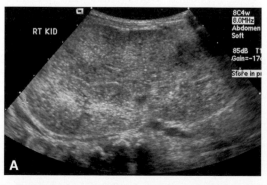 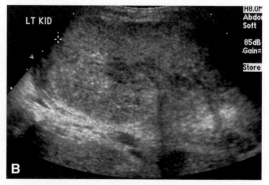

Fig. 5. Newborn who has bilaterally enlarged, echogenic kidneys consistent with ARPKD. The right kidney (*A*) measures 10 cm in length and the left kidney (*B*) measures 9.8 cm in length.

never occur in the absence of liver cysts, whereas in VHL they are common. On US the cysts tend to be cortical in location and range in size from 0.5 to 3.0 cm. RCC in VHL disease may show solid renal masses without cystic components or predominantly cystic lesions with enhancing solid components that contain the RCC. US may be used for screening these patients, especially those younger than 18 years; however, CT and MR are more sensitive in detecting small enhancing solid masses [18].

Tuberous sclerosis

TS is a neurophakomatosis involving the skin and CNS that most commonly occurs sporadically in 60% of patients. This condition is also inherited as an autosomal dominant pattern and is characterized by hamartomatous growths in the CNS, eyes, skin, heart, liver, kidney, and adrenal glands. The major presenting symptom is seizures. CNS manifestations occur in up to 90% of patients. The classic clinical triad is mental retardation, seizures, and adenoma sebaceum. At least two genetic loci have been associated with TS, involving chromosome 9 and 16 [18]. The leading causes of death in TS are renal failure, cardiac tumors, increased intracranial pressure, and bleeding [29]. Renal manifestations occur in about half of patients who have TS and include cysts, angiomyolipomas (AML), tumors, and perirenal lymphangiomas. There is an increased incidence of clear cell carcinomas in patients who have TS, especially women. RCC occurs bilaterally in 43% of affected TS patients, and tumors occur at a younger age than sporadic RCC [18,30,31]. The risk for malignancy is lower in TS than in VHL disease [18]. On US, renal cysts are seen in the cortex and medulla [**Fig. 6**]. The renal cysts in TS appear at an earlier age than the cysts seen in APKD. Renal cysts are not the primary diagnostic feature of TS, however. Multiple renal AML are a primary diagnostic feature of TS, occur in about 15% of patients who have TS, and are more common in women. The rate of hemorrhage in TS-related AML is higher than in sporadic AML [32]. If TS is a consideration, the diagnosis can usually be confirmed on CNS imaging with subependymal hamartomas or giant cell astrocytomas.

Acquired cystic kidney disease associated with dialysis

Acquired cystic kidney disease consists of renal cysts found in individuals who have chronic renal failure who may have a history of dialysis, but do not have a history of hereditary cystic renal disease. Dunnill and colleagues [33] first described this process in 1977. The most important factor in developing

ACKDD is the duration of ESRD or maintenance dialysis [34]. ACKDD is seen in 8% to 13% of patients who have ESRD, 10% to 20% of patients who have a 1- to 3-year history of dialysis, 40% to 60% of patients who have history of 3 to 5 years of dialysis, and greater than 90% of patients who have a history of 5 to 10 years of dialysis. Cysts occur with equal frequency in patients receiving peritoneal or hemodialysis. The cysts are of tubular origin (arising from the proximal tubules), thought to be caused by nondialyzable mitogenic or cytogenic substances; tubular obstruction from fibrosis or oxalate crystals; and ischemia. There is a histologic continuum from cysts with single-layered epithelia to multilayered (atypical) cysts to renal adenoma and RCC. RCC occurs in a younger population in ACKDD patients compared with sporadic RCC, with a mean age at diagnosis of about 49 years as compared with 62 years for patients who do not have ESRD [35]. RCC in patients undergoing dialysis is seven times more common in men than women, in contrast to the 2/1 ratio in patients who do not have ESRD [36]. Criteria used to define ACKDD include the presence of three to five cysts in each kidney in a patient who has chronic renal failure, which are not related to inherited renal cystic disease. On US, multiple bilateral renal cysts involving the cortex and medulla are seen in the setting of medical renal disease [**Fig. 7**]. The cysts are usually small, many measuring 0.5 cm or less. Confirmation of the simple cystic nature may be difficult because of the small size [37]. The cysts may increase in size and number with time, and the overall size of the kidneys may increase. This appearance may resemble ADPKD. Complications associated with ACKDD include cyst infection or hemorrhage, renal calculi, erythocytosis, and solid neoplasms.

Multiloculated cystic renal masses

A multiloculated appearance can be seen in neoplastic disease such as renal cell carcinoma, multilocular cystic nephroma, Wilms' tumor, and solid tumors with central necrosis, which are Bosniak category III lesions. Multiloculated renal masses can be seen in renal cystic disease such as localized renal cystic disease, septated cyst, and segmental multicystic dysplastic kidney. Inflammatory disease such as echinococcosis, segmental XGP, and abscess can appear as a multiloculated cystic renal mass. An organizing hematoma and vascular malformation can also appear as a multiloculated cystic renal mass.

Multicystic dysplastic kidney

The pathogenesis of multicystic dysplastic kidney (MCDK) is complete ureteral obstruction early in

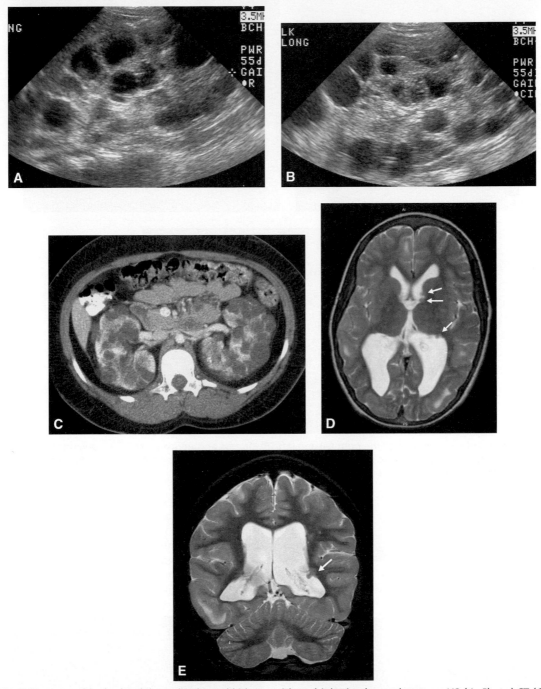

Fig. 6. Ten-year-old who has bilateral enlarged kidneys with multiple simple renal cysts on US (*A, B*) and CT (*C*). The right kidney measures 11 cm in length and the left kidney measures 11.5 cm in length. MR of the brain demonstrated multiple subependymal nodules protruding into the lateral ventricle on axial (*D*) and coronal (*E*) T2-weighted images.

fetal life before the eighth to tenth week, or incomplete ureteral obstruction occurring later in fetal life between the 10th and 36th week. Contralateral renal anomalies, most commonly uretero pelvic junction (UPJ) obstruction, occur in 33% of patients.

Imaging characteristics vary depending on age of the patient at diagnosis. Fetal US may show large cysts with no intercommunication between cysts, absence of identifiable cortical parenchyma, or central sinus structures [**Fig. 8**]. The MCDK may calcify or

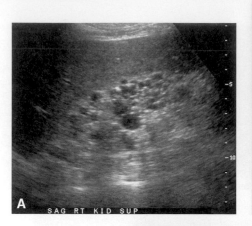
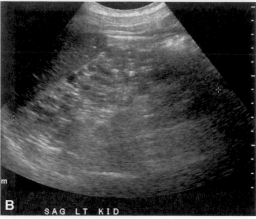
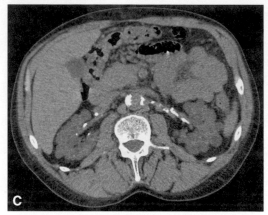

Fig. 7. Longitudinal US images of the right (*A*) and left (*B*) kidneys and noncontrast CT (*C*) demonstrate marked increased cortical echogenicity and loss of cortical-medullary distinction in this patient who has ESRD and multiple bilateral simple renal cysts consistent with acquired renal cystic disease.

may not be identifiable in a few patients who have been followed [38].

Multilocular cystic nephroma

Multilocular cystic nephroma (MLCM) is a benign, nonhereditary cystic neoplasm with a bimodal pre-

sentation that has greater incidence in males younger than 2 years and in women during the fifth to eighth decades. MLCN consists of multiple epithelially lined cysts that do not communicate. MLCN is usually a benign neoplasm; however, metastases have been reported [5,39]. US will show a mass containing multiple cysts or internal septations

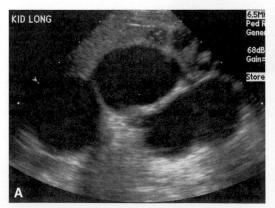
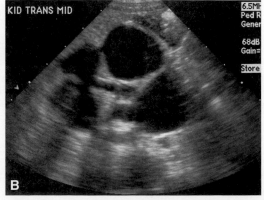

Fig. 8. Longitudinal (*A*) and transverse (*B*) images of the kidney show multiple large renal cysts with absence of central sinus structures and no identifiable cortical parenchyma consistent with multicystic dysplastic kidney.

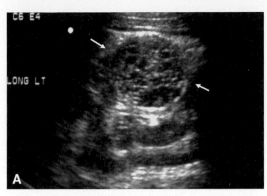 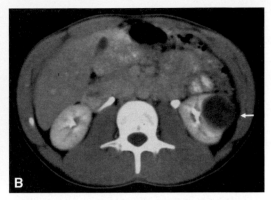

Fig. 9. Longitudinal US (*A*) and CT (*B*) images demonstrating a predominantly cystic mass with multiple internal septations, proven at surgery to be a multilocular cystic nephroma. Note the better representation of the lesion's internal architecture at US.

[Fig. 9]. It is not possible to conclusively distinguish MLCN from multiloculated RCC radiologically, and these are usually surgical lesions.

Summary

US plays an important role in evaluation of the kidney in cases of medical renal disease because of lower cost, ready availability, lack of radiation, and lack of need for iodinated contrast material. The primary role of US in evaluating benign cystic renal disease is the distinction of a simple cyst from a solid mass, and in defining the characteristics of a complex cyst.

Acknowledgments

The author would like to acknowledge Raymond B. Dyer, MD, for his editorial assistance.

References

[1] Kissane JM. Congenital malformations. In: Hepinstall RH, editor. Pathology of the kidney. Boston: Little, Brown; 1973. p. 69–119.

[2] Schmidt T, Holh C, Haage P, et al. Diagnostic accuracy of phase-inversion tissue harmonic imaging versus fundamental B-mode sonography in the evaluation of focal lesions of the kidney. AJR Am J Roentgenol 2003;180:1639–47.

[3] Bosniak MA. The current radiological approach to renal cysts. Radiology 1986;158:1–10.

[4] Leder RA. Radiological approach to renal cysts and the Bosniak classification system. Curr Opin Urol 1999;9(2):129–33.

[5] Hartman DS, Choyke PL, Hartman MS. A practical approach to the cystic renal mass. Radiographics 2004;24:S101–15.

[6] Bosniak MA. The small (<3 cm) renal parenchymal tumor: detection, diagnosis, and controversies. Radiology 1991;179:307–17.

[7] Zeman RK, Cronan JJ, Rosenfield AT, et al. Imaging approach to the suspected renal mass. Radiol Clin North Am 1985;23(3):503–29.

[8] Israel GM, Bosniak MA. Follow-up CT of moderately complex cystic lesions of the kidney (Bosniak category IIF). AJR Am J Roentgenol 2003;181:627–33.

[9] Israel GM, Bosniak MA. Calcification in cystic renal masses: is it important in diagnosis? Radiology 2003;226:47–52.

[10] Harisingani MG, Maher MM, Gervais DA, et al. Incidence of malignancy in complex cystic renal masses (Bosniak category III): should imaging-guided biopsy precede surgery? AJR Am J Roentgenol 2003;180:755–8.

[11] Rha SE, Byun JY, Jung SE, et al. The renal sinus: pathologic spectrum and multimodality imaging approach. Radiographics 2004;24:S117–31.

[12] Hidalgo H, Dunnick NR, Rosenburg ER, et al. Parapelvic cysts: appearance on CT and sonography. AJR Am J Roentgenol 1982;138:667–71.

[13] Chan JCM, Kodroff MB. Hypertension and hematuria secondary to parapelvic cyst. Pediatrics 1980;65:821–3.

[14] Gardner KD. Juvenile nephronophthiasis and renal medullary cystic disease. In: Gardner KD, editor. Cystic disease of the kidney. New York: John Wiley & Sons; 1976. p. 173–85.

[15] Wise SW, Hartman DS. Medullary cystic disease of the kidney. In: Pollack HM, McClennan BL, editors. Clinical urography: an atlas and textbook of urologic imaging. 2nd edition. Philadelphia: W.B. Saunders Company; 2000. p. 1398–403.

[16] Resnick JS, Hartman DS. Medullary cystic disease of the kidney. In: Polack HM, editor. Clinical urology: an atlas and textbook of urologic imaging. Philadelphia: W.B. Saunders Company; 1990. p. 1178–84.

[17] Rego JD, Laing FG, Jeffrey RB. Ultrasonic diagnosis of medullary cystic disease. J Ultrasound Med 1983;2:433–6.

[18] Choyke PL. Inherited cystic diseases of the kidney. Radiol Clin North Am 1996;34(5):925–46.

[19] Dalgaard OZ. Bilateral polycystic disease of the

kidney: A follow-up of 284 patients and their families. Acta Med Scand 1957;157(S328):1–255.

[20] Grampsas SA, Chandhoke PS, Fan J, et al. Anatomic and metabolic risk factors for nephrolithiasis in patients with autosomal dominant polycystic kidney disease. Am J Kidney Dis 2000; 36(1):53–7.

[21] Fick GM, Gabow PA. Natural history of autosomal dominant polycystic kidney disease. Annu Rev Med 1994;45:23–9.

[22] Bear JC, McManamon P, Morgan J, et al. Age at clinical onset and at ultrasound detection of adult polycystic kidney disease. Data for genetic counseling. Am J Med Genet 1984;18:45–53.

[23] Parfrey PS, Bear JC, Morgan J, et al. The diagnosis and prognosis of autosomal dominant polycystic kidney disease. N Engl J Med 1990;323:1085–90.

[24] Dimitrakov JD, Dimitrakov DI. Autosomal recessive polycystic kidney disease. Clinical and genetic profile. Folia Med (Plovdiv) 2003;45:5–7.

[25] Harris PC, Rosetti S. Molecular genetics of autosomal recessive polycystic kidney disease. Mol Genet Metab 2004;81:75–85.

[26] Sano T, Horiguchi H. Von Hippel-Lindau disease. Microsc Res Tech 2003;60:159–64.

[27] Kaelin Jr WG. The von Hippel-Lindau tumor suppressor gene and kidney cancer. Clin Cancer Res 2004;10:6290S–5S.

[28] Richard S, David P, Marsot-Dupuch K, et al. Central nervous system hemangioblastomas, endolymphatic sac tumors, and von Hippel-Lindau disease. Neurosurg Rev 2000;23:1–22.

[29] Gomez MR. Tuberous sclerosis. New York: Raven Press; 1988.

[30] Torres VE. Systemic manifestations of renal cystic disease. In: Gardner KD, Bernstein J, editors. The cystic kidney. Dordrecht (The Netherlands): Kluwer Academic Publishers; 1990. p. 207.

[31] Zimmerhackl LB, Rehm M, Kaufmehl K, et al. Renal involvement in tuberous sclerosis complex: a retrospective survey. Pediatr Nephrol 1994;8:451–7.

[32] Hildebrandt F. Genetic renal disease in children. Curr Opin Pediatr 1995;7:182–91.

[33] Dunnill MS, Millard PR, Oliver D. Acquired cystic kidney disease of the kidneys: a hazard of long-term intermittent maintenance haemodialysis. J Clin Pathol 1977;30:868–77.

[34] Levine E, Slusher SL, Grantham JJ, et al. Natural history of acquired cystic kidney disease in dialysis patients: a prospective longitudinal CT study. AJR Am J Roentgenol 1991;156:501–6.

[35] Port FK, Ragheb NE, Schwartz AG, et al. Neoplasms in dialysis patients: a population-bases study. Am J Kidney Dis 1989;14:119–23.

[36] Matson MA, Cohen EP. Acquired cystic kidney disease: occurrence, prevalence, and renal cancers. Medicine 1990;69:217–26.

[37] Allan PL. Ultrasonography of the native kidney in dialysis and transplant patients. J Clin Ultrasound 1992;20:557–67.

[38] Strife JF, Souza AS, Kirks DR, et al. Multicystic Dysplastic kidney in children: US follow-up. Radiology 1993;186:785–8.

[39] Madewell JE, Goldman SM, Davis CJ, et al. Multilocular cystic nephroma: a radiographic-pathologic correlation of 58 patients. Radiology 1983;146:309–21.

ULTRASOUND
CLINICS

Ultrasound Clin 1 (2006) 25–41

Sonography in Benign and Malignant Renal Masses

Raj Mohan Paspulati, MD[a,*], Shweta Bhatt, MD[b]

Ultrasonography is often the initial modality for imaging of the kidneys, although contrast-enhanced CT is the established imaging modality for the diagnosis of renal tumors. Despite technical limitations, a large percentage of renal tumors can be characterized by ultrasonography. Cystic and solid renal parenchymal mass lesions can be well differentiated by ultrasonography. Technical advances in the gray-scale and color-flow Doppler (CFD) ultrasound have improved the sensitivity in detection of small renal tumors. Gray-scale and CFD ultrasonography can demonstrate the vascular

invasion in selected groups of patients who have renal cell carcinoma (RCC). Contrast-enhanced Doppler ultrasonography appears promising as a cost-effective, noninvasive imaging technique in the characterization and follow-up of indeterminate renal mass lesions. As nephron-sparing surgery is being increasingly used in the management of small RCC, intraoperative ultrasound (US) has become a useful tool in guiding the surgeon. This article reviews the gray-scale and CFD features of benign and malignant renal masses encountered in radiology practice.

[a] Department of Radiology, University Hospitals of Cleveland, Case Western Reserve University, 11100 Euclid Avenue, Cleveland, OH 44106, USA
[b] Department of Radiology, University of Rochester Medical Center, 601 Elmwood Avenue, Box 648, Rochester, NY 14642, USA
* Corresponding author.
E-mail address: paspulati@uhrad.com (R.M. Paspulati).

Normal sonographic anatomy of the kidney

The kidneys are bean-shaped retroperitoneal organs with their medial aspects parallel to the lateral margin of the adjacent psoas muscles. The normal orientation of the kidneys is such that the upper pole is medial and anterior to the lower pole. The right kidney is 1 to 2 cm inferior in position as compared with the left kidney because of the location of the liver superior to the right kidney. The renal size varies with the age, sex, and body habitus. The measurement of renal volume is a more effective way of assessing the renal size, though measurement of renal length is more practical in regular practice [1]. The normal adult kidney measures 10 to 12 cm in length, 4 to 5 cm in width, and 2.5 to 3 cm in thickness. A discrepancy of more than 2 cm between the lengths of two kidneys is considered significant and needs further evaluation. The liver and hepatic flexure of the colon are situated anterior to the right kidney. The spleen lies anterosuperior to the left kidney and the rest of the left kidney is related anteriorly with the colon.

On ultrasonography of a normal kidney, there is good differentiation of the renal capsule, cortex, medulla, and central sinus complex [**Fig. 1**]. The renal capsule is visible as an echogenic line because of the interface between the echogenic perinephric fat and renal cortex. The renal parenchyma is composed of outer cortex and inner medulla (pyramids). The renal cortex is echogenic as compared with the medulla, but is iso- to hypoechoic as compared with the normal hepatic or splenic parenchyma. The extension of renal cortex toward the renal sinus between the renal pyramids forms the columns of Bertin. The central sinus is composed of fat, fibrous tissue, renal vessels, and lymphatic vessels. It has highest echogenicity because of the adipose tissue, and its size increases with the age of the person.

Sonographic technique

Sonographic evaluation of the right kidney is ideally performed from an anterior oblique approach

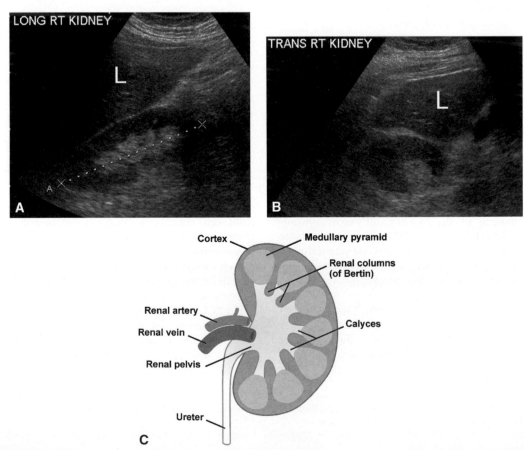

Fig. 1. Normal kidney. Longitudinal (*A*) and transverse (*B*) gray-scale US of the normal right kidney (calipers show the maximum longitudinal dimension of the kidney). (*C*) The schematic representation of the sagittal section of the kidney. L, liver.

using liver as an acoustic window, whereas the left kidney is scanned through a posterior oblique approach. The lower pole of the right kidney may be imaged using a more posterior approach. The upper pole of the left kidney is often best seen through an intercostal approach using spleen as a window. In addition to supine position, decubitus, prone, or upright positions may provide better images of the kidneys [2]. An appropriate transducer frequency ranging from 2.5 to 5 MHz should be used, depending on the body habitus. Time gain compensation and adjustment of other scanning parameters will allow a uniform acoustic pattern throughout the image [3]. Renal echogenicity should be compared with the echogenicity of the liver and spleen [2]. The renal parenchyma of a normal adult kidney is hypoechoic to the liver and spleen. The sonographic examination of the kidneys should include long axis and transverse views of the upper poles, midportions, and the lower poles, with assessment of the cortex and central sinus. Maximum measurement of renal length should be recorded for both kidneys [2]. Kidneys and the perirenal regions should be assessed for abnormalities. CFD and Power Doppler (PD) are used to differentiate vascular from nonvascular structures.

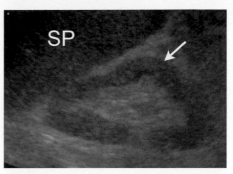

Fig. 2. Dromedary hump. Longitudinal gray-scale sonogram of the left kidney demonstrates the dromedary hump (*arrow*). SP, spleen.

Pseudolesions of kidney

There are various developmental variants of the kidney that need to be identified on sonography to avoid misdiagnosis as renal neoplasm or other renal pathology [Table 1].

Dromedary hump

Dromedary hump is a common renal variation usually seen as a focal bulge on the lateral border of the left kidney [**Fig. 2**]. It is a result of adaptation

of the renal surface to the adjacent spleen. It can be easily differentiated from a renal mass because of its similar echotexture to that of adjacent renal parenchyma on gray-scale ultrasound. CFD and PD will demonstrate similar perfusion to that of adjacent renal parenchyma.

Persistent fetal lobulation

Persistent fetal lobulation is another common renal variant that can be mistaken for renal scarring, a consequence of chronic infective process of the kidneys. Persistent fetal lobulation can be differentiated from scarred kidneys by the location of the renal surface indentations, which do not overlie the medullary pyramids as in true renal scarring [4], but overlie the space between the pyramids [**Fig. 3**]. The underlying medulla and the cortex are normal.

Prominent column of Bertin (hypertrophy)

Prominent column of Bertin is a prominent cortical tissue that is present between the pyramids and projects into the renal sinus [**Fig. 4**]. If not identified as a normal variant, it may be mistaken for an

Table 1: Renal pseudotumors	
Pseudotumor	**Diagnostic imaging features**
Congenital normal variants	
Dromedary hump	Focal bulge in the lateral contour of left kidney with echotexture similar to renal parenchyma
Persistent fetal lobulation	Renal surface indentations overlying the space between the pyramids
Prominent column of Bertin	Continuity with the normal cortex; echotexture and vascular perfusion similar to the normal cortex
Junctional parenchymal defect	Characteristic location in the anterosuperior and posteroinferior surface of the kidney and demonstration of continuity with the central sinus
Hypoechoic renal sinus fat	No distinct margin and normal vessels traversing the sinus
Inflammatory lesions	Diagnosis is based on the proper clinical context
Focal bacterial nephritis	
Renal abscess	

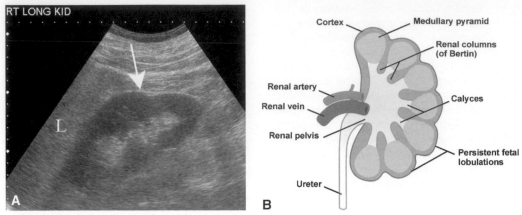

Fig. 3. Persistent fetal lobulations. Longitudinal (*A*) gray-scale sonogram of the right kidney demonstrates persistent fetal lobulation (*arrow*). L, liver. Schematic (*B*) appearance of persistent fetal lobulations (note fetal lobulations may be single or multiple).

intrarenal tumor. Sonography can accurately identify it by depicting its continuity with the renal cortex and a similar echo pattern as the renal parenchyma. CFD and PD imaging can further assist by depicting a similar vascular pattern as that of normal renal tissue [5,6]. Prominent columns of

Bertin are usually seen in the middle third of the kidney and are more common on the left side [5].

Junctional parenchymal defect

Junctional parenchymal defect (JPD) is another variant commonly mistaken for a cortical scar or

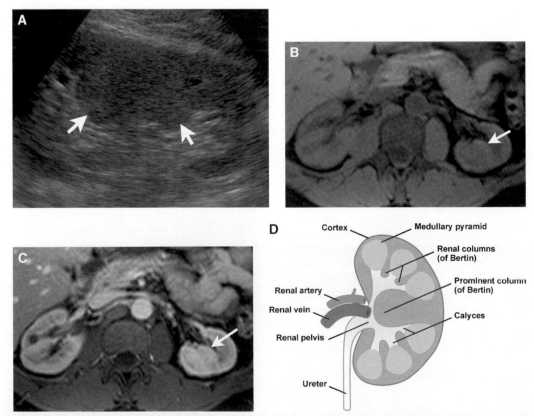

Fig. 4. Prominent column of Bertin. (*A*) Longitudinal gray-scale US of the left kidney demonstrates a prominent column of Bertin (*arrows*) mimicking an isoechoic renal mass. MRI was performed to confirm ultrasound findings. T1 flash fat-sat (*B*) and gadolinium-enhanced (*C*) MRI images of the kidneys reveal a prominent column of Bertin (*arrows*) seen in continuity with the renal cortex. (*D*) Schematic drawing of a prominent column of Bertin.

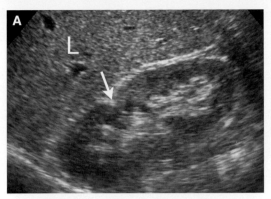

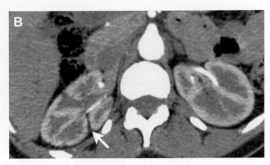

Fig. 5. Junctional parenchymal defect. (*A*) Longitudinal gray-scale US of the right kidney demonstrates a notch in the lateral border (*arrow*). L, liver. (*B*) Contrast-enhanced CT of the kidneys in another patient demonstrates the junctional parencymal defect (*arrow*).

a hyperechogenic renal tumor. JPD is a linear or triangular hyperechoic structure in the anterosuperior or posteroinferior surface of the kidney [**Fig. 5**]. These are caused by normal extensions of the renal sinus at the junction of the embryonic renunculi. These are differentiated from pathologic lesions by their characteristic location and demonstrate continuity with the central sinus by an echogenic line called interrenicular septum [7–9].

Hypoechoic renal sinus

The echogenicity of the renal sinus may vary from echogenic to anechoic. Hypoechoic renal sinus may mimic a mass lesion [10]. Absence of a well-defined margin and demonstration of normal vessels traversing the renal sinus by CFD will aid in differentiating a hypoechoic renal sinus from a mass lesion [10].

Inflammatory mass lesions

Acute focal bacterial nephritis and renal abscess may present as renal mass lesions indistinguishable from a renal tumor by ultrasonography and contrast-enhanced CT. The clinical presentation will aid in differentiating these inflammatory pseudotumors from RCC [11–13].

Benign renal tumors

Angiomyolipoma

Angiomyolipoma (AML) is a hamartoma and has variable amounts of mature adipose tissue, smooth muscle, and thick-walled blood vessels. Eighty percent of the AMLs are sporadic in occurrence and 20% of them are associated with tuberous sclerosis (TS). Presence of subependymal nodules and giant cell astrocytoma are sine qua non of TS, but not AML. On the contrary, 80% of the patients who have TS develop AMLs [14,15]. Patients who have

TS develop AMLs at a much younger age, and these tend to be multiple, bilateral, and larger than in sporadic cases. AMLs in patients who have TS are more likely to grow and become symptomatic [15,16]. The presence of estrogen and progesterone receptors in angiolipomas has been reported, and such AMLs are more common in women and in TS. These AMLs tend to grow during pregnancy and present with hemorrhage [17,18]. Small AMLs are asymptomatic and are incidental findings on imaging. AMLs smaller than 4 cm are symptomatic and are at increased risk for spontaneous hemorrhage [16,19]. Massive retroperitoneal hemorrhage from AML, also known as Wunderlich's syndrome, has been found in 10% of patients.

The characteristic sonographic appearance of AML is a well-defined hyperechoic mass [**Fig. 6**]. This increased echogenicity is attributed to the fat content, multiple interfaces, heterogeneous cellular architecture, and multiple vessels within the tumor [20,21]. However, there is significant overlap between the imaging features of AML and RCC. Small RCCs can be hyperechoic and indistinguishable from an AML on sonography. Acoustic shadowing, hypoechoic rim, and intratumoral cystic changes are some of the sonographic features found to be helpful in differentiating an AML from RCC. Hypoechoic rim and intratumoral cystic changes are seen only in RCC, whereas acoustic shadowing is observed with AML [**Fig. 7**] [22–24]. PD of AML may reveal focal intratumoral flow and a penetrating flow pattern [25]. The demonstration of intratumoral fat on CT confirms the diagnosis of an AML. The CT appearance of an AML also depends on the relative proportion of smooth muscle and vascular components of the tumor. Rarely, RCCs can demonstrate fat attenuation caused by entrapment of the perinal or renal sinus fat, lipid necrosis, or osseous metaplasia [26]. The characteristic intratumoral fat cannot be detected in 4.5% of AMLs,

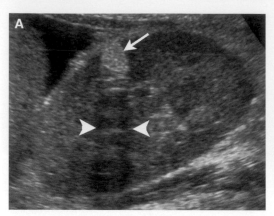 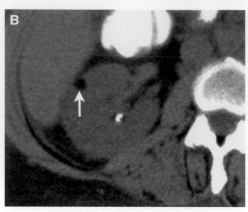

Fig. 6. Angiomyolipoma. (*A*) Longitudinal gray-scale US of the right kidney demonstrates an echogenic mass (*arrow*) with posterior acoustic shadowing (*arrowheads*). (*B*) Corresponding CT (excretory phase) confirms this lesion to be an angiomyolipoma, seen as a fat attenuation lesion (*arrow*) with a household unit of -8.

and will have high attenuation on an unenhanced CT scan. This finding has been attributed to minimal fat content or immature fat [25,27]. These AMLs with low fat content demonstrate homogeneous and prolonged enhancement on a contrast-enhanced scan, which distinguishes them from an RCC [25,28]. These AMLs with minimal fat are isoechoic with renal parenchyma on sonography [25]. The demonstration of micro- or macroaneurysms at angiography is reported to be characteristic of an AML [29].

The risk for spontaneous rupture and hemorrhage of an AML is related to the tumor size and the size of microaneurysms. AMLs larger than 4 cm and those with microaneurysms larger than 5 mm are reported to be at increased risk for spontaneous rupture [16,30,31]. Management options of AMLs include observation, embolization, and partial or total nephrectomy. Prophylactic transcatheter embolization of AMLs larger than 4 cm is reported to prevent tumor growth and spontaneous rupture

[19,31,32]. Kothary and colleagues [33] have described a high recurrence rate of AMLs after embolization in patients who have TS, and recommend long-term surveillance of these patients following embolization.

Renal adenoma

Renal cell adenoma is considered to be a benign counterpart of RCC, though the true nature and potential of this tumor is a subject of much debate. The size criterion used by many pathologists in distinguishing an adenoma from RCC is based on the initial observation by Bell, that renal cortical glandular tumors of smaller than 3 cm rarely metastasize [34,35]. There are no histopathologic, histochemical, immunologic, or imaging characteristics that distinguish a benign adenoma from an RCC [36]. Most pathologists consider these small renal cortical tumors to be premalignant or potentially malignant and believe that tumor size is not a valid differentiating criterion [37]. The widespread use of US and CT has resulted in the incidental detection of these tumors.

Oncocytoma

Renal oncocytoma is a benign tumor of renal tubular origin (renal tubular epithelium is also called *oncocyte*). It has the male predominance and age incidence similar to RCC. They are asymptomatic and are discovered as incidental findings on imaging [38]. They are well-defined tumors of variable size and can be as large as 20 cm [35]. The preoperative differentiation of oncocytomas from RCC is invaluable, but is often difficult because of overlap of imaging features. The characteristic central stellate scar on cross-sectional imaging and spoke-wheel pattern of enhancement on an angiogram are infrequently seen in oncocytomas and can also be

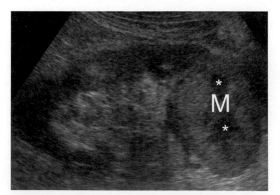

Fig. 7. RCC. Longitudinal gray-scale sonogram of the left kidney demonstrates a hyperechoic mass (M) arising from the lower pole with areas of intra tumoral cystic changes (*asterisk*).

seen in RCC [39–41]. Oncocytomas can be hypo-echoic, isoechoic, or hyperechoic to the renal pa-renchyma on sonography. MRI is reported to be superior to CT and US in identifying the imaging features of a small tumor [42]. The radiologic fea-tures, which are helpful in distinguishing an onco-cytoma from RCC, include well-defined margins, homogeneous enhancement without hemorrhage, calcification or necrosis, presence of a central stel-late scar, and spoke-wheel pattern of arterial en-hancement. There are few reports of bilateral and multicentric oncocytomas [43,44]. Renal oncocy-toma and RCC can coexist in the same or contra-lateral kidney [45,46]. Dechet and colleagues [47] have reported coexistent RCC in 10% of a total 138 cases of oncocytomas. Imaging-guided biopsy of renal tumors is indicated whenever there is radio-logic suspicion of an oncocytoma [48–50].

Leiomyoma

Renal leiomyoma is a rare benign tumor of smooth muscle origin. These tumors are either peripheral, arising from the renal capsule, or central in para-pelvic location. They are more common in women between the second and fifth decades of life. Most renal leiomyomas are asymptomatic, with inciden-tal detection on routine diagnostic imaging. These are well-defined tumors and are indistinguishable from RCC by imaging. Renal leiomyomas have variable appearance on imaging: from that of an entirely solid, to a mixed solid/cystic, to an entirely cystic lesion. Renal leiomyomas appear as well-defined hypoechoic solid mass lesions on ultra-sonography. The peripheral lesions may extend into the retroperitoneum and can resemble primary retroperitoneal sarcomas. The central lesions will have a mass effect over the collecting system and renal vasculature. They are most often avascular or hypovascular on angiogram [51–53].

Hemangioma

Hemangiomas are uncommon benign tumors of the kidney that can present with macroscopic he-maturia. They are commonly located in the renal pyramids and renal pelvis, and are classified into capillary and cavernous hemangiomas. The vascu-lar spaces are small in capillary hemangioma and large in cavernous hemangiomas. They are predomi-nantly smaller than 1 cm, but occasionally present as large mass lesions [54]. Gray-scale US features a nonspecific solid mass, and CT demonstrates a well-defined low-density mass without significant enhancement [55,56]. Larger lesions may cause dis-placement of the renal vessels and collecting sys-tem. Angiography may demonstrate a hypovascular or hypervascular mass [57,58].

Juxtaglomerular tumor (reninoma)

Juxtaglomerular tumors are benign, renin-producing tumors of the kidney that arise from the afferent ar-terioles of the glomerulus. These tumors were first described by Robertson and colleagues in 1967 [59]. They are twice as common in women as in men. In a young patient who has hypertension, the presence of a renal mass, elevated serum renin levels, and hypokalemia should raise a suspicion of reninoma. The tumor is either hypo- or hyper-echoic on sonography and appears as a well-defined hypodense solid mass on a contrast-enhanced CT. Angiography demonstrates a hypovascular mass with normal renal arteries. Renal vein sampling demonstrates elevated renin levels in reninomas, but renin is also elevated in renal artery stenosis. Surgical resection of the tumor results in reversal of hypertension and hypokalemia [60–62].

Hemangiopericytoma

Hemangiopericytomas are rare renal tumors with a malignant potential that arise from the pericytes. Tumor-induced hypoglycemia is characteristic of hemangiopericytoma and has been attributed to the production of insulin-like growth factors by the tumor. There are no distinguishing radiologic features of hemangiopericytoma from RCC or other mesenchymal tumors of the kidney [63–65].

Renal cell carcinoma

RCC is the most common primary malignancy of the kidney. It accounts for 2% of all malignancies. There has been a steady increase of 38% in the incidence of RCC between 1974 and 1990 [66]. The survival rates have also improved from 52% between 1974 and 1976 to 58% between 1983 and 1996 [66]. This trend has been attributed to the improved imaging technique and early diagnosis. Smith and colleagues [67] have reported that only 5.3% of the tumors between 1974 and 1977 were 3 cm or smaller as compared with 25.4% during 1982 to 1985. Of these small tumors in the later group, 96.7% were incidentally discovered by ultra-sonography and CT. Most RCCs that are amenable for surgical cure by either partial nephrectomy or nephron-sparing surgery are incidentally detected by the increased use of cross-sectional imaging. Ultrasonography, being the primary imaging mo-dality of the kidneys, is useful for screening and detection of small RCCs [68,69].

The RCCs are classified histologically into four main types [Table 2]. These include clear cell carci-noma, papillary carcinoma, chromophobe carci-noma, and collecting duct carcinoma. The clear cell carcinomas are the most common type, ac-

Table 2: Classification of renal cell carcinoma

Subtype	Incidence	Grade	Imaging features
Clear (conventional) cell carcinoma	70%–80%	Low-grade tumor	Poor enhancement
Papillary type	10%–15%		
Type 1		Low-grade tumor	Poor enhancement
Type 2		Aggressive tumor	Intense enhancement
Chromophobe type	4%–5%	–	
Collecting duct type	<1%	Aggressive tumor with poor prognosis	–
Medullary carcinoma	<1%	Aggressive tumor with poor prognosis and common in sickle cell trait	–

counting for 70% of the RCCs. The papillary type is the second most common type, accounting for 10% to 15% of the RCCs. The papillary type is subclasssified into type 1 and type 2 tumors. The type 2 papillary tumors are more aggressive than type 1. Clear cell and papillary tumors arise from the proximal tubular epithelium. The chromophobe carcinomas account for 5% of the RCCs and arise from cells of distal tubule. The collecting duct carcinomas are the least common type, arise from collecting duct epithelium, and are the most aggressive of all RCCs. The medullary carcinoma is a subtype of collecting duct carcinoma that is more common in patients who have sickle cell trait. Imaging cannot differentiate the different histologic types of RCC. The incidence of RCC is increased in acquired cystic disease of the kidney (ACDK). Clear cell carcinoma is the most common type of RCC associated with ACDK. The incidence of papillary type of RCC in ACDK is also higher than in the general population [70,71].

Hereditary renal cell carcinoma

RCCs are predominantly sporadic in occurrence and only 4% of them are familial in nature. The different types of hereditary RCCs are displayed in Table 3. The hereditary RCCs are characterized by autosomal dominant inheritance, presentation at a young age (third to fifth decades), and multifocal and bilateral tumors [72].

Clinical presentation of renal cell carcinoma

The classic clinical triad of hematuria, abdominal pain, and abdominal mass is seen in less than 10% of patients. About 20% to 40% present with paraneoplastic syndrome, which includes anemia, fever, hypertension, hypercalcemia, and hepatic dysfunction [73–75]. RCC can be associated with Stauffer syndrome, which is characterized by nonmetastatic intrahepatic cholestasis. This syndrome is a tumor-induced inflammatory response and is reversible after resection of the tumor [76–78]. About 2% of

Table 3: Hereditary renal cell carcinoma

Syndrome	Inheritance	Predominant renal tumor	Other renal lesions	Associated abnormalities
Von Hippel-Lindau	AD	Clear cell carcinoma	Cysts	Hemangioblastomas Retinal angiomas Pancreatic cysts Neuroendocrine tumors of pancreas Phaeochromocytoma
Hereditary papillary RCC	AD	Papillary type 1	None	None
Hereditary leiomyoma RCC	AD	Papillary type 2	None	Cutaneous and uterine leiomyomas
Birt-Hogg-Dubé	AD	Chromophobe carcinoma	Other types of RCC	Fibrofolliculomas Lung cysts Pneumothorax
Familial renal oncocytoma	–	Oncocytoma	None	–
Medullary carcinoma	–	Medullary carcinoma	None	Sickle cell trait

Abbreviation: AD, autosomal dominant.

the male patients present with left-sided varicocele because of renal vein involvement [79].

Imaging strategies of renal cell carcinoma

The goal of imaging is detection, diagnosis, and staging of RCC. Ultrasonography, CT, and MRI have variable sensitivity in detecting and staging RCC. Ultrasonography is less sensitive in detecting small renal lesions, especially those that do not deform the contour of the kidney. The sensitivity of CT and ultrasonography for detection of lesions 3 cm and less is 94% and 79%, respectively [80]. CT and MRI have nearly 100% accuracy in the diagnosis of RCC [81]. Ultrasonography is also less accurate than CT and MRI in staging of RCC. The accuracy of CT and MRI in staging of RCC ranges from 67% to 96%. Catalano and colleagues [82] have reported 96% sensitivity, 93% specificity, and 95% accuracy of multidetector CT (MDCT) in evaluating Robson stage I RCC. Robson and tumor, nodes, and metastases (TNM) staging of RCC are outlined in Table 4.

Despite these limitations, ultrasonography is still the initial imaging modality for screening and characterization of renal mass lesions. Ultrasonography is also useful in characterizing indeterminate renal mass lesions detected by CT, such as atypical cystic lesions, hypovascular solid mass lesions, and AMLs with minimal fat component [83].

Sonographic findings of renal cell carcinomas

The sonographic spectrum of RCCs varies from hypoechoic to hyperechoic solid mass lesions [**Fig. 8**]. RCCs 3 cm and smaller are predominantly hyperechoic and must be differentiated from AMLs [84,85]. The hyperechoic appearance is reported to be caused by papillary, tubular, or microcystic architecture; minute calcification; intratumoral hemorrhage; cystic degeneration; or fibrosis [24]. The presence of an anechoic rim caused by a pseudocapsule and intratumoral cystic changes can aid in differentiation of hyperechoic RCC from AML [24,86]. Several investigators have reported acoustic shadowing as a useful sign of AML [22,23]. Small isoechoic RCCs and those located at the poles can be missed by ultrasonography [26]. The isoechoic RCCs must be differentiated from pseudotumors, which include prominent column of Bertin, dromedary hump, persistent fetal lobulation, and compensatory hypertrophy. Careful attention to the morphology on gray-scale US will differentiate pseudotumors from a mass lesion. Power Doppler and contrast-enhanced sonography are useful in differentiating pseudotumors from true renal mass lesions by demonstrating similar vascularity of the pseudotumors to that of adjacent normal renal cortex [87,88]. Power Doppler and contrast-enhanced sonography will demonstrate the vascularity of a renal mass, but cannot differentiate an RCC from an AML [87,88].

Approximately 15% of the RCCs are cystic in nature and may result from extensive necrosis of a tumor, or represent a primary cystic renal carcinoma [89]. Histologically, the cystic RCCs are predominantly of clear cell type. RCCs with extensive necrosis are more aggressive as compared with the primary multilocular cystic RCCs [90,91]. Multilocular cystic RCC (MCRCC) is an uncommon subtype of RCC and constitutes about 3% of all RCCs. MCRCCs have a benign clinical course and may benefit from nephron-sparing surgery [92]. Cross-sectional imaging with US and CT of MCRCC will demonstrate well-defined, multilocular cystic mass with thin septations. Dystrophic calcification and mural nodules are less common and MCRCC should be included in the differential diagnosis of all multilocular cystic renal mass lesions in adults [93]. Small MCRCCs of less than 3 cm are hyperechoic on US and can mimic solid mass lesions, but show minimal enhancement on contrast-enhanced CT or MRI [94]. Contrast-enhanced Doppler US is reported to improve the diagnostic accuracy of malignant cystic renal mass by demonstrating the

Robson stage	Tumor description	TNM stage
I	Tumor confined within renal capsule	
	Tumor < 2.5 cm	T1
	Tumor > 2.5 cm	T2
II	Tumor extension to perinephric fat or adrenal gland	T3a
III-A	Renal vein involvement or infradiaphragmatic IVC involvement	T3b
	Supradiaphragmatic IVC involvement	T3c
III-B	Regional lymph node metastases	N1–N3
III-C	Venous involvement and lymph node metastases	
IV-A	Invasion of adjacent organs beyond the Gerota's fascia	T4
IV-B	Distant metastases	

Table 4: **Staging of renal cell carcinoma**

Abbreviations: IVC, inferior vena cava; TNM, tumor, nodes, metastases.

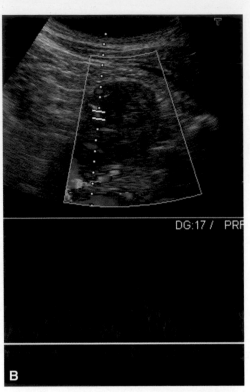

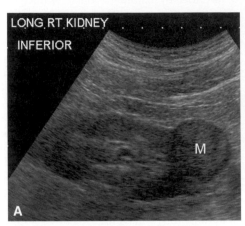

Fig. 8. RCC. Longitudinal gray-scale (*A*) and CFD (*B*) sonography of the right kidney demonstrates an iso- to hypoechoic mass arising from the lower pole, which shows presence of vascularity consistent with a RCC.

vascularity of the intracystic septations and mural nodules [95].

CT and MRI are the standard imaging methods for staging of RCC. However, US is useful in detecting the venous invasion and for demonstrating the cranial extent of the inferior vena cava (IVC) thrombus. Overall accuracy, sensitivity, and specificity of CFD for detecting the tumor involvement of renal vein and IVC is 93%, 81%, and 98%, respectively [96]. McGahan and colleagues [97] have reported a 100% sensitivity in the detection of renal vein involvement as compared with 89% sensitivity for IVC involvement by CFD sonography. Hence, US may be used as a complementary imaging modality when CT findings are equivocal in the assessment of venous extension of the tumor. The tumor thrombus is seen as an echogenic intraluminal mass causing distension of the vein. CFD will demonstrate flow around a bland thrombus and vascularity within a tumor thrombus. Use of US contrast agents is reported to improve the accuracy not only in demonstrating the extent of the thrombus but also in differentiating a tumor from a bland thrombus.

The prognosis of RCC will depend on the stage, histologic type, and grade of the tumor. The 5-year survival rates of TNM stages I, II, III, and IV are reported to be 91%, 74%, 67%, and 32%, respectively [98]. The presence of a sarcomatoid component is reported to have poor outcome [99].

Malignant uroepithelial tumors of the renal collecting system

Malignant uroepithelial tumors of the renal pelvis constitute about 5% of all the urinary tract neoplasms [100]. 90% of them are transitional cell carcinomas (TCC), 5% to 10% are squamous cell carcinomas, and less than 1% are adenocarcinomas [101,102].

Transitional carcinoma of renal pelvis

TCCs of the renal pelvis have similar epidemiologic features to those of bladder and ureter. The risk factors include exposure to chemicals in petroleum, rubber, and dye industries; analgesic abuse; and chronic inflammations. TCC is one of the several extracolonic manifestations of hereditary nonpolyposis colorectal cancer (HNPCC)/Lynch syndrome [103]. The mean age of presentation of TCC is 68 years with a higher rate of incidence in men than women. Painless hematuria is the characteristic clinical presentation of TCC [104]. Three morphologic forms of TCC are described, including focal intraluminal mass, mural thickening with narrowing of lumen, and an infiltrating mass in the renal sinus [105–107]. The excretory urogram has been the primary imaging modality for the diagnosis of TCC and is being replaced by CT or MR urogram [108,109]. These imaging modalities have the advantage of evaluating the entire urinary tract, which is crucial in the assessment of TCC.

Sonography demonstrates a poorly defined hypo- or hyperechoic mass in the renal sinus with or without pelvicaliectasis. The mass lesions are initially intraluminal and later invade the renal sinus fat and renal parenchyma. Infiltrating tumors of the renal parenchyma tend to preserve the reniform shape of the kidney [106,110].

Squamous cell carcinoma and adenocarcinoma

Squamous cell carcinoma is the second most common malignant uroepithelial tumor of the renal collecting system [**Fig. 9**]. Chronic irritation of the uroepithelium is the etiologic factor, which leads to squamous or columnar metaplasia of the transitional epithelium. Renal calculi with long-standing hydronephrosis and inflammation are important predisposing factors for squamous cell

carcinoma and adenocarcinoma of the renal pelvis [101,102,111]. The clinical presentation ranges from painless hematuria to nonspecific flank pain caused by hydronephrosis [101]. Squamous cell carcinomas are more aggressive than TCC and the tumor manifests as an infiltrating mass involving the collecting system, renal sinus fat, and renal parenchyma [112]. It is often difficult to differentiate squamous cell carcinoma of the renal pelvis from xanthogranulomatous pyelonephritis by imaging [113,114].

Renal metastases

The frequency of renal metastases is reported to vary from 7% to 13% based on autopsy findings [115,116]. More frequent use of cross-sectional imaging has resulted in an increase in the detection of renal metastases [117,118]. In patients who have a known history of malignancy, renal metastases are three times more common than primary renal tumors and are usually asymptomatic [115,116]. The tumors that most commonly metastasize to

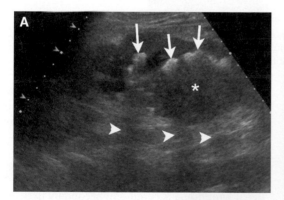

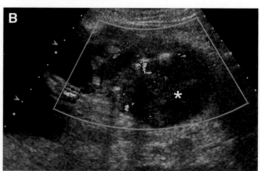

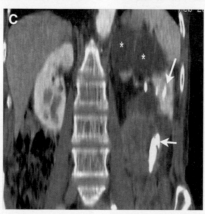

Fig. 9. Squamous cell carcinoma. Longitudinal gray-scale (*A*) and CFD (*B*) US of the left kidney demonstrates an enlarged kidney with areas of chunky calcification (*arrows*) with posterior acoustic shadowing (*arrowheads*). There is increased vascularity in the mass with large areas of necrosis (*asterisk*). Corresponding contrast-enhanced coronal CT (*C*) confirms the presence of calcification (*arrows*) and necrosis (*asterisk*). This tumor was pathologically confirmed to be a squamous cell carcinoma.

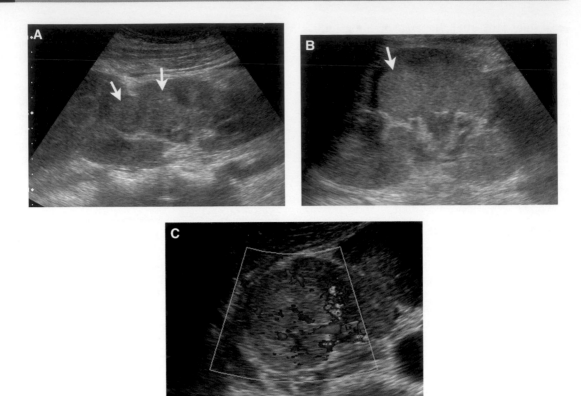

Fig. 10. Hyperechoic renal metastasis. Patient is a known case of esophageal carcinoma. Longitudinal gray-scale US of the right (A) and the left (B) kidney demonstrate multiple hyperechoic mass lesions (arrows). Tranverse CFD image (C) of the right kidney reveals increased vascularity.

the kidney are carcinoma of the lung, breast, and gastrointestinal tract, and melanoma [**Fig. 10**] [115,119]. The most common manifestation is bilateral, multiple renal mass lesions, though they can present with unilateral and solitary lesions. Renal metastases can be well-defined focal mass lesions or infiltrating in nature [117,120].

The most common sonographic appearance is hypoechoic, cortical mass lesions without through-transmission [**Fig. 11**] [121,122]. CT has higher sensitivity and accuracy than US in the detection of renal metastases [121–123]. In patients who have a known extrarenal primary malignancy, tissue sampling is necessary to differentiate metastases from a synchronous primary RCC [124].

Renal lymphoma

Renal lymphoma is commonly secondary to hematogeneous dissemination or contiguous extension from a retroperitoneal nodal disease. Primary lymphoma is rare as there is no lymphoid tissue in the

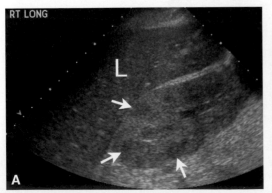
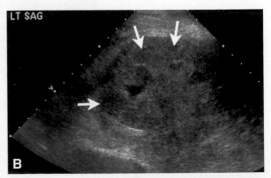

Fig. 11. Hypoechoic renal metastasis. Longitudinal gray-scale ultrasound of the right (A) and left (B) kidneys demonstrate multiple hypoechoic masses (arrows) in the renal parenchyma consistent with metastasis. L, liver.

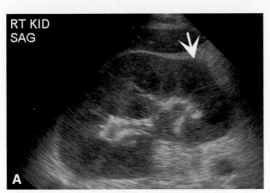
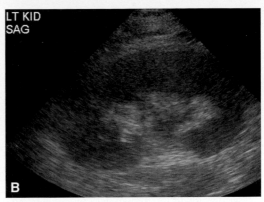

Fig. 12. Lymphoma. Longitudinal gray-scale US of the right (*A*) and the left (*B*) kidneys demonstrates bilaterally enlarged kidneys (R, 15.6 cm; L, 14.8 cm). In addition, right kidney also demonstrates a focal mass (*arrow*) in patient who has known non–Hodgkins lymphoma.

kidney [125,126]. Though the reported incidence of renal involvement on autopsy ranges from 30% to 60%, the actual detection by imaging is only 3% to 8% [127]. The kidney is most commonly involved by the non–Hodgkin's B-cell type of lymphoma [128–130]. There is a wide spectrum of renal involvement of lymphoma. Unilateral or bilateral multiple renal mass lesions are the most common type of renal lymphoma. Bilateral renal involvement is reported to occur in 50% to 72% of lymphomas [**Fig. 12**]. Other manifestations include solitary renal mass, diffuse infiltration of the renal parenchyma, contiguous invasion from retroperitoneal disease, and isolated perinephric mass [127]. In the diffuse infiltrative form, there is proliferation of lymphoma within the interstitium of the renal parenchyma, resulting in enlarged kidneys with preservation of the reniform shape [131]. The renal mass lesions are homogenously hypoechoic on ultrasonography and are hypodense on a contrast-enhanced CT [131–133]. Spontaneous hemorrhage, cystic changes, and calcification are uncommon and are usually secondary to prior treatment [127].

Summary

CT is the gold standard for the detection and characterization of renal mass lesions and in staging of RCC. Despite its limitations, ultrasonography is often the first imaging modality of the kidneys and plays an important role in the diagnosis of renal tumors. Technical advances in the gray-scale ultrasonography have improved the detection of small RCCs. CFD and contrast-enhanced Doppler ultrasonography are useful in characterization of renal tumors and in the identification of pseudotumors.

As nephron-sparing surgery is now an established technique in the management of small

RCC, intraoperative US has a key role in guiding the surgeon.

References

[1] Emamian SA, Nielsen MB, Pedersen JF, et al. Kidney dimensions at sonography: correlation with age, sex, and habitus in 665 adult volunteers. AJR Am J Roentgenol 1993;160:83–6.

[2] Grant EG, Barr LL, Borgstede J, et al. AIUM standard for the performance of an ultrasound examination of the abdomen or retroperitoneum. American Institute of Ultrasound in Medicine. J Ultrasound Med 2002;21:1182–7.

[3] Hagen-Ansert SL, Levzow B. Kidneys and adrenal glands. 3rd edition. St. Louis (MO): Mosby; 1993.

[4] Marchal G, Verbeken E, Oyen R, et al. Ultrasound of the normal kidney: a sonographic, anatomic and histologic correlation. Ultrasound Med Biol 1986;12:999–1009.

[5] Lafortune M, Constantin A, Breton G, et al. Sonography of the hypertrophied column of Bertin. AJR Am J Roentgenol 1986;146:53–6.

[6] Ascenti G, Zimbaro G, Mazziotti S, et al. Contrast- enhanced power Doppler US in the diagnosis of renal pseudotumors. Eur Radiol 2001; 11:2496–9.

[7] Tsushima Y, Sato N, Ishizaka H, et al. US findings of junctional parenchymal defect of the kidney. Nippon Igaku Hoshasen Gakkai Zasshi 1992;52:436–42.

[8] Carter AR, Horgan JG, Jennings TA, et al. The junctional parenchymal defect: a sonographic variant of renal anatomy. Radiology 1985;154: 499–502.

[9] Hoffer FA, Hanabergh AM, Teele RL. The interrenicular junction: a mimic of renal scarring on normal pediatric sonograms. AJR Am J Roentgenol 1985;145:1075–8.

[10] Seong CK, Kim SH, Lee JS, et al. Hypoechoic normal renal sinus and renal pelvis tumors: sonographic differentiation. J Ultrasound Med 2002;21:993–9 [quiz 1001–2].

[11] Schmidt H, Fischedick AR, Wiesmann W, et al. Acute focal bacterial nephritis. Rofo 1986;145: 245–9.

[12] Lee JK, McClennan BL, Melson GL, et al. Acute focal bacterial nephritis: emphasis on gray scale sonography and computed tomography. AJR Am J Roentgenol 1980;135:87–92.

[13] Soulen MC, Fishman EK, Goldman SM, et al. Bacterial renal infection: role of CT. Radiology 1989;171:703–7.

[14] Casper KA, Donnelly LF, Chen B, et al. Tuberous sclerosis complex: renal imaging findings. Radiology 2002;225:451–6.

[15] Ewalt DH, Sheffield E, Sparagana SP, et al. Renal lesion growth in children with tuberous sclerosis complex. J Urol 1991;160:141–5.

[16] Steiner MS, Goldman SM, Fishman EK, et al. The natural history of renal angiomyolipoma. J Urol 1993;150:1782–6.

[17] L'Hostis H, Deminiere C, Ferriere JM, et al. Renal angiomyolipoma: a clinicopathologic, immunohistochemical, and follow-up study of 46 cases. Am J Surg Pathol 1999;23:1011–20.

[18] Hatakeyama S, Habuchi T, Ichimura Y, et al. Rapidly growing renal angiomyolipoma during pregnancy with tumor thrombus into the inferior vena cava: a case report. Nippon Hinyokika Gakkai Zasshi 2002;93:48–51.

[19] Dickinson M, Ruckle H, Beaghler M, et al. Renal angiomyolipoma: optimal treatment based on size and symptoms. Clin Nephrol 1998;49: 281–6.

[20] Hartman DS, Goldman SM, Friedman AC, et al. Angiomyolipoma: ultrasonic-pathologic correlation. Radiology 1981;139:451–8.

[21] Scheible W, Ellenbogen PH, Leopold GR, et al. Lipomatous tumors of the kidney and adrenal: apparent echographic specificity. Radiology 1978; 129:153–6.

[22] Siegel CL, Middleton WD, Teefey SA, et al. Angiomyolipoma and renal cell carcinoma: US differentiation. Radiology 1996;198:789–93.

[23] Zebedin D, Kammerhuber F, Uggowitzer MM, et al. Criteria for ultrasound differentiation of small angiomyolipomas (< or = 3 cm) and renal cell carcinomas. Rofo 1998;169:627–32.

[24] Yamashita Y, Ueno S, Makita O, et al. Hyperechoic renal tumors: anechoic rim and intratumoral cysts in US differentiation of renal cell carcinoma from angiomyolipoma. Radiology 1993;188:179–82.

[25] Jinzaki M, Tanimoto A, Narimatsu Y, et al. Angiomyolipoma: imaging findings in lesions with minimal fat. Radiology 1997;205:497–502.

[26] Helenon O, Merran S, Paraf F, et al. Unusual fat-containing tumors of the kidney: a diagnostic dilemma. Radiographics 1997;17:129–44.

[27] Sant GR, Heaney JA, Ucci Jr AA, et al. Computed tomographic findings in renal angiomyolipoma: an histologic correlation. Urology 1984; 24:293–6.

[28] Kim JK, Park SY, Shon JH, et al. Angiomyo-

lipoma with minimal fat: differentiation from renal cell carcinoma at biphasic helical CT. Radiology 2004;230:677–84.

[29] Silbiger ML, Peterson Jr CC. Renal angiomyolipoma: its distinctive angiographic characteristics. J Urol 1971;106:363–5.

[30] Zagoria RJ, Dyer RB, Assimos DG, et al. Spontaneous perinephric hemorrhage: imaging and management. J Urol 1991;145:468–71.

[31] Yamakado K, Tanaka N, Nakagawa T, et al. Renal angiomyolipoma: relationships between tumor size, aneurysm formation, and rupture. Radiology 2002;225:78–82.

[32] Mourikis D, Chatziioannou A, Antoniou A, et al. Selective arterial embolization in the management of symptomatic renal angiomyolipomas. Eur J Radiol 1999;32:153–9.

[33] Kothary N, Soulen MC, Clark TW, et al. Renal angiomyolipoma: long-term results after arterial embolization. J Vasc Interv Radiol 2005; 16:45–50.

[34] Harrison RB, Dyer R. Benign space-occupying conditions of the kidneys. Semin Roentgenol 1987;22:275–83.

[35] Davis Jr CJ. Pathology of renal neoplasms. Semin Roentgenol 1987;22:233–40.

[36] Bennington JL. Proceedings: Cancer of the kidney–etiology, epidemiology, and pathology. Cancer 1973;32:1017–29.

[37] Bosniak MA. The small (less than or equal to 3.0 cm) renal parenchymal tumor: detection, diagnosis, and controversies. Radiology 1991; 179:307–17.

[38] Licht MR. Renal adenoma and oncocytoma. Semin Urol Oncol 1995;13:262–6.

[39] Quinn MJ, Hartman DS, Friedman AC, et al. Renal oncocytoma: new observations. Radiology 1984;153:49–53.

[40] Jasinski RW, Amendola MA, Glazer GM, et al. Computed tomography of renal oncocytomas. Comput Radiol 1985;9:307–14.

[41] Ambos MA, Bosniak MA, Valensi QJ, et al. Angiographic patterns in renal oncocytomas. Radiology 1978;129:615–22.

[42] De Carli P, Vidiri A, Lamanna L, et al. Renal oncocytoma: image diagnostics and therapeutic aspects. J Exp Clin Cancer Res 2000;19:287–90.

[43] Mead GO, Thomas Jr LR, Jackson JG. Renal oncocytoma: report of a case with bilateral multifocal oncocytomas. Clin Imaging 1990;14: 231–4.

[44] Zhang G, Monda L, Wasserman NF, et al. Bilateral renal oncocytoma: report of 2 cases and literature review. J Urol 1985;133:84–6.

[45] Kavoussi LR, Torrence RJ, Catalona WJ. Renal oncocytoma with synchronous contralateral renal cell carcinoma. J Urol 1985;134:1193–6.

[46] Nishikawa K, Fujikawa S, Soga N, et al. Renal oncocytoma with synchronous contralateral renal cell carcinoma. Hinyokika Kiyo 2002;48: 89–91.

[47] Dechet CB, Bostwick DG, Blute ML, et al. Renal

oncocytoma: multifocality, bilateralism, meta-chronous tumor development and coexistent renal cell carcinoma. J Urol 1999;162:40–2.

[48] Rodriguez CA, Buskop A, Johnson J, et al. Renal oncocytoma: preoperative diagnosis by aspiration biopsy. Acta Cytol 1980;24:355–9.

[49] Nguyen GK, Amy RW, Tsang S. Fine needle aspiration biopsy cytology of renal oncocytoma. Acta Cytol 1985;29:33–6.

[50] Alanen KA, Tyrkko JE, Nurmi MJ. Aspiration biopsy cytology of renal oncocytoma. Acta Cytol 1985;29:859–62.

[51] Steiner M, Quinlan D, Goldman SM, et al. Leiomyoma of the kidney: presentation of 4 new cases and the role of computerized tomography. J Urol 1990;143:994–8.

[52] Kanno H, Senga Y, Kumagai H, et al. Two cases of leiomyoma of the kidney. Hinyokika Kiyo 1992;38:189–93.

[53] Protzel C, Woenckhaus C, Zimmermann U, et al. Leiomyoma of the kidney. Differential diagnostic aspects of renal cell carcinoma with increasing clinical Relevance. Urologe A 2001;40: 384–7.

[54] Yazaki T, Takahashi S, Ogawa Y, et al. Large renal hemangioma necessitating nephrectomy. Urology 1985;25:302–4.

[55] Fujii Y, Ajima J, Oka K, et al. Benign renal tumors detected among healthy adults by abdominal ultrasonography. Eur Urol 1995;27: 124–7.

[56] Stanley RJ, Cubillo E, Mancilla Jimenez R, et al. Cavernous hemangioma of the kidney. Am J Roentgenol Radium Ther Nucl Med 1975;125: 682–7.

[57] Gordon R, Rosenmann E, Barzilay B, et al. Correlation of selective angiography and pathology in cavernous hemangioma of the kidney. J Urol 1976;115:608–9.

[58] Cubillo E, Hesker AE, Stanley RJ. Cavernous hemangioma of the kidney: an angiographic-pathologic correlation. J Can Assoc Radiol 1973; 24:254–6.

[59] Roswell RH. Renin-secreting tumors. J Okla State Med Assoc 1990;83:57–9.

[60] Dunnick NR, Hartman DS, Ford KK, et al. The radiology of juxtaglomerular tumors. Radiology 1983;147:321–6.

[61] Haab F, Duclos JM, Guyenne T, et al. Renin secreting tumors: diagnosis, conservative surgical approach and long-term results. J Urol 1995; 153:1781–4.

[62] Niikura S, Komatsu K, Uchibayashi T, et al. Juxtaglomerular cell tumor of the kidney treated with nephron-sparing surgery. Urol Int 2000; 65:160–2.

[63] Weiss JP, Pollack HM, McCormick JF, et al. Renal hemangiopericytoma: surgical, radiological and pathological implications. J Urol 1984; 132:337–9.

[64] Matsuda S, Usui M, Sakurai H, et al. Insulin-like growth factor II-producing intra- abdominal hemangiopericytoma associated with hypoglycemia. J Gastroenterol 2001;36:851–5.

[65] Chung J, Henry RR. Mechanisms of tumor-induced hypoglycemia with intraabdominal hemangiopericytoma. J Clin Endocrinol Metab 1996;81:919–25.

[66] Motzer RJ, Bander NH, Nanus DM. Renal-cell carcinoma. N Engl J Med 1996;335:865–75.

[67] Smith SJ, Bosniak MA, Megibow AJ, et al. Renal cell carcinoma: earlier discovery and increased detection. Radiology 1989;170:699–703.

[68] Filipas D, Spix C, Schulz-Lampel D, et al. Screening for renal cell carcinoma using ultrasonography: a feasibility study. BJU Int 2003; 91(7):595–9.

[69] Tsuboi N, Horiuchi K, Kimura G, et al. Renal masses detected by general health checkup. Int J Urol 2000;7:404–8.

[70] Ishikawa I, Kovacs G. High incidence of papillary renal cell tumours in patients on chronic haemodialysis. Histopathology 1993;22:135–9.

[71] Sasagawa I, Nakada T, Kubota Y, et al. Renal cell carcinoma in dialysis patients. Urol Int 1994; 53:79–81.

[72] Choyke PL, Glenn GM, Walther MM, et al. Hereditary renal cancers. Radiology 2003;226: 33–46.

[73] Steffens MG, de Mulder PH, Mulders PF. Paraneoplastic syndromes in three patients with renal cell carcinoma. Ned Tijdschr Geneeskd 2004; 148:487–92.

[74] Gold PJ, Fefer A, Thompson JA. Paraneoplastic manifestations of renal cell carcinoma. Semin Urol Oncol 1996;14:216–22.

[75] Kim HL, Belldegrun AS, Freitas DG, et al. Paraneoplastic signs and symptoms of renal cell carcinoma: implications for prognosis. J Urol 2003;170:1742–6.

[76] Gil H, de Wazieres B, Desmurs H, et al. Stauffer's syndrome disclosing kidney cancer: another cause of inflammatory syndrome with anicteric cholestasis. Rev Med Interne 1995;16: 775–7.

[77] Sarf I, el Mejjad A, Dakir M, et al. Stauffer syndrome associated with a giant renal tumor. Prog Urol 2003;13:290–2.

[78] Dourakis SP, Sinani C, Deutsch M, et al. Cholestatic jaundice as a paraneoplastic manifestation of renal cell carcinoma. Eur J Gastroenterol Hepatol 1997;9:311–4.

[79] Ritchie AW, Chisholm GD. The natural history of renal carcinoma. Semin Oncol 1983;10: 390–400.

[80] Amendola MA, Bree RL, Pollack HM, et al. Small renal cell carcinomas: resolving a diagnostic dilemma. Radiology 1988;166:637–41.

[81] Zagoria RJ, Wolfman NT, Karstaedt N, et al. CT features of renal cell carcinoma with emphasis on relation to tumor size. Invest Radiol 1990; 25:261–6.

[82] Catalano C, Fraioli F, Laghi A, et al. High-resolution multidetector CT in the preoperative

evaluation of patients with renal cell carcinoma. AJR Am J Roentgenol 2003;180:1271–7.

[83] Helenon O, Correas JM, Balleyguier C, et al. Ultrasound of renal tumors. Eur Radiol 2001; 11:1890–901.

[84] Yamashita Y, Takahashi M, Watanabe O, et al. Small renal cell carcinoma: pathologic and radiologic correlation. Radiology 1992;184:493–8.

[85] Forman HP, Middleton WD, Melson GL, et al. Hyperechoic renal cell carcinomas: increase in detection at US. Radiology 1993;188:431–4.

[86] Coleman BG, Arger PH, Mulhern Jr CB, et al. Gray-scale sonographic spectrum of hypernephromas. Radiology 1980;137:757–65.

[87] Jinzaki M, Ohkuma K, Tanimoto A, et al. Small solid renal lesions: usefulness of power Doppler US. Radiology 1998;209:543–50.

[88] Ascenti G, Zimbaro G, Mazziotti S, et al. Usefulness of power Doppler and contrast- enhanced sonography in the differentiation of hyperechoic renal masses. Abdom Imaging 2001; 26:654–60.

[89] Hartman DS, Davis Jr CJ, Johns T, et al. Cystic renal cell carcinoma. Urology 1986;28:145–53.

[90] Brinker DA, Amin MB, de Peralta-Venturina M, et al. Extensively necrotic cystic renal cell carcinoma: a clinicopathologic study with comparison to other cystic and necrotic renal cancers. Am J Surg Pathol 2000;24:988–95.

[91] Murad T, Komaiko W, Oyasu R, et al. Multilocular cystic renal cell carcinoma. Am J Clin Pathol 1991;95:633–7.

[92] Nassir A, Jollimore J, Gupta R, et al. Multilocular cystic renal cell carcinoma: a series of 12 cases and review of the literature. Urology 2002;60:421–7.

[93] Kim JC, Kim KH, Lee JW. CT and US findings of multilocular cystic renal cell carcinoma. Korean J Radiol 2000;1:104–9.

[94] Yamashita Y, Miyazaki T, Ishii A, et al. Multilocular cystic renal cell carcinoma presenting as a solid mass: radiologic evaluation. Abdom Imaging 1995;20:164–8.

[95] Kim AY, Kim SH, Kim YJ, et al. Contrast-enhanced power Doppler sonography for the differentiation of cystic renal lesions: preliminary study. J Ultrasound Med 1999;18:581–8.

[96] Habboub HK, Abu-Yousef MM, Williams RD, et al. Accuracy of color Doppler sonography in assessing venous thrombus extension in renal cell carcinoma. AJR Am J Roentgenol 1997;168: 267–71.

[97] McGahan JP, Blake LC, deVere White R, et al. Color flow sonographic mapping of intravascular extension of malignant renal tumors. J Ultrasound Med 1993;12:403–9.

[98] Tsui KH, Shvarts O, Smith RB, et al. Prognostic indicators for renal cell carcinoma: a multivariate analysis of 643 patients using the revised 1997 TNM staging criteria. J Urol 2000;163: 1090–5.

[99] Cheville JC, Lohse CM, Zincke H, et al. Sarco-matoid renal cell carcinoma: an examination of underlying histologic subtype and an analysis of associations with patient outcome. Am J Surg Pathol 2004;28:435–41.

[100] Leder RA, Dunnick NR. Transitional cell carcinoma of the pelvicalices and ureter. AJR Am J Roentgenol 1990;155:713–22.

[101] Blacher EJ, Johnson DE, Abdul-Karim FW, et al. Squamous cell carcinoma of renal Pelvis. Urology 1985;25:124–6.

[102] Stein A, Sova Y, Lurie M, et al. Adenocarcinoma of the renal pelvis. Report of two cases, one with simultaneous transitional cell carcinoma of the bladder. Urol Int 1988;43:299–301.

[103] Sijmons RH, Kiemeney LA, Witjes JA, et al. Urinary tract cancer and hereditary nonpolyposis colorectal cancer: risks and screening options. J Urol 1998;160:466–70.

[104] Nocks BN, Heney NM, Daly JJ, et al. Transitional cell carcinoma of renal pelvis. Urology 1982;19:472–7.

[105] Yousem DM, Gatewood OM, Goldman SM, et al. Synchronous and metachronous transitional cell carcinoma of the urinary tract: prevalence, incidence, and radiographic detection. Radiology 1988;167:613–8.

[106] Wong-You-Cheong JJ, Wagner BJ, Davis CJ. Transitional cell carcinoma of the urinary tract: radiologic-pathologic correlation. Radiographics 1998;18:123–42.

[107] Baron RL, McLennan BL, Lee JKT, et al. Computed tomography of transitional cell carcinoma of the renal pelvis and ureter. Radiology 1982; 144:125–30.

[108] Kawashima A, Vrtiska TJ, LeRoy AJ, et al. CT urography. Radiographics 2004;24:35–54.

[109] Joffe SA, Servaes S, Okon S, et al. Multi-detector row CT urography in the evaluation of hematuria. Radiographics 2003;23(6):1441–55.

[110] Subramanyam BR, Raghavendra BN, Madamba MR. Renal transitional cell carcinoma: sonographic and pathologic correlation. J Clin Ultrasound 1982;10:203–10.

[111] Kobayashi S, Ohmori M, Akaeda T, et al. Primary adenocarcinoma of the renal pelvis. Report of two cases and brief review of literature. Acta Pathol Jpn 1983;33:589–97.

[112] Wimbish KJ, Sanders MM, Samuels BI, et al. Squamous cell carcinoma of the renal pelvis: case report emphasizing sonographic and CT appearance. Urol Radiol 1983;5:267–9.

[113] Kenney PJ. Imaging of chronic renal infections. AJR Am J Roentgenol 1990;155:485–94.

[114] Kim J. Ultrasonographic features of focal xanthogranulomatous pyelonephritis. J Ultrasound Med 2004;23:409–16.

[115] Choyke PL, White EM, Zeman RK, et al. Renal metastases: clinicopathologic and radiologic correlation. Radiology 1987;162:359–63.

[116] Bhatt GM, Bernardino ME, Graham Jr SD. CT diagnosis of renal metastases. J Comput Assist Tomogr 1983;7:1032–4.

[117] Mitnick JS, Bosniak MA, Rothberg M, et al. Metastatic neoplasm to the kidney studied by computed tomography and sonography. J Comput Assist Tomogr 1985;9:43–9.

[118] Becker WE, Schellhammer PF. Renal metastases from carcinoma of the lung. Br J Urol 1986; 58:494–8.

[119] Volpe JP, Choyke PL. The radiologic evaluation of renal metastases. Crit Rev Diagn Imaging 1990;30:219–46.

[120] Hartman DS, Davidson AJ, Davis Jr CJ, et al. Infiltrative renal lesions: CT- sonographic-pathologic correlation. AJR Am J Roentgenol 1988;150:1061–4.

[121] Paivanalo M, Tikkakoski T, Merikanto J, et al. Radiologic findings in renal metastases. Aktuelle Radiol 1993;3:360–5.

[122] Dalla Palma L, Pozzi Mucelli RS, Zuiani C. Ultrasonography and computerized tomography in the diagnosis of renal metastasis. Radiol Med (Torino) 1991;82:95–100.

[123] Honda H, Coffman CE, Berbaum KS, et al. CT analysis of metastatic neoplasms of the kidney. Comparison with primary renal cell carcinoma. Acta Radiol 1992;33:39–44.

[124] Pickhardt PJ, Lonergan GJ, Davis Jr CJ, et al. From the archives of the AFIP. Infiltrative renal lesions: radiologic-pathologic correlation. Armed Forces Institute of Pathology. Radiographics 2000;20:215–43.

[125] Fernandez-Acenero MJ, Galindo M, Bengoechea O, et al. Primary malignant lymphoma of the kidney: case report and literature review. Gen Diagn Pathol 1998;143:317–20.

[126] Porcaro AB, D'Amico A, Novella G, et al. Primary lymphoma of the kidney. Report of a case and update of the literature. Arch Ital Urol Androl 2002;74:44–7.

[127] Heiken JP, Gold RP, Schnur MJ, et al. Computed tomography of renal lymphoma with ultrasound correlation. J Comput Assist Tomogr 1983;7:245–50.

[128] Cohan RH, Dunnick NR, Leder RA, et al. Computed tomography of renal lymphoma. J Comput Assist Tomogr 1990;14:933–8.

[129] Ferry JA, Harris NL, Papanicolaou N, et al. Lymphoma of the kidney. A report of 11 cases. Am J Surg Pathol 1995;19:134–44.

[130] Richards MA, Mootoosamy I, Reznek RH, et al. Renal involvement in patients with non-Hodgkin's lymphoma: clinical and pathological features in 23 cases. Hematol Oncol 1990;8:105–10.

[131] Hartman DS, Davidson AJ, Davis Jr CJ, et al. Infiltrative renal lesions: CT-sonographic-pathologic correlation. AJR Am J Roentgenol 1988;150:1061–4.

[132] Horii SC, Bosniak MA, Megibow AJ, et al. Correlation of CT and ultrasound in the evaluation of renal lymphoma. Urol Radiol 1983;5:69–76.

[133] Sheeran SR, Sussman SK. Renal lymphoma: spectrum of CT findings and potential mimics. AJR Am J Roentgenol 1998;171:1067–72.

ULTRASOUND CLINICS

Ultrasound Clin 1 (2006) 43–54

Prostate Ultrasound: Past, Present, and Future

Sarah E. McAchran, MD, Martin I. Resnick, MD*

- Ultrasonographically guided biopsy
- Benign prostatic hyperplasia
- Prostate volume
- Prostatic abscess
- Future
- Summary
- References

The first application of ultrasound in medical diagnosis occurred in 1942 when Karl Dussik [1] placed transducers on patients' craniums and recorded the through-transmission of the sound beam in an attempt to localize a brain tumor. In 1949, the first successful pulse echo system, which could record echoes from tissue interfaces, was developed by Douglas Howry and W. Roderic Bliss at the University of Colorado School of Medicine [2]. In 1951, Wild and Neal [3] of St. Martin's Hospital reported that A-mode display ultrasonography was capable of showing differences between normal and abnormal tissues. The following year, Wild and Reid [4] published the first two-dimensional echograms of biologic tissues (kidney cortex and myoblastoma of the thigh). In 1963, Takahashi and Ouchi [5] were the first investigators to report the use of ultrasound to image the prostate by way of an abdominal approach, but unfortunately these A-mode display images were difficult to interpret and not clinically useful. One year later, these investigators successfully obtained tomographic pictures of the prostate with the use of a transrectal probe equipped with a radial scanning device [6]. Although resolution was improved, the images also were of poor quality and of no clinical value.

Watanabe and associates [7], using a chair device, are credited with obtaining the first clinically useful transrectal ultrasonographic images of the prostate in 1967 [Fig. 1]. Remarkable improvement in ultrasonography of the prostate was obtained with the use of a transrectal radial probe with a special concave 3.5-MHz transducer covered with a water-filled balloon [8]. A B-mode display was used and reproducible transverse prostate images were visualized on a black and white screen. Transrectal ultrasound scanning was also evaluated by VonMicsky [9], a gynecologist who developed an ultrasound scanning device in conjunction with a sigmoidoscope to visualize pelvic structures.

The first reports of investigators in the United States using transrectal ultrasound for evaluation of prostate came in 1972, and the images shown in the cathode ray tube were recorded with a Polaroid camera [Fig. 2] [10,11]. These initial reports were the culmination of several experiments that were conducted beginning in 1968 at the Bowman Gray School of Medicine under the direction of William H. Boyce [12–14], who described these early developments. Initially studies were performed with skin-coupled B-mode transducers through the perineum and other portals before the final decision was made to use an intrarectal balloon-coupled rotational array transducer. It was mounted on a stable tripod, adjustable in height to the cystoscopic table, and capable of fixation at virtually any angle selected by the operator as the

Department of Urology, University Hospitals of Cleveland, 11100 Euclid Avenue, Cleveland, OH 44106-5046, USA
* Corresponding author.
E-mail address: martin.resnick@case.edu (M.I. Resnick).

1556-858X/06/$ – see front matter © 2005 Elsevier Inc. All rights reserved.
ultrasound.theclinics.com

doi:10.1016/j.cult.2005.09.003

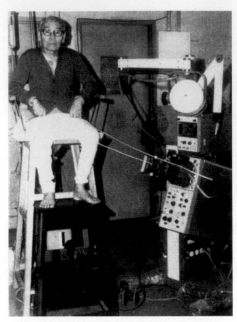

Fig. 1. Early chair device with a rectal probe for prostate imaging. Refinements in instrumentation simplified the examination, but all studies continued using the chair device. (*From* Resnick MI. Ultrasonography of the prostate and testes. J Ultrasound Med 2003;22: 869–77; with permission.)

planned position of reference [**Fig. 3**]. The probe had a ratchet and a scale, which permitted the planned position to become zero on the scale. The ratchet then moved the transducer a precise distance (1–5 mm) along the axis of the probe, permitting serial tomograms of the prostate and related structures. These "loaf-of-bread" slices permitted a three-dimensional reconstruction of the prostate gland [**Fig. 4**].

The first transducer was the 3.5-MHz generator receiver mounted at 90° from the long axis of the probe [**Fig. 5**]. A single 360° sweep at a precise rate was made for each activation of an electronic motor, providing highly reproducible static sonograms. A plastic sheet protected the balloon from contact with the rotating element. The balloon covered the entire insertable probe and was filled with fluid through a tube in the probe shaft.

In 1968 and 1969, work progressed on construction of prototype equipment and attempts to solve the apparently simple problems of air bubbles; detection of highly absorptive interrectal interfaces; and establishment of reliable points of reference (anatomic and ultrasonographic). More difficult problems included those of focusing, energy control, and permanent records from a cathode ray tube. Placing the patient in the knee-chest position ultimately eliminated the air bubble problem. However, there was no electronic conversion ca-

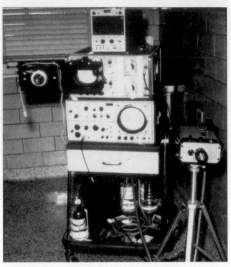

Fig. 2. Early transrectal equipment with a cathode ray tube and tripod device to position the probe. Early studies used fluoroscopy to document probe position and to correlate anatomic structures visualized with ultrasonographic images. (*From* Resnick MI. Ultrasonography of the prostate and testes. J Ultrasound Med 2003;22:869–77; with permission.)

pability, and it was essential to have a roadmap orientation of the sonogram to cystoscopic, fluoroscopic, radiologic, and physical examination of the patient. Several coupling agents and techniques were investigated, but none was satisfactory. Virtually everything done was repeated in all reasonable variations, modes, and patient positions.

In late 1969 and early 1970, the equipment was assembled in the Urology Department, and a proto-

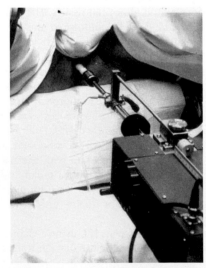

Fig. 3. Patient in the lithotripsy position with the probe in place. The probe is mounted on a tripod with a planned position indicator. (*From* Resnick MI. Ultrasonography of the prostate and testes. J Ultrasound Med 2003;22:869–77; with permission.)

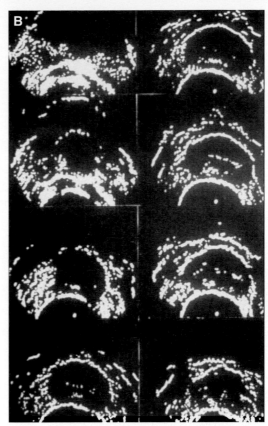

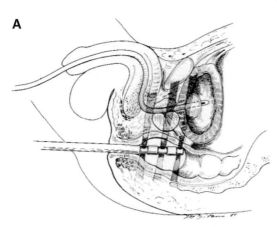

Fig. 4. (*A*) Diagram showing successive cephalad and caudad movement of the probe for imaging the prostate in the transverse plane. (*B*) Typical examination. Serial scans at 4-mm intervals beginning at the urinary bladder (*upper left*) and progressing to the apex of the prostate are shown. The patient is in the lithotomy position, and the rectum is at the bottom of each scan. (*From* Resnick MI. Ultrasonography of the prostate and testes. J Ultrasound Med 2003;22:869–77; with permission.)

col was developed for standardized examinations. Examinations were performed on patients who had well-defined urologic disease who required fluoroscopic examinations, radiographic examinations, or both, and cystoscopic evaluations. In addition to Dr. William Boyce, Dr. William King, Dr. Mark Wilkiemeyer, and James Willard conducted these early investigations. Dr. James Martin, Dr. William

McKinney, and Dr. Fred Kremkau also lent their radiologic and ultrasonic experience to these early studies. In 1972, a scan converter and video screen with a capacity of 8 to 10 shades of gray were obtained, with considerable improvement in image quality [**Fig. 6**]. For the three ensuing years from

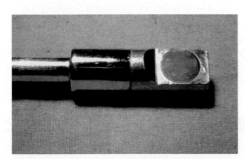

Fig. 5. Initial studies were performed with a 3.5-MHz transducer mounted on a rotating probe. (*From* Resnick MI. Ultrasonography of the prostate and testes. J Ultrasound Med 2003;22:869–77; with permission.)

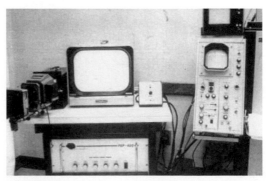

Fig. 6. First scan converter and video display, 1972. The capacity was 8 to 10 shades of gray. (*From* Resnick MI. Ultrasonography of the prostate and testes. J Ultrasound Med 2003;22:869–77; with permission.)

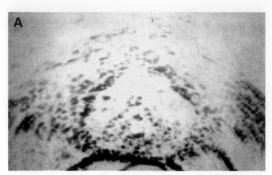
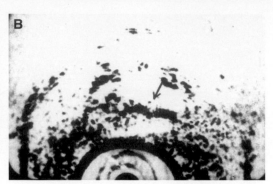

Fig. 7. (*A*) Scan of prostate with benign hyperplasia using a 3.5-MHz transducer. (*B*) Scan of prostate with malignancy (*arrow*) using a 3.5-MHz transducer. (*From* Resnick MI. Ultrasonography of the prostate and testes. J Ultrasound Med 2003;22:869–77; with permission.)

1972 to 1975, many studies were performed to assess urologic diseases of the pelvis. Data were recoded using 35-mm filmstrips, and the first clinical research program began in 1972 studying patients who had localized carcinoma of the prostate. Recognition of advanced stages of prostate cancer was noted, but early stage disease could not be detected. Furthermore, it was noted that the locations of histologic cancer in radical prostatectomy specimens were often at variance with the sonographic impressions [**Fig. 7**].

In 1975, gray-scale equipment with more than 18 shades of gray was acquired, and studies ensued addressing early diagnosis of prostate cancer; accurate staging of cancer of the bladder and prostate; and monitoring the response of prostate cancer to therapy. The National Prostate Cancer Project of the National Cancer Institute funded much of this work, with Dr. Martin Resnick as the principle investigator. The studies recognized that higher-frequency transducers were required, and with the assistance of Dr. Ronald Heilman, higher-frequency transducers of up to 7 MHz were used. Gray-scale quality was further enhanced by increasing the number of shades of gray produced by the scan converter, and the use of higher-frequency transducers improved the resolution of ultrasonographic imaging considerably [**Figs. 8 and 9**].

The introduction of electronic real-time imaging in the early 1980s further enhanced the quality of ultrasonographic images [**Fig. 10**] [15]. Shortly thereafter, the clinical applications of transrectal ultrasonography of the prostate began to expand, as evidenced by the dramatic increase in publications on transrectal ultrasonography of the prostate in the medical literature during the mid-1980s. Most investigators concluded that the transrectal techniques were preferable to the transabdominal, transperineal, and transurethral techniques when visualizing the prostate because of more consistent and reproducible imaging. These alternative techniques often provided poor definition of the prostate margins depending on the approach and were dependent on bladder distension to improve image quality. Currently, transrectal techniques are used almost exclusively. The future of prostate ultrasound will involve improvements in image processing; application of color and power Doppler imaging; the development and use of ultrasonographic contrast agents; and the application of three-dimensional imaging. All of these methods promise to enhance the reliability and applicability of this examination and are discussed later.

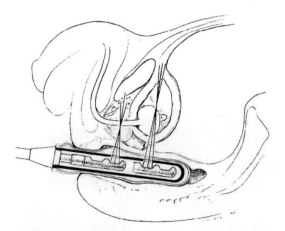

Fig. 8. Transrectal probe with 3.5- and 5.0-MHz transducers to enhance imaging of the prostate. Only one frequency was used at a time. (*From* Resnick MI. Ultrasonography of the prostate and testes. J Ultrasound Med 2003;22:869–77; with permission.)

Ultrasonographically guided biopsy

The office-based performance of ultrasound-guided prostate biopsies has become the primary modality used to diagnose prostate adenocarcinoma in patients who have an increased prostate-specific antigen (PSA) or abnormal digital rectal examination.

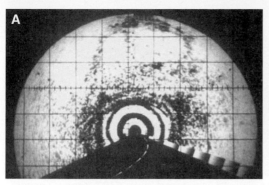
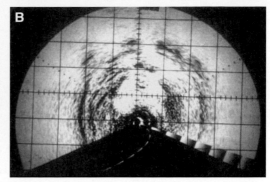

Fig. 9. (*A*) Scan of the prostate with benign hyperplasia using a 5.0-MHz transducer. (*B*) Scan of the prostate with benign hyperplasia using a 3.5-MHz transducer. (*From* Resnick MI. Ultrasonography of the prostate and testes. J Ultrasound Med 2003;22:869–77; with permission.)

The first investigators to use transrectal ultrasonographic guidance performed a biopsy by way of the transperineal route with the use of a radial scanner equipped with a special puncture attachment containing holes aligned parallel to the transducer [**Fig. 11**] [16]. Interestingly, Holm and colleagues [17] were the first to report the use of this technique for the placement of radioactive seeds within the prostate for treating localized cancer of the prostate. This method of seed implantation continues today. Other investigators have used the longitudinal linear array transducer to perform the biopsy by way of the perineal route [18–20]. Popularized by Lee and associates [21–24], more recently transrectal ultrasonographic guidance has been used to perform transrectal biopsies and has become the standard in today's practice. Transrectal techniques are preferred over transperineal approaches because the path of the needle is shorter and deviation of the needle within the prostate is less likely to occur, thus making positioning easier and more accurate. The procedure is quicker because there is no skin preparation, and local anesthesia, although not required, is being used with increasing frequency and has considerably reduced pain associated with the procedure. Although the risk for infection is greater with a transrectal approach, the use of prophylactic antibiotics has resulted in an infection rate of approximately 1%. Improvements in biopsy needles and the use of spring-loaded biopsy guns have improved prostate tissue samples and have also lessened patient discomfort.

The descriptions of prostate anatomy by Dr. John McNeal [25,26] had a considerable impact on the technique of prostate biopsy. McNeal described the prostate as being composed of three glandular zones (peripheral, transitional, and central) and the periurethral glands. The peripheral zone accounts for approximately 75% of the glandular tissue of the normal prostate and is the most frequent site of origin of carcinoma. With aging there is appreciable growth of the transition zone, which predominantly gives rise to benign prostatic hyperplasia. Initially McNeal's concept of zonal anatomy had little usefulness in the clinical sphere or in

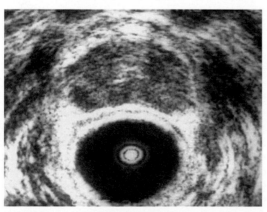

Fig. 10. Scan of the prostate, 3.5-MHz transducer with improved gray-scale imaging. (*From* Resnick MI. Ultrasonography of the prostate and testes. J Ultrasound Med 2003;22:869–77; with permission.)

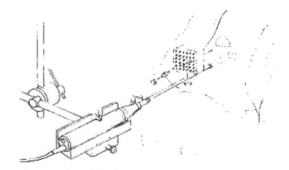

Fig. 11. Biopsy technique as described by Holm and colleagues. A similar technique is used for brachytherapy. (*From* Resnick MI. Ultrasonography of the prostate and testes. J Ultrasound Med 2003;22:869–77; with permission.)

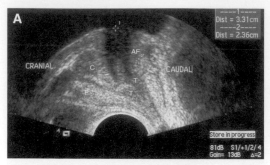 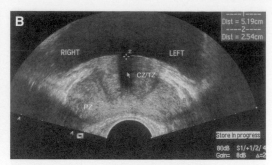

Fig. 12. (A) Normal prostate, sagittal view. C, central zone; P, peripheral zone; T, transitional zone; AF, anterior fibromuscular stroma. (B) Normal prostate, transverse view. PZ, peripheral zone; CZ/TZ, central zone/transitional zone.

diagnostic imaging; however, with the development of cross-sectional imaging techniques, the zonal concept of anatomy became useful because it not only permitted interpretation of sonographic images of the internal structure of the prostate but also assisted in guiding prostate biopsy [**Fig. 12**]. Cooner and colleagues [27] also brought attention to the importance of zonal anatomy in the interpretation of ultrasonographic images and recognized the potential value of prostate ultrasonography in the detection and diagnosis of early cancer of the prostate.

Exhaustive research has been aimed at determining the sonographic appearance of prostate cancer. Early investigators demonstrated that tumors can appear as hypoechoic areas in the peripheral zone [**Fig. 13**]; therefore, it was hoped that transrectal ultrasound would be able to locate malignant lesions for biopsy and serve as a noninvasive screening tool. Unfortunately, ultrasound proved to be fairly disappointing in both regards [28]. The sonographic appearance of prostate cancer is varied, and early stage lesions tend to be indistinct from normal prostate tissue. As PSA screening has evolved and has led to the detection of early stage, low-volume cancers, the strategy of first recognizing the lesion on radiologic examination and then obtaining a biopsy of the lesion is not practical. Therefore, the true use of transrectal ultrasound resides in its ability to enable sampling of all relevant areas of the prostate, including those that appear ultrasonically normal [29].

The normal prostate appears homogeneous with a stipple gray echogenicity and a well-defined, echogenic, continuous capsule. The zonal anatomy can usually be identified. A distinct layer of echogenic fibrous tissue separates the transition zone from the central and peripheral zones. In transverse images the prostate appears symmetric with a semilunar shape. The periurethral tissue can be identified as hypoechoic and centrally located, whereas the peripheral zone tissue has a fine, homogeneous echo pattern. In longitudinal or sagittal images, the relationship of the prostate to the bladder neck, seminal vesicles, and normal prostatic urethra is easily identified [**Figs. 14 and 15**]. In the midline the urethra will appear as a curved structure within the central portion of the gland. Oriented horizontally in the transverse plane, the seminal vesicles are paired, symmetric, crescent-shaped structures that appear less echogenic than the prostate and are separated from the prostate base by hyperechoic fatty tissue.

The practice of systematic, sextant biopsies was described by Hodge and colleagues [30] in 1989 and remains the foundation of the prostate biopsy procedure today. The technical aspects of transrectal ultrasound-guided prostate biopsy are straightforward. Before the procedure, patients should discontinue all anticoagulants. Recent studies have demonstrated that prebiopsy cleansing enemas do not significantly reduce the incidence of postprocedure infection and can be abandoned [31]. Traditionally 2 to 3 days of prophylactic antibiotics have been prescribed but recent studies have demonstrated that a single dose of a long-acting fluoroquinolone 1 hour before the procedure is sufficient antibiotic coverage and does not increase the postprocedure infection rate of 1% [32–34].

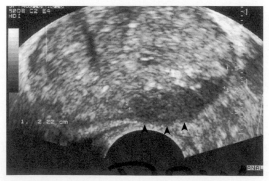

Fig. 13. Prostate cancer appearing as a peripheral, hypoechoic lesion.

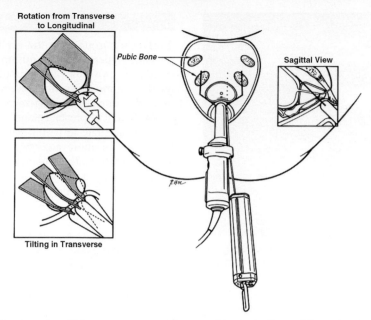

Fig. 14. Prostatic ultrasound and biopsy, transverse. The sound beam is directed from the tip of the biplanar, or end-fire probe. Manipulating the probe in the anterior—posterior direction will image the prostate in the transverse section from the apex to the base, as shown. (*From* Torp-Pedersen ST, Lee F. Transrectal biopsy of the prostate guided by transrectal ultrasound. Urol Clin N Am 1989;16(4):703–12; with permission.)

With the patient in either the lateral decubitus or dorsal lithotomy position, the well-lubricated transrectal probe is guided into the rectum above the anal verge and a thorough sonographic examination of the prostate is performed. Biplane, multiplane, and end-fire endorectal probes with a frequency range from 6 to 8 MHz are used to image the prostate and adjacent structures, including the seminal vesicles and urethra. Suspicious, hypoechoic areas should be recorded.

Periprostatic nerve blockade has recently been studied as a localized and uncomplicated method of decreasing the pain associated with prostate biopsy [35–39]. Under ultrasound guidance a sterile 5-inch 22-gauge spinal needle is passed through the biopsy needle port and positioned at the prostate base at the junction between the prostate and seminal vesicle—the site of the neurovascular bundle. Before injecting 2.5 cm^3 of 1% lidocaine, the syringe is aspirated to ensure that intravascular in-

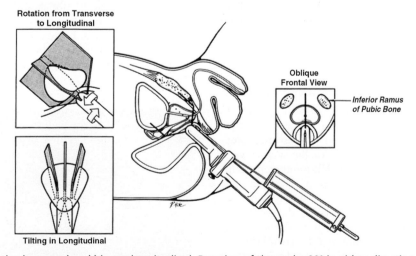

Fig. 15. Prostatic ultrasound and biopsy, longitudinal. Rotation of the probe 90° in either direction will reach the longitudinal plane. Angling the probe from left to right in this plane will image the lateral borders of the prostate. (*From* Torp-Pedersen ST, Lee F. Transrectal biopsy of the prostate guided by transrectal ultrasound. Urol Clin N Am 1989;16(4):703–12; with permission.)

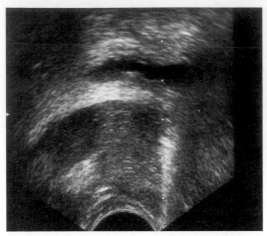

Fig. 16. The dotted line represents the needle guide, and overlies the corresponding echogenic trail of the needle.

jection will not occur, as this can cause seizures. Periprostatic nerve blockade is performed bilaterally.

A sterile 18-gauge biopsy needle is placed into a spring-loaded biopsy gun and advanced through the needle guide attached to the ultrasound probe. Using a marker line, available with most modern ultrasound view monitors, any suspicious lesion can be biopsied in either the sagittal or longitudinal plane [**Fig. 16**]. The rest of the prostate should then be sampled in a systematic fashion, encompassing the full length of the peripheral zone laterally and anteriorly. There is considerable debate over the number and location of core biopsies necessary to detect prostate cancer, but the evidence suggests that an extended biopsy technique, including 10 to 12 cores and more laterally placed biopsies, improves detection over the traditional sextant technique [29,35,36].

Benign prostatic hyperplasia

Benign prostatic hyperplasia (BPH) is present in 50% of 50-year-old men, and the percentage increases with aging. Some men will remain asymptomatic, whereas others will develop symptoms of bladder outlet obstruction. Ultrasonographically, BPH is seen as the proliferation of transition zone tissues, with compression of the adjacent peripheral zone [**Fig. 17**]. Occasionally, the peripheral gland is so compressed that it is almost totally displaced. The echotexture of the hyperplastic tissue is mixed, with regions of increased echogenicity that may be foci of corpora amylacea. Corpora amylacea lack the distal acoustic shadows that are seen with true calcifications.

Prostate volume

Prostate ultrasound for the evaluation of benign prostatic hyperplasia has minimal clinical utility, except in providing an accurate volume assessment. Volume determination may help in planning the surgical management of the disease. Measurement of prostate gland volume using ultrasound is accurate to within 5% of its true weight [40]. It is far more accurate than estimation by digital palpation. The length, width, and height of the prostate are measured using the transverse and longitudinal orientations. The volume of the prostate is then estimated using the formula for an ellipsoid. Planimetry, which measures the surface area of the prostate at regular intervals throughout the gland and is used to determine gland volume, is the most accurate means of volume measurement. This method accommodates individual variations in prostate shape. With its superior accuracy, planimetry is used when planning brachytherapy treatment for prostate cancer.

Prostate volume is also used in the calculation of PSA density, where serum PSA is interpreted in relation to prostate size. PSA density may help the clinician judge whether a PSA increase is caused by BPH or malignancy. PSA density is calculated according to the formula: PSA density = PSA (ng/cm^3)/prostate volume (cm^3). A PSA density of 0.15 or greater is considered suspicious for cancer [41,42].

Prostatic abscess

Acute and chronic prostatitis are conditions that are diagnosed by history, physical examination, and urinalysis. The role of ultrasound is reserved for situations in which acute prostatitis is complicated by a prostatic abscess. Intravenous antibiotics may penetrate the prostatic tissue poorly, and ultimately ultrasound-guided drainage may be indicated.

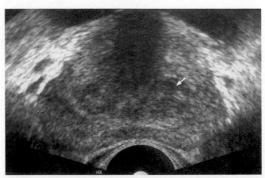

Fig. 17. Benign prostatic hyperplasia. The small arrow indicates the hyperplastic transition zone.

Sonographically, the prostatic abscess presents as a complex collection of cystic and solid elements within the parenchyma. The internal echoes represent cellular debris and necrotic material. It may have a frankly fluid-looking appearance, or may be more difficult to appreciate if it has more of the characteristics of soft tissue. Where visualized, a prostatic abscess may be drained by transrectally guided transperineal or transrectal placement of a wide-bore needle, or it may be resected transuretherally [43].

Future

The roles of three-dimensional, color, and power Doppler ultrasound and the value of ultrasound contrast materials for the evaluation of prostate cancer are the subject of much current research [44]. For tumors to grow, they require a blood supply. This blood supply has been typified by low, slow flow. Power Doppler enables these small tumor vessels to be imaged by ultrasound in real time [37]. Color Doppler analysis is performed during transrectal ultrasound with a probe capable of color and pulsed Doppler. Increased flow in the peripheral gland is considered abnormal and suggestive of malignancy [38]. However, interpretation of this increased flow is not always straightforward, and the use of color Doppler ultrasound to increase sensitivity and specificity of transrectal ultrasound remains to be proven [39,45].

Where color Doppler analysis may prove most beneficial is in the planning of interstitial laser treatment for BPH. With this treatment, a laser fiber is placed into the prostate transurethrally and allowed to heat the tissue to a predetermined temperature for a predetermined length of time. This heating causes the destruction of prostate cells in an area surrounding the fiber, thereby widening the voiding channel and improving symptoms of urinary obstruction. The size and shape of the area destroyed may strongly depend on the vascular flow in that area. Therefore, using color Doppler ultrasound to accurately quantify prostatic blood flow may help to select the optimal thermal dose necessary to achieve the desired improvement in voiding parameters and symptoms [39]. Furthermore, preoperative ultrasound with color Doppler analysis may help to select patients who would be optimal candidates for this type of procedure.

Three recent studies have used intravenous ultrasound contrast in an attempt to enhance color Doppler ultrasound of the prostate [46–48]. Ultrasound contrast agents are injectable liquids that yield circulating microbubbles measuring 1 to 5 μm. These small air bubbles increase the echo density of the blood, resulting in enhanced visualization of the vasculature and better spatial resolution of the ultrasound image [39]. They have been used to characterize renal vascularity and renal masses [49]. The study from Thomas Jefferson University performed contrast injection and color Doppler ultrasound in the office setting, demonstrating encouraging improvement in biopsy sensitivity from 38% to 65% without substantial loss of specificity [48].

Similarly, three-dimensional ultrasound of the prostate can be easily performed in the office setting [50]. A three-dimensional endorectal volume transducer is substituted for the conventional two-dimensional ultrasound probe and can be coupled to a commercially available ultrasound unit. Automatic, planimetric volume scanning allows for nearly immediate reconstruction and display of sectional anatomy in orthogonal and oblique planes. It remains to be proven, but three-dimensional ultrasound may be superior in depicting tumor

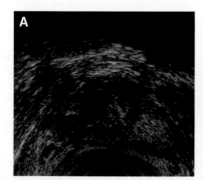 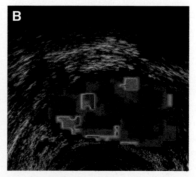

Fig. 18. Example of analysis of ultrasound image to obtain probability of malignancy. (*A*) Gray-scale ultrasound image used for color coding. (*B*) Probability of malignancy. Red represents high probability and blue represents low probability (*From* Aarnink RG, Beerlage HP, De La Rosette JJ, et al. Transrectal ultrasound of the prostate: innovations and future applications. J Urol 1998;159:1568–79; with permission.)

presence and extraglandular extent of disease. Furthermore, it allows more accurate repeated measurement than does two-dimensional imaging. This capability can be useful when accurate volume assessments are required for dosimetry planning for radiation therapy or for estimating prostate-specific antigen levels [51].

Although the above innovations deal with the acquisition of ultrasound images, other areas of research are focused on the interpretation of these images. Computerized interpretation of ultrasound images of the prostate may reveal information not perceptible to the human eye. Abnormal structures may have subtle changes in texture that can be quantified on a structural, statistical, or spectral basis. Using a neural network, these subtle changes can be translated into color-coded images, where different colors indicate different probabilities of malignancy [**Fig. 18**] [52]. This method may help to overcome the low predictive value of transrectal ultrasound for the clinical diagnosis of prostate cancer by better discriminating malignant from benign. In one study from Memorial Sloan Kettering comparing prostate biopsy guided by traditional B-mode ultrasound with prostate biopsy using spectrum analysis, the use of spectrum analysis significantly improved the sensitivity and specificity of prostate cancer detection [53].

It is no great leap to see how this would also improve planning for brachytherapy for prostate cancer. Because current prostatic imaging methods cannot accurately identify cancerous regions within the prostate, the whole prostate is irradiated, causing the inherent increase in the potential side effects of radiation. Guidance for radiation therapy using the described tissue characterization methods would allow more effective targeting of cancerous tissue and spare noncancerous tissue. Similarly, this type of imaging could be applied to the evaluation of men who have a rising PSA following definitive treatment for prostate cancer. Spectrum analysis–based tissue characterization techniques have already shown promise for noninvasively monitoring intraocular cancer treated with ^{60}cobalt plaque therapy [54].

Summary

Since its inception 60 years ago, there have been profound advances in the field of prostatic ultrasound. Its major usefulness remains in the areas of volume measurement and biopsy guidance; however, ongoing research into refinements of image acquisition and processing promise to expand on these applications. Equally brisk progress can be expected in the next 60 years.

References

[1] Dussik K. Uber die Moglichkeit hochfrequente mechanische Schwingungen als diagnostisches Hilfsmittel zu verwenden [The use of high frequency ultrasound as a diagnostic tool]. Z Ges Neurol Psychiatr 1942;174:153 [in German].

[2] Martin J. History of ultrasound. In: Resnick MI, editor. Ultrasound in urology. Baltimore (MD): Williams & Wilkins; 1984. p. 1–12.

[3] Wild JJ, Neal D. Use of high-frequency ultrasonic waves for detecting changes of texture in living tissues. Lancet 1951;1:655–7.

[4] Wild JJ, Reid JM. Application of echo-ranging techniques to the determination of structure of biological tissues. Science 1952;115:226–30.

[5] Takahashi H, Ouchi T. The ultrasonic diagnosis in the field of biology. In: Japanese medicine and ultrasonics: the first report, Vol 7. 1963.

[6] Takahashi H, Ouchi T. The ultrasonic diagnosis in the field of urology. In: Proceedings of the Fourth Meeting of the Japanese Society of Ultrasonics in Medicine 1964;2:35.

[7] Watanabe H, Kato H, Kato T, et al. Diagnostic application of ultrasonography to the prostate. Nippon Hinyokika Gakkai Zasshi 1968;59:273–9.

[8] Watanabe H, Kaiho H, Tanaka M, et al. Diagnostic application of ultrasonotomography to the prostate. Invest Urol 1971;8:548–59.

[9] VonMicksy L. Gynecologic ultrasonography. In: VonMicsky L, editor. Diagnostic ultrasound. St. Louis (MO): CV Mosby Co.; 1974. p. 207–41.

[10] Boyce W. Advances in urologic surgery. Med World News 1972;13:29–31.

[11] Boyce W. New test for prostate cancer. In: Health bulletin: official publication of the North Carolina State Board of Health, Vol 87. :Raleigh (NC): North Carolina State Board of Health; 1972. p. 6.

[12] Boyce W. History of prostatic ultrasonography. In: Resnick M, editor. Prostatic ultrasonography. Philadelphia: BC Decker Inc.; 1990. p. 1–15.

[13] King WW, Wilkiemeyer RM, Boyce WH, et al. Current status of prostatic echography. JAMA 1973;226:444–7.

[14] Boyce WH, McKinney WM, Resnick MI, et al. Ultrasonography as an aid in the diagnosis and management of surgical diseases of the pelvis: special emphasis on the genitourinary system. Ann Surg 1976;184:477–89.

[15] Waterhouse RL, Resnick MI. The use of transrectal prostatic ultrasonography in the evaluation of patients with prostatic carcinoma. J Urol 1989;141:233–9.

[16] Holm HH, Gammelgaard J. Ultrasonically guided precise needle placement in the prostate and the seminal vesicles. J Urol 1981;125:385–7.

[17] Holm HH, Juul N, Pedersen JF, et al. Transperineal 125iodine seed implantation in prostatic cancer guided by transrectal ultrasonography. J Urol 1983;130:283–6.

[18] Rifkin MD, Kurtz AB, Goldberg BB. Sonographically guided transperineal prostatic biopsy:

preliminary experience with a longitudinal linear-array transducer. AJR Am J Roentgenol 1983; 140:745–7.

[19] Fornage BD, Touche DH, Deglaire M, et al. Real-time ultrasound-guided prostatic biopsy using a new transrectal linear-array probe. Radiology 1983;146:547–8.

[20] Abe M, Hashimoto T, Matsuda T, et al. Prostatic biopsy guided by transrectal ultrasonography using real-time linear scanner. Urology 1987; 29:567–9.

[21] Lee F, Littrup P, Torp-Pedersen S, et al. Transrectal US of prostate cancer with use of transrectal guidance and an automatic biopsy system [abstract]. Radiology 1987;165:215.

[22] Cooner WH, Mosley BR, Rutherford Jr CL, et al. Clinical application of transrectal ultrasonography and prostate specific antigen in the search for prostate cancer. J Urol 1988;139:758–61.

[23] Stamey T, Hodge K. Ultrasound visualization of prostate anatomy and pathology. Monogr Urol 1988;9:55–63.

[24] Torp-Pedersen S, Lee F, Littrup PJ, et al. Transrectal biopsy of the prostate guided with transrectal US: longitudinal and multiplanar scanning. Radiology 1989;170:23–7.

[25] McNeal JE. Normal and pathologic anatomy of prostate. Urology 1981;17:11–6.

[26] McNeal J. The prostate gland: morphology and pathology. Monogr Urol 1983;4:3–33.

[27] Cooner WH, Mosley BR, Rutherford Jr CL, et al. Prostate cancer detection in a clinical urological practice by ultrasonography, digital rectal examination and prostate specific antigen. J Urol 1990; 143:1146–52.

[28] Shinohara K, Wheeler TM, Scardino PT. The appearance of prostate cancer on transrectal ultrasonography: correlation of imaging and pathological examinations. J Urol 1989;142:76–82.

[29] Klein EA, Zippe CD. Transrectal ultrasound guided prostate biopsy–defining a new standard. J Urol 2000;163:179–80.

[30] Hodge KK, McNeal JE, Terris MK, et al. Random systematic versus directed ultrasound guided transrectal core biopsies of the prostate. J Urol 1989;142:71–4.

[31] Carey JM, Korman HJ. Transrectal ultrasound guided biopsy of the prostate. Do enemas decrease clinically significant complications? J Urol 2001;166:82–5.

[32] Terris MK, McNeal JE, Stamey TA. Ultrasonography and biopsy of the prostate. In: Walsh PC, Retik AB, Vaughan ED, et al, editors. Campbell's urology. 8th edition. Philadelphia: WB Saunders; 2002. p. 3038–54.

[33] Aron M, Rajeev TP, Gupta NP. Antibiotic prophylaxis for transrectal needle biopsy of the prostate: a randomized controlled study. BJU Int 2000;85:682–5.

[34] Griffith BC, Morey AF, Ali-Khan MM, et al. Single dose levofloxacin prophylaxis for prostate biopsy in patients at low risk. J Urol 2002;168:1021–3.

[35] Scherr DS, Eastham J, Ohori M, et al. Prostate biopsy techniques and indications: when, where, and how? Semin Urol Oncol 2002;20:18–31.

[36] Eskew LA, Bare RL, McCullough DL. Systematic 5 region prostate biopsy is superior to sextant method for diagnosing carcinoma of the prostate. J Urol 1997;157:199–202.

[37] Cochlin DL, Dubbins PA, Goldberg BB, et al. Urogenital ultrasound: a text atlas. Philadelphia: JB Lippincott Co.; 1994.

[38] Rifkin MD, Sudakoff GS, Alexander AA. Prostate: techniques, results, and potential applications of color Doppler US scanning. Radiology 1993; 186:509–13.

[39] Aarnink RG, Beerlage HP, De La Rosette JJ, et al. Transrectal ultrasound of the prostate: innovations and future applications. J Urol 1998; 159:1568–79.

[40] Hastak SM, Gammelgaard J, Holm HH. Transrectal ultrasonic volume determination of the prostate–a preoperative and postoperative study. J Urol 1982;127:1115–8.

[41] Horstman W, Watson L. Ultrasound of the genitourinary tract. In: Resnick MI, Older RA, editors. Diagnosis of genitourinary disease. 2nd edition. New York: Thieme; 1997.

[42] Benson MC, Whang IS, Olsson CA, et al. The use of prostate specific antigen density to enhance the predictive value of intermediate levels of serum prostate specific antigen. J Urol 1992; 147:817–21.

[43] Kinahan TJ, Goldenberg SL, Ajzen SA, et al. Transurethral resection of prostatic abscess under sonographic guidance. Urology 1991;37:475–7.

[44] Goldman SM, Sandler CM. Genitourinary imaging: the past 40 years. Radiology 2000;215: 313–24.

[45] Halpern EJ, Frauscher F, Strup SE, et al. Prostate: high-frequency Doppler US imaging for cancer detection. Radiology 2002;225:71–7.

[46] Roy C, Buy X, Lang H, et al. Contrast enhanced color Doppler endorectal sonography of prostate: efficiency for detecting peripheral zone tumors and role for biopsy procedure. J Urol 2003; 170:69–72.

[47] Frauscher F, Klauser A, Volgger H, et al. Comparison of contrast enhanced color Doppler targeted biopsy with conventional systematic biopsy: impact on prostate cancer detection. J Urol 2002;167:1648–52.

[48] Halpern EJ, Rosenberg M, Gomella LG. Prostate cancer: contrast-enhanced us for detection. Radiology 2001;219:219–25.

[49] Robbin ML, Lockhart ME, Barr RG. Renal imaging with ultrasound contrast: current status. Radiol Clin North Am 2003;41:963–78.

[50] Hamper UM, Trapanotto V, DeJong MR, et al. Three-dimensional US of the prostate: early experience. Radiology 1999;212:719–23.

[51] Downey DB, Fenster A, Williams JC. Clinical utility of three-dimensional US. Radiographics 2000;20:559–71.

[52] Huynen AL, Giesen RJ, de la Rosette JJ, et al. Analysis of ultrasonographic prostate images for the detection of prostatic carcinoma: the automated urologic diagnostic expert system. Ultrasound Med Biol 1994;20:1–10.

[53] Balaji KC, Fair WR, Feleppa EJ, et al. Role of advanced 2 and 3-dimensional ultrasound for detecting prostate cancer. J Urol 2002;168: 2422–5.

[54] Lizzi L, Kalisz D, Coleman F, et al. Very-high frequency ultrasonic imaging and spectral assays of the eye. In: Lees S, Ferrara LA, editors. Acoustical imaging. New York: Plenum Press; 1998. p. 107–12.

ULTRASOUND
CLINICS

Ultrasound Clin 1 (2006) 55–66

Sonographic Evaluation of Testicular Torsion

Vikram S. Dogra, MD*, Shweta Bhatt, MD, Deborah J. Rubens, MD

Broadband high-frequency transducer sonography has become the gold standard for the evaluation of patients who have acute scrotal pain. High-frequency transducer sonography can not only help delineate the anatomic details of the testes but also aids in evaluating testicular perfusion. Testicular perfusion can be studied with the help of color or power Doppler sonography. Evaluation of testicular perfusion aids in the diagnosis of testicular torsion. This article reviews the gray-scale and color flow Doppler features of testicular torsion, including the partial torsion and torsion-detorsion syndrome.

Sonographic anatomy

The postnatal human testis is intraperitoneal. The adult human testis is also intraperitoneal but may appear extraperitoneal. The apparent discrepancy between the adult testis being intraperitoneal or extraperitoneal is likely to result from differences in the relative size of the tunica vaginalis between infant boys and elderly men [1]. Testes are bilaterally symmetrical and housed within the scrotum.

Testes are ovoid in shape with medium-level echoes and measure 5×3×2 cm each. Tunica albuginea is the fibrous covering of the testicle and is covered by the tunica vaginalis. The tunica albuginea can be seen with a high-frequency transducer as an echogenic line [Fig. 1]. Septa extend from the tunica albuginea into the testicle, dividing the testis into 250 to 400 lobules. The posterior surface of the tunica albuginea is reflected into the interior of the testis, forming the incomplete septum known as the mediastinum testis. Sonographically, the mediastinum testis is seen as an echogenic band running in a cephalocaudal direction [Fig. 2]. Each lobule consists of one to three seminiferous tubules supporting the Sertoli cells and the spermatocytes that give rise to sperm. The seminiferous tubules open through the tubuli recti into dilated spaces called the rete testis within the mediastinum [Fig. 3]. The rete testis drains into the epididymis through 10 to 15 efferent ductules. The epididymis, consisting of a head, body, and tail, is located superior to and is contiguous with the posterior aspect of the testis. The tail of the epididymis continues as the vas deferens.

University of Rochester School of Medicine and Dentistry, 601 Elmwood Ave, Rochester, NY 14642, USA
* Corresponding author.
E-mail address: Vikram_Dogra@URMC.Rochester.Edu (V.S. Dogra).

doi:10.1016/j.cult.2005.09.006

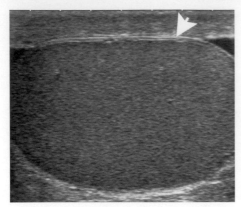

Fig. 1. Longitudinal sonogram of the testis reveals homogeneous medium-level echoes. The arrow points to the tunica albuginea.

Arterial blood supply to the testes is derived from the testicular artery, a branch of the abdominal aorta. The superior epididymal artery, a branch of the testicular artery, predominantly supplies the epididymis. The cremasteric artery, which is a branch of the inferior epigastric artery, predominantly supplies the peritesticular tissue and anastomoses with the deferential artery. The deferential artery, a branch of the superior vesicle artery, supplies the vas deferens [**Fig.** 4]. There are variable anastomoses between the posterior epididymal, deferential, and cremasteric arteries. A transmediastinal arterial branch of the testicular artery is present in approximately half of normal testes; it courses through the mediastinum to supply the capsular arteries and is usually accompanied by a large vein [**Fig.** 5] [2].

Sonographic technique

Scrotal US is performed with the patient in the supine position and the scrotum supported by a towel placed between the thighs. Optimal results are obtained with a 10 to 14-MHz, high-frequency, linear-array transducer. Scanning is performed with

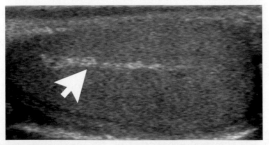

Fig. 2. Longitudinal sonogram of the testis reveals an echogenic band (*arrow*) consistent with mediastinum testis.

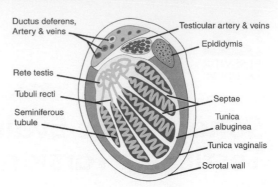

Fig. 3. Diagrammatic representation of the testis in cross-section.

the transducer in direct contact with the skin; however, a stand-off pad can be used for evaluation of superficial lesions if necessary.

The testes are examined in at least two planes: the longitudinal and transverse axes. The size and echogenicity of each testis and of the epididymis are compared with those on the opposite side. Scrotal skin thickness is evaluated. Color Doppler and pulsed Doppler parameters are optimized to display low-flow velocities and to demonstrate blood flow in the testes and surrounding scrotal structures. Bilateral testicular spectral Doppler tracings must be recorded. Power Doppler US may also be used to demonstrate intratesticular blood flow in patients who have an acute scrotum. In patients being evaluated for an acute scrotum, the asymptomatic side should be scanned initially to set the gray-scale and color Doppler gain settings to allow comparison with the affected side, remembering that testicular torsion can be a bilateral process in 2% of patients [3]. Transverse images with portions of each testis on the same image should be acquired in gray-scale and color Doppler modes. Additional techniques, such as use of the Valsalva maneuver or upright positioning, can be used as needed for venous evaluation.

Normal spectral Doppler

The proper interpretation of velocity waveforms requires an understanding of the normal waveform characteristics of a given vessel, and of the physiologic status of the circulation subtended by the vessel. The normal spectral waveform of the testicular artery and artery supplying the epididymis is a low-resistance, high-flow pattern [**Fig.** 6] [4], whereas that of the cremasteric artery supplying the scrotal wall has a high-resistance, low-flow pattern [**Fig.** 7] [4].

Quantification of outflow resistance may be achieved by determining the resistive index (RI). In the testes of a normal healthy volunteer, the RI is

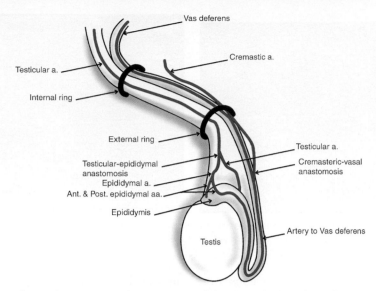

Fig. 4. Diagrammatic representation of the testicular blood supply.

rarely less than 0.5 [2]. It is the most widely used parameter and is defined as the peak systolic velocity minus the end diastolic velocity, divided by the peak systolic velocity.

Clinical presentation

In 1776, Hunter provided the first description of testicular torsion [5]. The chances of torsion of the testis or its appendage developing by the age of 25 years is about 1 in 160 [6]. Testicular torsion can occur at any age; however, it is most frequent in adolescent boys. Most testicular torsion occurs in young patients, with 66% occurring between 12 and 18 years of age and peak incidence occurring at 14 years [7].

Patients who have acute testicular torsion present after a sudden onset of pain followed by nausea, vomiting, and a low-grade fever. Physical examination reveals a swollen, tender, and inflamed hemiscrotum. It is difficult to distinguish the testis from the epididymis because of localized swelling. For this reason, the condition is frequently misdiagnosed as epididymitis. The cremasteric reflex is usually absent [8,9], and the pain cannot be relieved by elevating the scrotum [5]. In an adult in a standing position, the normal testis hangs in a near-vertical position, whereas the torsed testis will tend to hang in a near-horizontal position [10].

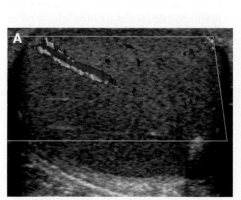

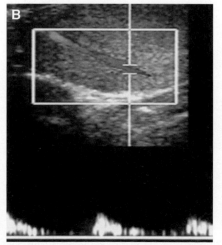

Fig. 5. (A) Transverse oblique sonogram reveals a transmediastinal artery. (B) Demonstrates the arterial waveform of the low-resistance pattern.

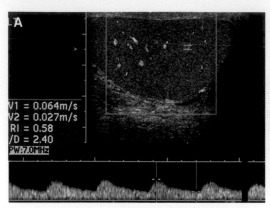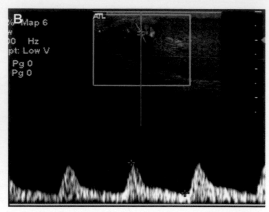

Fig. 6. Longitudinal sonogram: (*A*) demonstrates the low-resistance, high-flow pattern of the intratesticular artery, (*B*) demonstrates a similar pattern obtained from within the epididymis because anterior and posterior epididymal arteries originate from the testicular artery.

Elevation and transverse location of the testis with an anteriorly rotated epididymis associated with loss of the ipsilateral cremasteric reflex strongly suggests testicular torsion [11].

Testicular torsion

Extravaginal torsion

Two types of torsion have been described: extravaginal and intravaginal. Extravaginal testicular torsion occurs exclusively in newborns. Torsion occurs outside the tunica vaginalis when the testes and gubernacula are not fixed and are free to rotate [12]. The affected neonate presents with swelling, discoloration of the scrotum on the affected side, and a firm, painless mass in the scrotum [13]. The testis is typically infarcted and necrotic at birth. US findings include an enlarged heterogeneous testis,

ipsilateral hydrocele, skin thickening, and no color Doppler flow signal in the testis or spermatic cord [Fig. 8] [14]. In children, power Doppler US is more sensitive than color Doppler US for detection of intratesticular blood flow. In one study [15], power Doppler US demonstrated intratesticular blood flow in 66 (97%) of 68 testes, whereas color Doppler US demonstrated intratesticular blood flow in 60 (88%) of the testes. Both techniques combined depicted blood flow in all 68 (100%) testes. Color Doppler US and scintigraphy are comparable with regard to the diagnosis of torsion in adolescent and adult populations [16]. Scintigraphy remains a reasonable alternative to color flow Doppler for evaluation of acute scrotal pain and should be used when color Doppler US sensitivity for low-velocity, low-volume testicular blood flow is inadequate and the diagnosis of torsion remains in question.

Intravaginal torsion

Intravaginal torsion occurs within the tunica vaginalis and is the most frequent type of testicular torsion seen in 80% of the population [17]. The predisposing factors include a long mesorchium or a bell-clapper deformity in which the tunica vaginalis completely encircles the epididymis, distal spermatic cord, and testis rather than attaching to the posterolateral aspect of the testis. This deformity leaves the testis free to swing and rotate within the tunica vaginalis, much like a clapper inside a bell [18]. The bell-clapper deformity can be diagnosed by US in the presence of moderate hydrocele [Fig. 9]. In most cases, the bell-clapper deformity is bilateral. A 12% prevalence of bell-clapper deformity was found in one autopsy series [19], thereby suggesting that it is a more common deformity than intravaginal testicular torsion. Testicular torsion, caused by long mesorchium, is associated

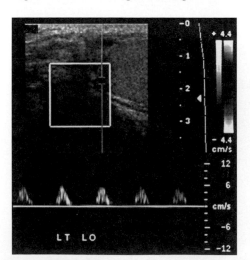

Fig. 7. Cremasteric artery at the periphery of the epididymis reveals a high-resistance, low-flow pattern of spectral waveform.

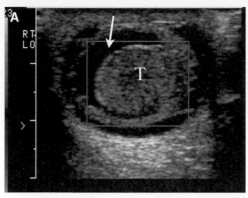 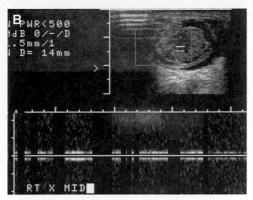

Fig. 8. (A) Sonogram of the testis in a newborn reveals the absence of blood flow within the testis (T) and the presence of a small hydrocele (*arrow*). (B) Corresponding spectral Doppler tracing further demonstrates the absence of blood flow (only noise is observed).

with cryptorchism [**Fig. 10**]. The most frequently found anatomical relation between the testis and the epididymis in patients who have testicular torsion is type I (epididymis united to the testis by its head and tail) [17].

Gray-scale features

In testicular torsion, venous obstruction occurs first, followed by obstruction of arterial flow, and ultimately by testicular ischemia. The extent of testicular ischemia depends on the degree of torsion, which ranges from 180° to 720° or greater. The testicular salvage rate depends on the degree of torsion and the duration of ischemia. A nearly 100% salvage rate exists within the first 6 hours after the onset of symptoms, a 70% rate within 6 to 12 hours, and a 20% rate within 12 to 24 hours [20].

US findings vary with the duration and degree of rotation of the spermatic cord. Gray-scale images are nonspecific for testicular torsion [21] and often appear normal if the torsion has just occurred

[**Fig. 11**]. Testicular swelling and decreased echogenicity are the most commonly encountered findings 4 to 6 hours after the onset of torsion. At 24 hours after the onset, the testis has a heterogeneous echotexture secondary to vascular congestion, hemorrhage, and infarction. This condition is referred to as late or missed torsion [**Fig. 12**]. The gray-scale features are summarized in Box 1. An enlarged hypoechoic epididymal head may be visible because the artery supplying the epididymis is often involved in the torsion [22]. In a recent prospective study [23], a spiral twisting of the spermatic cord at the external inguinal ring was seen in 14 of 23 cases of torsion. The twisting induced an abrupt change in the course, size, and shape of the spermatic cord below the point of torsion and appeared as a round or oval homogeneous extratesticular mass with or without blood flow that could be traced cephalad to the normal spermatic cord. In the setting of testicular torsion, normal testicular echogenicity is a strong predictor of testicular viability [24]. Other indicators of testicular torsion include the presence of scrotal wall thickening and reactive hydrocele.

Color flow Doppler

Testicular perfusion can be evaluated by color Doppler, power Doppler, or spectral Doppler sonography. Color Doppler sonography can reliably demonstrate intratesticular flow [25]. Power Doppler sonography uses the integrated power of the Doppler signal to depict the presence of blood flow. Higher power gains are more likely with power Doppler sonography than with standard color Doppler sonography, thereby resulting in increased sensitivity for detecting blood flow. Power Doppler sonography is valuable in scrotal sonography because of its increased sensitivity to low-flow states and its independence from the Doppler angle correction [26]. Pulsed Doppler sonography is a useful method to

Fig. 9. Bell-Clapper Deformity in a 10-year-old male. Sonogram reveals hydrocele (*arrow*) encircling the distal third of the spermatic cord (*asterisk*). The child underwent a bilateral orchiopexy. T, Testis.

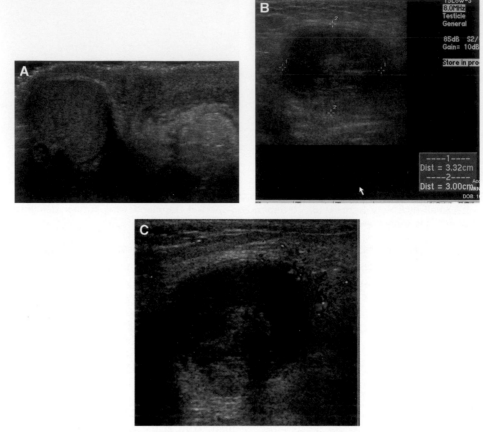

Fig. 10. Testicular torsion in a cryptorchid testis. (*A*) Transverse gray-scale sonogram demonstrates the right testis and empty left scrotal sac. (*B*) Transverse sonogram in the left inguinal region reveals a hypoechoic testis (within calipers) with no color flow (*C*).

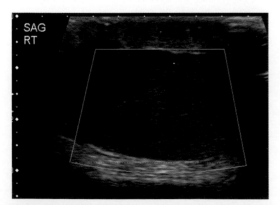

Fig. 11. Color flow Doppler of the right testis in the longitudinal plane reveals absent color flow with normal gray-scale echotexture, suggestive of early testicular torsion.

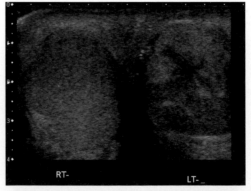

Fig. 12. Gray-scale sonogram of both testes in the transverse plane demonstrates a normal gray-scale appearance of the right testis. Left testis has heterogeneous echotexture with areas of increased echogenicity representing hemorrhage. This type of appearance favors testicular torsion of more than at least 6 hours.

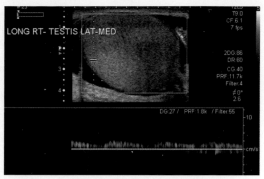

identify flow in the testis using the time–velocity spectrum to quantify blood flow [27]. The spectral waveform of the intratesticular arteries characteristically has a low-resistance pattern [28] with a mean RI of 0.62 (range, 0.48–0.75) [25]; however, this is not true for testicular volumes less than 4 cm^3 as are often found in prepubertal boys when diastolic arterial flow may not be detectable [29].

Because gray-scale US findings are often normal in the early phases of torsion, the Doppler component of the examination is essential. The absence of testicular flow on color and power Doppler US is considered diagnostic of ischemia, provided that the scanner is optimized for detection of slow flow, is limited to the use of a small color-sampling box, and is adjusted for the lowest repetition frequency and the lowest possible threshold setting [30]. The threshold should be set just above the level for detection of color noise.

The role of color Doppler and power Doppler US in the diagnosis of acute testicular torsion is well established [31–33]. Using the absence of identifiable intratesticular flow as the only criterion for detecting testicular torsion, color Doppler US was 86% sensitive, 100% specific, and 97% accurate in the diagnosis of torsion and ischemia in painful scrotum [**Fig. 13**] [16]. As it is sometimes possible to record a small arterial signal in one part of the

Fig. 14. Testicular torsion. A 28-year-old man presented with sudden onset of scrotal pain of 5-hours duration. Power Doppler examination revealed absent blood flow in the right testis except for a tiny arterial signal at the periphery. Please note the decreased echogenicity of the right testis. Despite the presence of minimal peripheral arterial flow, a diagnosis of testicular torsion was advanced. The patient underwent surgical exploration and was found to have bell-clapper deformity. Untwisting of the testis did not result in return of normal blood flow to the testis. Patient had to undergo orchiectomy.

testis [**Fig. 14**] [34,35] in the appropriate clinical setting and age group, this should not dissuade one from making the diagnosis of testicular torsion. The presence of hypervascularity in paratesticular tissue is a characteristic finding of an infarcted testis [**Fig. 15**] [36]. Color flow Doppler features of testicular torsion are summarized in Box 2.

Unilateral testicular torsion has bilateral effects and is a form of ischemia-reperfusion injury. Treatment of torsion by detorsion alone does not prevent testicular damage and may result in infertility [37]. If nonsalvagable, the necrotic testis is removed to decrease the risk for an autoimmune reaction to the residual testis [38].

Partial testicular torsion

Torsion is not an all-or-nothing phenomenon but may be complete, incomplete, or transient. Cases of partial or transient torsion present a diagnostic challenge. The ability of color and power Doppler sonography to definitively diagnose partial testicular torsion remains uncertain. The role of spectral Doppler US analysis is not well established with regard to the diagnosis of partial torsion, but the findings may be useful [39]. There are no studies that validate the role of spectral Doppler US in partial torsion; however, there are findings from sporadic case reports [19,40] that suggest its usefulness. Asymmetry in resistive indices with decreased diastolic flow or diastolic flow reversal may be seen [**Fig. 16**]. The presence of color or power Doppler

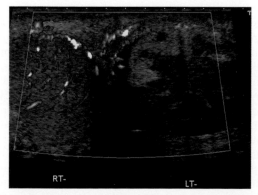

Fig. 13. Testicular torsion. Power Doppler reveals absent flow in the left testis and a normal power Doppler appearance in the right testis.

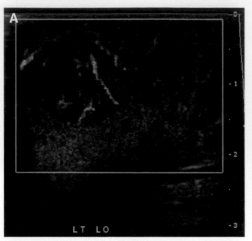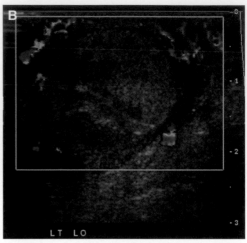

Fig. 15. Increased paratesticular blood flow. Color flow Doppler of the left testis demonstrates increased paratesticular blood flow (*A*) with absent blood flow within the left testis (*B*), consistent with testicular infarction.

signal in a patient who has the clinical manifestation of torsion does not exclude torsion [19,40].

Torsion-detorsion syndrome

Acute and intermittent sharp testicular pain and scrotal swelling, interspersed with long intervals without symptoms, are characteristic of torsion-detorsion. This type of presentation should arouse the suspicion of torsion-detorsion syndrome [41]. Physical findings may include horizontal or very mobile testes; an anteriorly located epididymis; or bulkiness of the spermatic cord from partial twisting [41,42]. Horizontal testicular position, even in the absence of pain at the time of physical examination, is a strong indication for exploration and bilateral testicular fixation [43]. If scanned when asymptomatic or immediately after detorsion, the affected testis may demonstrate increased blood flow [**Fig. 17**]. The testis may be enlarged, and focal infarcts may or may not be present.

If the suspicion for torsion-detorsion is high, a bell-clapper deformity can be expected on exploration and prophylactic orchiopexy should be performed bilaterally [44,45].

Box 2: Color flow Doppler patterns in testicular torsion

Absent arterial and venous flow
Increased RI on affected side (diminished or reversed diastolic flow)
Decreased flow velocity difficult to measure because of small vessels/angle correction, but may be subjectively inferred by the relative difficulty in finding small, low-amplitude flow on the symptomatic side

---

Mimics of testicular torsion

Testicular infarction without torsion of the spermatic cord is a rare lesion, generally idiopathic and spontaneous. Absence or decrease of color flow within the testis is not always because of testicular torsion and can result from vasculitis, protein S, or antithrombin III deficiency [46]. Patients who have polyarteritis nodosa can present with acute scrotum [47,48]. Other causes of decreased testicular perfusion include large hydroceles [**Fig. 18**] and extratesticular hematomas [49].

Idiopathic testicular infarcts also present with acute pain, and testicular torsion is the main suspect [50]. These patients have a focal area of decreased echogenicity, usually anteriorly near the upper pole. The conditions resulting in decreased blood flow to the testis are listed in Box 3.

Testicular appendigeal torsion

Five testicular appendages are formed during the development of the male genitourinary tract; these are the remnants of the degenerating mesonephric and paramesonephric ducts. The testicular and epididymal appendages, found at the upper pole of the testis and at the head of the epididymis, respectively, are the most common [**Fig. 19**] [51]. Approximately 91% to 95% of twisted testicular appendices involve the appendix testis and occur most often in boys 7 to 14 years old. Patients who have torsion of the appendix testis and appendix epididymis present with acute scrotal pain, but there are usually no other physical symptoms and the cremasteric reflex can still be elicited. The classic finding on physical examination is a small, firm, palpable nodule on the superior aspect of the

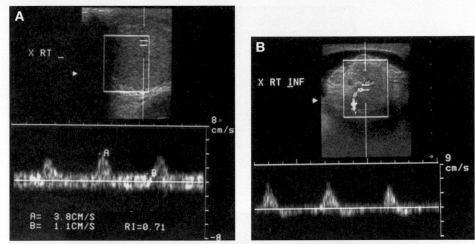

Fig. 16. Partial testicular torsion. (*A*) Right testis spectral Doppler evaluation reveals decreased diastolic blood flow. (*B*) In the same testis, the diastolic waveform can be seen below the baseline. This appearance is suggestive of increased resistance to the inflow of arterial blood. The patient underwent surgical exploration and partial torsion was confirmed. (*From* Dogra VS, Sessions A, Mevorach RA, et al. Reversal of diastolic plateau in partial testicular torsion. J Clin Ultrasound 2001;29:105–8; with permission.)

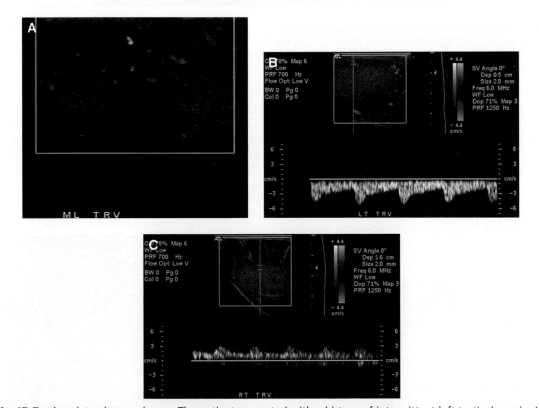

Fig. 17. Torsion-detorsion syndrome. The patient presented with a history of intermittent left testicular pain. He was asymptomatic at the time of examination. (*A*) Color flow Doppler in the transverse plane demonstrates increased blood flow to the left testis. Comparing spectral Doppler waveform of the left testis (*B*) with that of the right testis (*C*), it is evident that there is increased blood flow to the left testis.

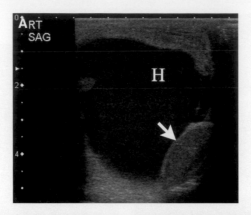

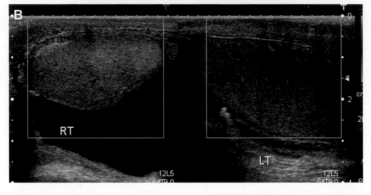

Fig. 18. Testicular torsion mimic. Patient who has right scrotal pain. (*A*) Gray-scale sonogram of the right testis demonstrates a large hydrocele (H) pushing and causing pressure on the testis (*arrow*). (*B*) Color Doppler evaluation of both testes side-by-side reveals decreased blood flow to the right testis. Blood flow returned to normal after hydrocelectomy.

testis; it exhibits a bluish discoloration through the overlying skin which is called the "blue dot" sign [52].

US appearance of torsion of the appendages of the testes is variable and may be isoechoic, hypoechoic, or hyperechoic to the testis or epididymis [**Fig. 20**] [53,54]. Reactive hydrocele and skin thickening are common in these cases. An appendix testis size of 5 mm or larger, spherical shape, and increased

periappendiceal blood flow are suggestive of a torsed appendix testis [54]. The identification of a testicular appendage larger than 5.6 mm is suggestive of torsion. Therefore, depending on a patient's clinical condition, such cases can be treated conservatively when an appendage larger than 5.6 mm is identified [55]. The role of US examination in tor-

---

Box 3: Conditions that may result in decreased blood flow in the testes

Poor technical parameters
Pediatric population (small testicular volume)
Hydrocele/hematoma
Vasculitis, such as polyarteritis nodosa
    and lupus
Marked scrotal edema, resulting in poor
    penetration of US beam
Epididymo-orchitis, resulting in testicular
    infarction (a rare complication)
Protein S and antithrombin III deficiency

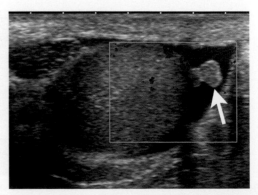

Fig. 19. Appendix testis. Sonogram demonstrates appendix of the testis (*arrow*). The presence of fluid facilitates this visualization.

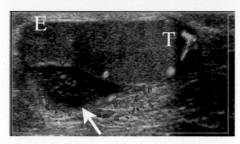

Fig. 20. Testicular appendigeal torsion. A 10-year-old man presented with testicular pain. Color flow Doppler demonstrates a hypoechoic mass with peripheral hyperemia (*arrow*) separate from epididymis (E). This hypoechoic mass resolved on follow-up. T, Testis.

sion of testicular appendages is to exclude testicular torsion and acute epididymo-orchitis.

Summary

As US is considered as the first step in evaluation of acute painful scrotum, it is important to optimize the scan parameters. Testicular torsion is a urologic emergency that can be accurately diagnosed by high-frequency transducer sonography in conjunction with appropriate clinical history and physical examination. Absence of color flow Doppler does not always signify testicular torsion as this could be secondary to vasculitis. Similarly, the presence of color flow does not exclude partial testicular torsion.

Acknowledgments

We would like to acknowledge our sincere thanks to Bonnie Hami, MA, for her editorial assistance in the preparation of this manuscript.

References

[1] Pham SB, Hong MK, Teague JA, et al. Is the testis intraperitoneal? Pediatr Surg Int 2005;21(4): 231–9.

[2] Dogra V, Bhatt S. Acute painful scrotum. Radiol Clin North Am 2004;42:349–63.

[3] Washowich TL. Synchronous bilateral testicular torsion in an adult. J Ultrasound Med 2001;20: 933–5.

[4] Dogra VS, Rubens DJ, Gottlieb RH, et al. Torsion and beyond: new twists in spectral Doppler evaluation of the scrotum. J Ultrasound Med 2004;23:1077–85.

[5] Noske HD, Kraus SW, Altinkilic BM, et al. Historical milestones regarding torsion of the scrotal organs. J Urol 1998;159:13–6.

[6] Williamson RC. Torsion of the testis and allied conditions. Br J Surg 1976;63:465–76.

[7] Haynes BE, Bessen HA, Haynes VE. The diagnosis of testicular torsion. JAMA 1983;249:2522–7.

[8] Nelson CP, Williams JF, Bloom DA. The cremasteric reflex: a useful but imperfect sign in testicular torsion. J Pediatr Surg 2003;38:1248–9.

[9] Rabinowitz R. The importance of the cremasteric reflex in acute scrotal swelling in children. J Urol 1984;132:89–90.

[10] Angell JC. Torsion of the testicle. A plea for diagnosis. Lancet 1963;1:19–21.

[11] Ciftci AO, Senocak ME, Tanyel FC, et al. Clinical predictors for differential diagnosis of acute scrotum. Eur J Pediatr Surg 2004;14:333–8.

[12] Backhouse KM. Embryology of testicular descent and maldescent. Urol Clin North Am 1982;9: 315–25.

[13] Hawtrey CE. Assessment of acute scrotal symptoms and findings. A clinician's dilemma. Urol Clin North Am 1998;25:715–23 [x.].

[14] Brown SM, Casillas VJ, Montalvo BM, et al. Intrauterine spermatic cord torsion in the newborn: sonographic and pathologic correlation. Radiology 1990;177:755–7.

[15] Barth RA, Shortliffe LD. Normal pediatric testis: comparison of power Doppler and color Doppler US in the detection of blood flow. Radiology 1997;204:389–93.

[16] Burks DD, Markey BJ, Burkhard TK, et al. Suspected testicular torsion and ischemia: evaluation with color Doppler sonography. Radiology 1990;175:815–21.

[17] Favorito LA, Cavalcante AG, Costa WS. Anatomic aspects of epididymis and tunica vaginalis in patients with testicular torsion. Int Braz J Urol 2004; 30:420–4.

[18] Dogra V. Bell-clapper deformity. AJR Am J Roentgenol 2003;180:1176–7.

[19] Dogra VS, Sessions A, Mevorach RA, et al. Reversal of diastolic plateau in partial testicular torsion. J Clin Ultrasound 2001;29:105–8.

[20] Patriquin HB, Yazbeck S, Trinh B, et al. Testicular torsion in infants and children: diagnosis with Doppler sonography. Radiology 1993;188:781–5.

[21] Horstman WG. Scrotal imaging. Urol Clin North Am 1997;24:653–71.

[22] Berman JM, Beidle TR, Kunberger LE, et al. Sonographic evaluation of acute intrascrotal pathology. AJR Am J Roentgenol 1996;166:857–61.

[23] Baud C, Veyrac C, Couture A, et al. Spiral twist of the spermatic cord: a reliable sign of testicular torsion. Pediatr Radiol 1998;28:950–4.

[24] Middleton WD, Middleton MA, Dierks M, et al. Sonographic prediction of viability in testicular torsion: preliminary observations. J Ultrasound Med 1997;16:23–7 [quiz 29–30].

[25] Siegel MJ. The acute scrotum. Radiol Clin North Am 1997;35:959–76.

[26] Hamper UM, DeJong MR, Caskey CI, et al. Power Doppler imaging: clinical experience and correlation with color Doppler US and other imaging modalities. Radiographics 1997;17:499–513.

[27] Scoutt LM, Zawin ML, Taylor KJ. Doppler US. Part II. Clinical applications. Radiology 1990; 174:309–19.

[28] Middleton WD, Melson GL. Testicular ischemia: color Doppler sonographic findings in five patients. AJR Am J Roentgenol 1989;152:1237–9.

[29] Paltiel HJ, Connolly LP, Atala A, et al. Acute scrotal symptoms in boys with an indeterminate clinical presentation: comparison of color Doppler sonography and scintigraphy. Radiology 1998;207:223–31.

[30] Wilbert DM, Schaerfe CW, Stern WD, et al. Evaluation of the acute scrotum by color-coded Doppler ultrasonography. J Urol 1993;149:1475–7.

[31] Lerner RM, Mevorach RA, Hulbert WC, et al. Color Doppler US in the evaluation of acute scrotal disease. Radiology 1990;176:355–8.

[32] Horstman WG, Middleton WD, Melson GL, et al. Color Doppler US of the scrotum. Radiographics 1991;11:941–57 [discussion 958].

[33] Middleton WD, Siegel BA, Melson GL, et al. Acute scrotal disorders: prospective comparison of color Doppler US and testicular scintigraphy. Radiology 1990;177:177–81.

[34] Luker GD, Siegel MJ. Color Doppler sonography of the scrotum in children. AJR Am J Roentgenol 1994;163:649–55.

[35] Prando D. Torsion of the spermatic cord: sonographic diagnosis. Ultrasound Q 2002;18:41–57.

[36] Luker GD, Siegel MJ. Scrotal US in pediatric patients: comparison of power and standard color Doppler US. Radiology 1996;198:381–5.

[37] Adivarekar PK, Bhagwat SS, Raghavan V, et al. Effect of Lomodex-MgSO(4) in the prevention of reperfusion injury following unilateral testicular torsion: an experimental study in rats. Pediatr Surg Int 2005;21:184–90.

[38] Donohue RE, Utley WL. Torsion of spermatic cord. Urology 1978;11:33–6.

[39] Fitzgerald SW, Erickson S, DeWire DM, et al. Color Doppler sonography in the evaluation of the adult acute scrotum. J Ultrasound Med 1992;11:543–8.

[40] Sanelli PC, Burke BJ, Lee L. Color and spectral doppler sonography of partial torsion of the spermatic cord. AJR Am J Roentgenol 1999;172:49–51.

[41] Stillwell TJ, Kramer SA. Intermittent testicular torsion. Pediatrics 1986;77:908–11.

[42] Lopez Aramburu MA, Arroyo Munoz JL, Amon Sesmero JH, et al. [Intermittent testicular torsion.] Arch Esp Urol 1996;49:1–4.

[43] Schulsinger D, Glassberg K, Strashun A. Intermittent torsion: association with horizontal lie of the testicle. J Urol 1991;145:1053–5.

[44] Schneck F, Bellinger MF. Abnormalities of the testes and scrotum and their surgical management. 8th edition. Philadelphia: Saunders; 2002.

[45] Kamaledeen S, Surana R. Intermittent testicular pain: fix the testes. BJU Int 2003;91:406–8.

[46] Ameur A, Zarzur J, Albouzidi A, et al. [Testicular infarction without torsion in cryptorchism.] Prog Urol 2003;13:321–3.

[47] Suty JM, Hubert J, Duquenne M, et al. [Bilateral testicular ischemia in vasculitis. Differential diagnosis with torsion and the value of color Doppler ultrasonography.] Prog Urol 1995;5:586–9.

[48] Leibovici D, Strauss S, Sharon A. [Acute, painful, swollen testis in polyarteritis nodosa: a diagnostic problem]. Harefuah 1999;136:938–9.

[49] Jacob M, Barteczko K. Contribution to the origin and development of the appendices of the testis and epididymis in humans. Anat Embryol (Berl) 2005;209(4):287–302.

[50] Fukuhara Y, Shiga Y, Omori Y, et al. [Idiopathic testicular infarction: a case report.] Hinyokika Kiyo 2005;51:129–31.

[51] Sellars ME, Sidhu PS. Ultrasound appearances of the testicular appendages: pictorial review. Eur Radiol 2003;13:127–35.

[52] Skoglund RW, McRoberts JW, Ragde H. Torsion of testicular appendages: presentation of 43 new cases and a collective review. J Urol 1970;104:598–600.

[53] Cohen HL, Shapiro MA, Haller JO, et al. Torsion of the testicular appendage. Sonographic diagnosis. J Ultrasound Med 1992;11:81–3.

[54] Yang DM, Lim JW, Kim JE, et al. Torsed appendix testis: gray scale and color Doppler sonographic findings compared with normal appendix testis. J Ultrasound Med 2005;24:87–91.

[55] Baldisserotto M, de Souza JC, Pertence AP, et al. Color Doppler sonography of normal and torsed testicular appendages in children. AJR Am J Roentgenol 2005;184:1287–92.

ULTRASOUND
CLINICS

Ultrasound Clin 1 (2006) 67–75

Sonography of Pediatric Urinary Tract Emergencies

Carlos J. Sivit, MD

- Ureteropelvic junction obstruction
- Renal vein thrombosis
- Urolithiasis
- Infected urachal remnant
- Hemorrhagic cystitis
- Acute renal failure
- Summary
- References

Urinary tract emergencies frequently result in acute signs and symptoms in the pediatric age group. The imaging evaluation of these conditions plays an important role in their diagnosis and management. The most compelling indication for emergent imaging in children who have suspected urinary tract emergencies is that nonemergent treatment may lead to irreversible loss of renal function. Sonography is typically the initial examination of choice in infants and children who have suspected emergencies of the urinary tract. Sonography provides a rapid initial screening method to assess the urinary tract without any pre-exam preparation and without ionizing radiation. This article focuses on the sonographic assessment of common urinary tract emergencies in children, including the typical clinical presentation and characteristic sonographic findings of such conditions.

Ureteropelvic junction obstruction

Ureteropelvic junction (UPJ) obstruction is the most common cause of urinary tract obstruction in the pediatric age group. There is controversy regarding the underlying cause. Multiple underlying factors have been proposed, including: (1) abnormal development of the proximal ureteral smooth muscle; (2) aberrant vessels, or bands crossing the upper ureter and renal pelvis; (3) delayed recana-

lization of the fetal ureter; or (4) abnormal ureteral peristalsis.

The widespread use of prenatal sonography has impacted how the diagnosis of UPJ obstruction is made. The condition is now often diagnosed in utero. However, it is still not unusual for the diagnosis to be made after birth. Infants and children who have a UPJ obstruction usually present with a palpable abdominal mass representing the enlarged kidney; flank or abdominal pain; hematuria; or symptoms related to urinary tract infection.

Sonography is typically the initial imaging examination of choice for the evaluation of suspected UPJ obstruction. The sonographic findings associated with a UPJ obstruction include dilatation of the intrarenal collecting system, including renal pelvis and calyces [Fig. 1] [1]. When the degree of dilatation is mild to moderate, it is typically easier to identify the fluid-filled areas within the kidney as the dilated collecting system. However, when the dilatation is severe, multiple cystic lesions of uniform size are noted, representing the dilated calyces [Fig. 2]. In these instances it is important to demonstrate communication between the cysts to identify the abnormality as dilated calices and differentiate the condition from a multicystic dysplastic kidney (MCDK) or renal dysplasia. The cysts in MCDK or renal dysplasia vary in size and will not communicate [Fig. 3]. Additionally, there is no

Department of Radiology, Rainbow Babies and Children's Hospital, 11100 Euclid Avenue, Cleveland, OH 44106-5056, USA
E-mail address: Sivit@uhrad.com

1556-858X/06/$ – see front matter © 2005 Elsevier Inc. All rights reserved.
ultrasound.theclinics.com

doi:10.1016/j.cult.2005.09.001

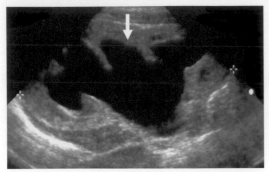

Fig. 1. UPJ obstruction. Longitudinal sonogram through the right kidney shows dilatation of the intrarenal collecting system (*arrow*). The right ureter was not dilated. The findings are consistent with a UPJ obstruction.

recognizable renal parenchyma in an MCDK. The ipsilateral ureter is typically not dilated in children who have a UPJ obstruction, although ureteral vesical junction (UVJ) may occasionally coexist and result in a dilated ureter [2]. The obstruction is bilateral in approximately one fourth of children.

Small amounts of fluid in the intrarenal collecting system resulting in a renal pelvis anteroposterior diameter of less than 10 mm in size may occasionally be seen in infants and young children in the absence of urinary tract obstruction [**Fig. 4**]. A renal pelvis diameter of less than 10 mm is characterized as mild pyelectasis and generally has no pathologic significance, particularly if the examination occurs after 48 hours of birth. The kidney may occasionally appear normal at sonography in neonates who have a UPJ obstruction, particularly if the examination is performed in the first day of life when urine production is low. Therefore, if the diagnosis is suspected on prenatal sonography, it is best to delay the postnatal sonogram until the infant is at least 48 to 72 hours old.

There is an increased prevalence of UPJ obstruction in children who have a horseshoe kidney. This condition is felt to be caused by the atypical location of the proximal ureters in horseshoe kidney. They are positioned more anteriorly, resulting in an increased risk for obstruction by crossing blood vessels. There may also be coexistent urolithiasis associated with UPJ obstruction caused by the associated urinary stasis [3]. A urinoma may occasionally be noted because of urine leakage secondary to a high-grade obstruction. Renal parenchymal thinning may also be noted because of secondary renal scarring. This scarring usually results following the development of acute pyelonephritis, which is prone to develop secondary to urine stasis. UPJ obstruction may also be associated with vesicoureteral reflux. Therefore, the imaging evaluation of children who have a UPJ obstruction should include a voiding cystourethrogram to evaluate for potential reflux. The diagnosis of UPJ obstruction is confirmed with diuretic renal scintigraphy, which will show delayed renal isotope excretion. Renal scintigraphy allows for assessment of severity of obstruction and quantification of residual renal function.

Renal vein thrombosis

Renal vein thrombosis most commonly presents in the neonatal period. However, it may be seen at any age. The clinical presentation includes a palpable mass representing enlarged kidney, renal insufficiency, hematuria, or hypertension. The pathophysiology of renal vein thrombosis differs between infants and older children. In infants the condition is typically associated with hemoconcentration attributable to dehydration, sepsis, and maternal diabetes mellitus. In this age group the thrombus formation is felt to start in the arcuate and interlobar venules and progress centrally to the

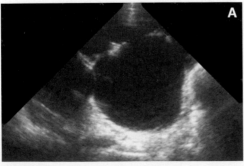
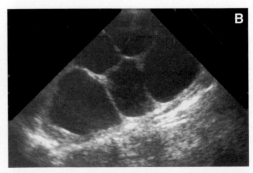

Fig. 2. Severe UPJ obstruction. Longitudinal sonogram through the right renal pelvis (*A*) and calyces (*B*) show marked dilatation of the intrarenal collecting system. Note that on the image through the calyces, the dilated calyces appear as large cysts. However, they are symmetrical in size and were noted to communicate by sonography. Also note the diminished renal parenchyma.

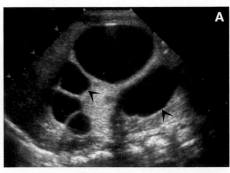 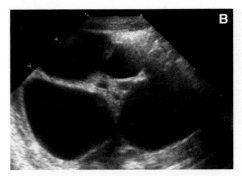

Fig. 3. Multicystic dysplastic kidney. Longitudinal (*A*) and transverse (*B*) views through the right kidney demonstrate multiple parenchymal cysts of varying size (*arrowheads*). They were not noted to communicate on real-time sonography. Additionally, there is no normal renal parenchyma visualized.

renal hilum. Renal vein thrombosis may also be seen in the neonatal age group in association with indwelling umbilical venous catheters. These neonates typically develop thrombi in the inferior vena cava with secondary extension into the renal vein. In older children renal vein thrombosis is associated with renal tumor, glomerulonephritis, or nephrotic syndrome and is felt to originate in the main renal vein or inferior vena cava.

Doppler sonography is the examination of choice for the evaluation of suspected renal vein thrombosis. The sonographic findings associated with renal vein thrombosis vary depending on the extent and duration of renal venous occlusion. Sonographic findings include the presence of filling defects in the main renal vein or inferior vena cava and absence or diminution of renal venous flow surrounding the thrombus [4]. The acute thrombus is usually echogenic. Occasionally, the thrombus may be hypoechoic and difficult to recognize at sonography. The venous outflow obstruction caused by renal vein thrombosis results in diminution of ipsilateral renal arterial flow. This diminution in turn results in narrowing of the systolic peak and reduction or reversal of diastolic flow with an elevated resistive index in the ipsilat-

eral renal artery [**Fig. 5**] [5]. Enlargement of the involved kidney with diffuse increase in parenchymal echogenicity or loss of corticomedullary differentiation is also typically seen in the acute period [**Fig. 6**].

The treatment of renal vein thrombosis is usually nonsurgical. It consists primarily of fluid and electrolyte management. Sonography is useful in the serial evaluation of children who have renal vein thrombosis to monitor progression of disease. The outcome associated with renal vein thrombosis is variable and dependent on extent and rapidity of venous occlusion. If renal vein occlusion by thrombus is incomplete, or if the thrombus develops slowly allowing time for development of collateral venous drainage, then there is typically diminished renal edema and increased renal arterial perfusion, resulting in a more favorable outcome. If the renal vein obstruction is complete, then renal ischemia develops followed by parenchymal atrophy. In severe cases, serial sonographic assessment 2 to 3 weeks following the initial event shows parenchymal echogenicity in the involved kidney gradually becoming heterogenous and renal size diminishing.

Urolithiasis

Urolithiasis represents the formation of macroscopic calcification within the urinary collecting system. It is not a disease but a complication of many different diseases. It is a common condition, with estimates that 12% of individuals will develop a calculi sometime during their lives [6]. The calculi are formed on the renal papillae by retention of lithogenic particles either by obstruction or adherence to damaged renal epithelium. Urolithiasis is a complication of many different disorders that result in the supersaturation of urine by calculi-promoting factors such as increased calcium or oxalate excretion. It is also associated with conditions that result in urine stasis. The most common

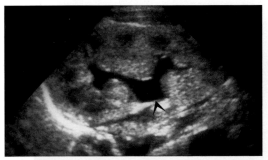

Fig. 4. Pyelectasis and caliectasis. Longitudinal sonogram through the right kidney in a 2-week-old infant shows a small amount of fluid (*arrowhead*) within the intrarenal collecting system without dilatation.

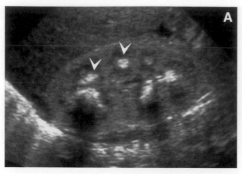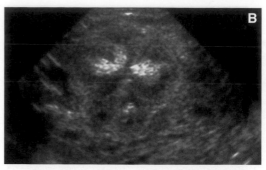

Fig. 9. Medullary nephrocalcinosis. Longitudinal (*A*) and transverse (*B*) views through the left kidney demonstrate increased medullary echogenicity (*arrowheads*) indicative of medullary nephrocalcinosis.

CT may provide improved definition of the extent of abscess and enhanced delineation of the anatomic relationship of the abscess to the bladder. The treatment of an infected urachal remnant typically involves surgical drainage. These infections usually do not respond to antibiotic therapy because of the diminished blood supply to the involved area.

Hemorrhagic cystitis

Hemorrhagic cystitis results from damage to the bladder transitional epithelium, resulting in diffuse bleeding. The cause may be multifactorial. The condition has been associated with drugs, infection, and toxins. Chemotherapeutic agents, particularly cyclophosphamide and busulfan, are the drugs most commonly associated with the condition. It has most frequently been reported following bone marrow transplantation, particularly in younger children [19]. It has been reported as early as 1 week and as late as 4 months following transplantation. Children who have hemorrhagic cystitis typically present with gross hematuria, dysuria,

suprapubic pain, and urinary frequency. The extent of hemorrhage may be severe and the condition may be life-threatening. It can result in impaired renal and bladder function. Treatment usually involves bladder irrigation, blood transfusions, and maintenance of adequate hydration. Endoscopic removal of blood clots is sometimes required, as the clots may result in bladder outlet obstruction.

Sonography is usually the initial modality in the evaluation of suspected hemorrhagic cystitis. Associated sonographic findings include focal [**Fig. 11**], multifocal [**Fig. 12**], or circumferential bladder wall thickening [**Fig. 13**] [19–21]. The normal bladder wall thickness should not exceed 3 mm for a distended bladder and 5 mm for a nondistended bladder [22]. Bladder wall thickening associated with hemorrhagic cystitis is most pronounced in the hypoechoic muscularis layer. The echogenic mucosal and submucosal layers are less involved. The bladder wall thickening may be polypoid in appearance and resemble a bladder wall mass. One sonographic finding that is helpful in distinguishing hemorrhagic cystitis from a true bladder wall mass is that bladder thickening with hemor-

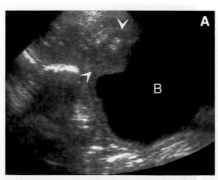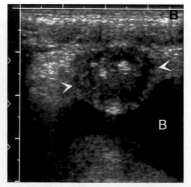

Fig. 10. Infected urachal remnant. (*A*) Longitudinal midline sonogram through the bladder shows a complex midline mass with mass effect on the superior aspect of the bladder (*arrowheads*). (*B*) Transverse midline sonogram immediately above the dome of the bladder in same child demonstrates a rounded, solid, complex mass (*arrowheads*). At surgery, an infected urachal remnant was noted. B, bladder.

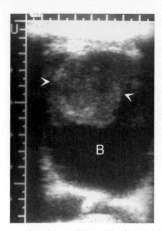

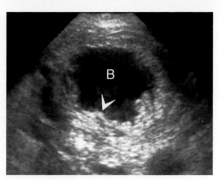

Fig. 13. Hemorrhagic cystitis with diffuse bladder wall thickening. Transverse sonogram through the bladder in a child who has hemorrhagic cystitis shows diffuse bladder wall thickening (*arrowhead*). B, bladder.

Fig. 11. Hemorrhagic cystitis with focal bladder wall thickening. Transverse sonogram through the bladder in a child who has hemorrhagic cystitis shows focal bladder wall thickening resembling a mass (*arrowheads*). B, bladder.

rhagic cystitis usually changes in contour and thickness with bladder wall filling, whereas a true bladder wall mass does not change. Echogenic clots may be noted within the bladder lumen. The bladder may also have a reduced capacity. In severe cases there may be complete contraction of the bladder without a visualized lumen. There may be associated hydronephrosis secondary to obstruction from bladder clots. In addition, the entire urothelial surface is at risk and lesions of the renal pelvis and ureter have been reported. Suburothelial thickening of the renal pelvis may be noted at sonography.

Sonography is a useful modality for the serial evaluation of children who have hemorrhagic cystitis in monitoring response to therapy. Serial follow-up by sonography typically demonstrates gradual improvement in bladder wall thickening associated with clinical improvement [23]. It also al-

lows for surveillance of bladder clots that can lead to obstruction.

Acute renal failure

Acute renal failure (ARF) is defined as the sudden loss of renal function with or without oliguria. It typically results from an ischemic–hypoxic or toxic event. ARF may result from prerenal, intrinsic, or postrenal causes [24]. Prerenal causes result from renal hypoperfusion usually secondary to volume depletion. The kidneys are intrinsically normal in prerenal failure and usually improve with restoration of renal perfusion. Intrinsic ARF results from acute tubular necrosis secondary to prolongued prerenal ARF or secondary to a primary renal insult. Postrenal ARF develops secondary to acute bilateral obstructive uropathy. It is caused by an acute elevation of intrarenal pressure resulting in reduction of renal blood flow.

Sonography is the examination of choice for the initial evaluation of infants and children who have ARF. The primary role of sonography is to detect

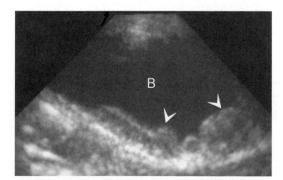

Fig. 12. Hemorrhagic cystitis with multifocal bladder wall thickening. Longitudinal sonogram through the bladder in a child who has hemorrhagic cystitis shows multifocal areas of bladder wall thickening (*arrowheads*). B, bladder.

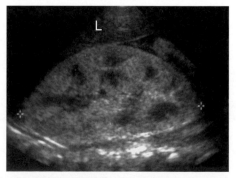

Fig. 14. Acute renal failure. Longitudinal sonogram through the right kidney in a child who has ARF demonstrates increased renal parenchymal echogenicity. Note that the renal parenchyma is hyperechoic relative to the liver. L, liver.

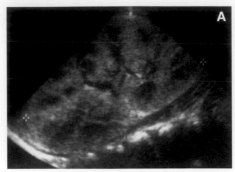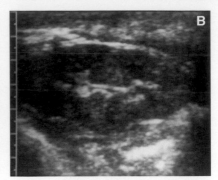

Fig. 15. Reversible acute renal failure. (*A*) Longitudinal sonogram through the right kidney in a child who has ARF shows increased renal parenchymal echogenicity. (*B*) Follow-up sonogram in the same child 3 months after restoration of normal renal function shows normal renal parenchymal echotexture.

obstructive uropathy resulting in postrenal ARF or intrinsic causes such as renal vein thrombosis. Renal sonography in children who have ARF typically demonstrates increased renal parenchymal echogenicity [**Fig. 14**] [25]. The normal renal parenchymal echogenicity in children over the age of 4 months is usually hypoechoic relative to that of liver or spleen. In most children who have ARF, the renal parenchymal echogenicity will be equal to or greater than liver or spleen. Correlation has been shown between increased renal parenchymal echogenicity and elevated blood urea nitrogen and serum creatinine values. Therefore, the sonographic finding of increased parenchymal echogenicity is significant in that it indicates the presence of renal disease that is usually associated with decreased renal function. However, increased renal parenchymal echogenicity is a nonspecific finding that may be seen with various diffuse parenchymal renal disorders that involve glomerular, tubular, interstitial, or vascular abnormalities [25,26]. This finding may also be noted with renal involvement in leukemia or lymphoma. The entity is generally described as medical renal disease. Furthermore, in children who have ARF, sonography cannot discriminate between reversible and irreversible renal insufficiency. Improvement in renal parenchymal echogenicity is often seen with improvement in renal function [**Fig. 15**].

Summary

Sonography plays an important role in the evaluation of pediatric urinary tract emergencies. Sonography is often the initial imaging examination of choice for evaluation of such conditions. The precise characterization of urinary tract pathology by sonography allows for prompt diagnosis and treatment. Therefore, it is important for the practicing radiologist to have an understanding of the typical sonographic findings associated with such conditions.

References

[1] Brown T, Mandell J, Lebowitz RL. Neonatal hydronephrosis in the era of sonography. AJR Am J Roentgenol 1987;148:959–63.

[2] McGrath MA, Estroff J, Lebowitz RL. The coexistence of obstruction at the UPJ and UVJ. AJR Am J Roentgenol 1987;149:403–6.

[3] Kraus SJ, Lebowitz RI, Royal SA. Renal calculi in children. Pediatr Radiol 1999;28:624–30.

[4] Helenon O, Rody FE, Correas J-M, et al. Color Doppler US of renal vascular disease in native kidneys. Radiographics 1995;15:833–54.

[5] Laplante S, Patriquin HB, Robitaille P, et al. Renal vein thrombosis in children: evidence of early flow recovery with Doppler US. Radiology 1993; 189:37–42.

[6] Dyer RB, Chen MYM, Zagoria RJ. Abnormal calcifications in the urinary tract. Radiographics 1998;18:1405–24.

[7] Santos-Victoriano M, Brouhard BH, Cunningham III RJ. Renal stone disease in children. Clin Pediatr (Phila) 1998;37:583–99.

[8] Haddad M, Sharif HS, Shahed MS, et al. Renal colic: Diagnosis and outcome. Radiology 1992; 184:83–8.

[9] Erwin BC, Carroll BA, Sommer FG. Renal colic: the role of ultrasound in initial evaluation. Radiology 1984;152:147–50.

[10] Bonner MP, Pollack HM. Urolithiasis in the lower urinary tract. Semin Roentgenol 1982;17: 140–8.

[11] Burge HJ, Middleton WD, McClennan RI, et al. Ureteral jets in healthy subjects and in patients with unilateral ureteral calculi: comparison with color Doppler US. Radiology 1991;180:437–42.

[12] Hernanz-Schulman M. Hyperechoic renal medullary pyramids in infants and children. Radiology 1991;181:9–11.

[13] Tamm EP, Silverman PM, Shuman WP. Evalua-

tion of the patient with flank pain and possible ureteral calculus. Radiology 2003;228:319–29.

[14] Smith RC, Verga M, McCarthy S, et al. Diagnosis of acute flank pain: value of unenhanced helical CT. AJR Am J Roentgenol 1966;166:97–101.

[15] Sommer FG, Jeffrey RB, Rubin GD, et al. Detection of ureteral calculi in patients with suspected renal colic: value of reformatted noncontrast helical CT. AJR Am J Roentgenol 1995; 165:509–13.

[16] Khati NJ, Enquist EG, Javitt MC. Imaging of the umbilicus and periumbilical region. Radiographics 1998;18:413–31.

[17] DiSantis DJ, Siegel MJ, Katz ME. Simplified approach to umbilical remnant abnormalities. Radiographics 1991;11:59–66.

[18] Cacciorelli AA, Kass EJ, Yang SS. Urachal remnants: Sonographic demonstration in children. Radiology 1990;174:473–5.

[19] Benya EC, Sivit CJ, Quinones RR. Abdominal complications after bone marrow transplantation in children: sonographic and CT findings. AJR Am J Roentgenol 1993;161:1023–7.

[20] Yang CC, Hurd DD, Case LD, et al. Hemorrhagic cystitis in bone marrow transplantation. Urology 1994;44:322–8.

[21] McCarville MB, Hoffer FA, Gingrich JR, et al. Imaging findings of hemorrhagic cystitis in pediatric oncology patients. Pediatr Radiol 2000;30: 131–8.

[22] Jequier S, Rousseau O. Sonographic measurements of the normal bladder wall in children. AJR Am J Roentgenol 1987;149:563–6.

[23] Cartoni C, Arcese W, Avvisati G, et al. Role of ultrasonography in the diagnosis and followup of hemorrhagic cystitis after bone marrow transplant. Bone Marrow Transplant 1993;12:463–7.

[24] Andreoli SP. Management of acute renal failure. In: Barratt TM, Avni ED, Harmon DE, editors. Pediatric nephrology. 4th edition. Baltimore (MD): Lippincott Williams & Wilkins; 1999. p. 119–34.

[25] Kraus RA. Increased renal parenchymal echogenicity: cases in pediatric patients. Radiographics 1990;10:1009–18.

[26] Platt JF, Rubin JM, Bowerman RA, et al. The inability to detect kidney disease on the basis of echogenicity. AJR Am J Roentgenol 1988;151: 317–9.

ULTRASOUND CLINICS

Ultrasound Clin 1 (2006) 77

Preface
Vascular Ultrasound

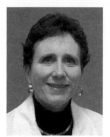

Deborah J. Rubens, MD
Guest Editor

Deborah J. Rubens, MD
Department of Imaging Sciences
University of Rochester Medical Center
601 Elmwood Avenue
Rochester, NY 14542-8648, USA

E-mail address:
deborah_rubens@urmc.rochester.edu

Rapid advancements in cross-sectional imaging systems over the past two decades have provided a wide array of diagnostic tools for the practicing radiologist. Advances in computer technology with faster processing and miniaturization have permitted tremendous anatomic imaging advances in CT, MR imaging, and ultrasound.

One of the unique capabilities of ultrasound is its elegant depiction of blood flow, both the real-time anatomic display, as well as the physiologic information of blood flow velocity and flow direction. In this inaugural issue of the *Ultrasound Clinics*, we felt it was important to dedicate part of the issue to this significant ultrasound feature. As such, we have selected topics that emphasize the foundation of vascular ultrasound, the technical aspects of Doppler imaging, and the basic principles of carotid artery imaging. In addition, subjects include advances in vascular Doppler imaging, including imaging of nonvascular structures, advanced waveform analysis, Doppler applications in gynecologic imaging, and new Doppler frontiers such as trans-cranial Doppler imaging and Doppler-guided interventional arterial therapy. The hope is to familiarize readers with the essentials of Doppler imaging in the modern ultrasound laboratory and to excite them with the future possibilities of this ever-changing and advancing technology.

My thanks to Dr. Vikram Dogra, editorial board member for the *Ultrasound Clinics*, for his commitment to ultrasound and ultrasound education. Thank you to Barton Dudlick for agreeing that ultrasound deserved its own *Clinics* series and for his editorial assistance, and thanks also to the staff at Elsevier for their help. Thank you especially to Margaret Kowaluk and Holly Stiner for graphics and manuscript preparation, respectively. Lastly, and most importantly, thanks to all of my collaborators and coauthors who contributed such outstanding articles. Each and every one of us is enthusiastic about the practice of vascular ultrasound and the its exciting future. We hope you will find our efforts valuable and stimulating as well.

doi:10.1016/j.cult.2005.10.002

ULTRASOUND
CLINICS

Ultrasound Clin 1 (2006) 79–109

Doppler Artifacts and Pitfalls

Deborah J. Rubens, MD*, Shweta Bhatt, MD,
Shannon Nedelka, MD, Jeanne Cullinan, MD

Thirty years ago, use of Doppler ultrasound (US) was limited to the vascular laboratory and was mainly used to interrogate the carotid arteries. Today, Doppler US has pervaded all of diagnostic US imaging, is the mainstay of venous diagnosis, and is used extensively throughout abdominal, pelvic, and obstetric imaging. In addition to continuous wave Doppler, pulsed wave (duplex) Doppler, color Doppler, and power Doppler are now available. Motion is imaged in high-velocity settings (ie, the aorta, carotid, and renal arteries) and in low flow states (portal vein thrombosis, calf veins, and so forth). Superficial structures (neck and arm vessels, testicular and ovarian vessels) and deep structures (hepatic and renal arteries) are imaged. To accomplish this range of diversity takes more than one knob on a machine. The image obtained, the particular organ being viewed, and the capabilities of the machine itself are governed by the intrinsic properties of US and Doppler. The physical properties of US give rise to several artifacts—some occur

in gray-scale and Doppler imaging and others are specific to Doppler, especially color or power Doppler. Knowing an artifact's typical location and appearance helps avoid misinterpretation and can actually be useful diagnostically [1]. Understanding how to generate a Doppler signal enables the examiner to better avoid day-to-day scanning pitfalls, which primarily fall into two clinical categories: too little flow or too much flow. This article addresses the machine parameters first, then the artifacts, and concludes with the operational issues (or pitfalls) as they apply to day-to-day scanning.

Understanding the technical challenge of Doppler ultrasound or setting up your equipment to get the best images and spectral tracings

The Doppler effect measures a change in the reflected sound frequency generated by motion of the source or the detector. The challenge lies in

Department of Radiology, University of Rochester Medical Center, 601 Elmwood Avenue, Rochester, NY 14642-8648, USA
* Corresponding author.
E-mail address: Deborah_Rubens@urmc.rochester.edu (D.J. Rubens)

doi:10.1016/j.cult.2005.09.009
ultrasound.theclinics.com

the detection of the signal and the accurate display of its direction and speed. Although the Doppler effect is commonly used to measure flowing blood, any tissue or fluid motion may generate a Doppler signal. That signal is a shift or difference in frequency between the transmitted and the received US pulse. The greatest difference or strongest signal is achieved when the motion is parallel to the US beam and no signal is generated when the motion is perpendicular to it.

Choosing the correct transducer frequency

Of all the technical parameters that can be controlled, the choice of transducer frequency is paramount because the intensity of the scattered sound varies in proportion to the fourth power of the Doppler frequency [2]. Higher frequencies are,

therefore, much more sensitive to flow but sometimes cannot penetrate deep enough without attenuation; thus, for superficial structures such as the testes, 7 to 10 MHz may be ideal, whereas for deep abdominal structures, such as the hepatic arteries or the portal vein, 3 MHz or lower may be needed. Often the choice of Doppler transducer frequency is empiric with a trial of different frequencies until the best compromise between penetration and signal strength is achieved [**Fig. 1**].

Doppler angle

Unlike in gray-scale US imaging whereby the best image is obtained perpendicular to the US beam, in Doppler US, the strongest signals (and best spectra) result when the motion is parallel to the beam. A Doppler angle of 90° does not display flow because no component of the frequency shift is directed

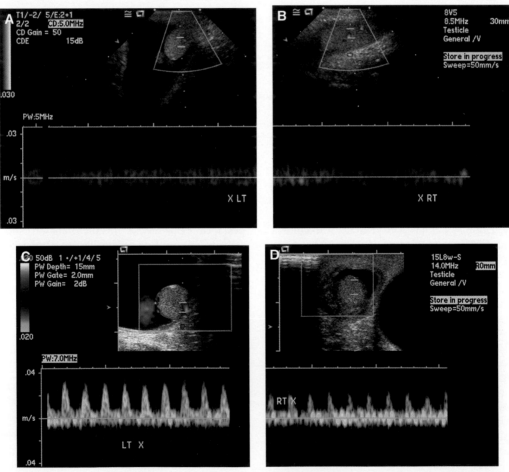

Fig. 1. Pseudotesticular torsion. Four-day-old infant presents with left hydrocele and testicular torsion is suspected. (*A, B*) Initial axial images of the symptomatic left (*A*) and asymptomatic right (*B*) sides at identical gain and scale settings show symmetric spectral Doppler patterns equal above and below the baseline but do not have typical vascular spectral Doppler waveform. This is noise. Note scanning frequency is 8.5 MHz and spectral Doppler frequency is 5 MHz. (*C, D*) Axial images from repeat examination with appropriate high frequency transducer shows normal symmetric arterial waveforms bilaterally. Note transducer frequency of 14 MHz and spectral Doppler frequency of 7 MHz.

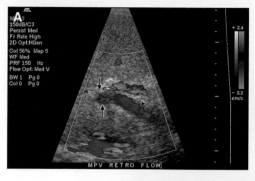
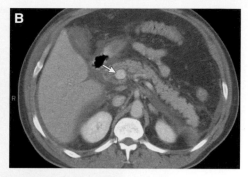
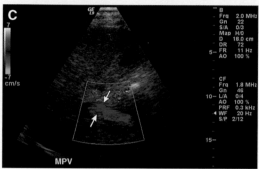

Fig. 2. Pseudothrombosis of main portal vein (MPV). (*A*) Color Doppler ultrasound (CDUS) of the MPV detects no flow in confluence of MPV (*arrows*) suggesting thrombosis of MPV. Note reversed flow in splenic vein (*arrowhead*) indicating portal hypertension and potentially slow-flow state in MPV. Wall filter set on medium, which may exclude low velocity flow and MPV segment which lacks flow is parallel to transducer surface, and therefore at 90° to Doppler beam. (*B*) Portal venous phase of subsequent contrast enhanced CT on the same day reveals completely patent MPV (*arrow*). (*C*) Repeat CDUS examination with different machine following day shows retrograde flow in MPV (*arrows*) and no apparent thrombus. Doppler angle has been improved (no longer 90°) and wall filter is corrected to low setting (20 Hz).

back toward the transducer [Fig. 2]. Any Doppler angle other than zero requires angle correction to adjust for the component of the signal not directed parallel to the beam. The larger the Doppler angle, the greater the correction is that needs to be done and the greater chance for error; therefore, the Doppler beam angle must always be kept as low as possible. Ideally, it should be less than 60° and always less than 70° because the errors associated with the angle correction increase up to 20% to 30% with higher Doppler angles [Fig. 3] [3].

Sample volume

The sample volume is the three-dimensional space from which the Doppler frequency shifts are measured. In color or power Doppler it is the color box, and in pulsed wave Doppler it is the cursor one places within the vessel. Although on the image the sample looks like a flat box, it has a third dimension in and out of the plane of the image, which may be much larger than anticipated (even 1 cm or more in thickness, depending on frequency and depth). Signals may be sampled and displayed from unwanted areas of a vessel (ie, too close to the vessel wall, giving more turbulence, and slower

velocities) or even from unwanted vessels (adjacent arteries or veins). In a large vessel, blood flow is not uniform across the vessel; it is generally slower near the wall (as a result of friction and turbulence) and faster in the center. Therefore, with spectral Doppler, too wide a sample (which encompasses the entire vessel lumen) includes the normal turbulence and slower velocities along the vessel margins, which result in spectral broadening (that may be incorrectly interpreted as poststenotic turbulence) [3]. If the spectral sample is too small and is not placed in the area of greatest flow, the resulting measured velocity is too low. If the sample volume is too small and the vessel is mobile, a discontinuous Doppler signal may result with loss of the diastolic signal in each cycle. The ideal sample volume size for routine survey of a vessel is about two thirds of the vessel width positioned in the center of the vessel [3] excluding as much of the unwanted clutter from near the vessel walls as possible [2].

Wall filters

The Doppler frequency shift can be detected from moving blood vessel walls and from the blood

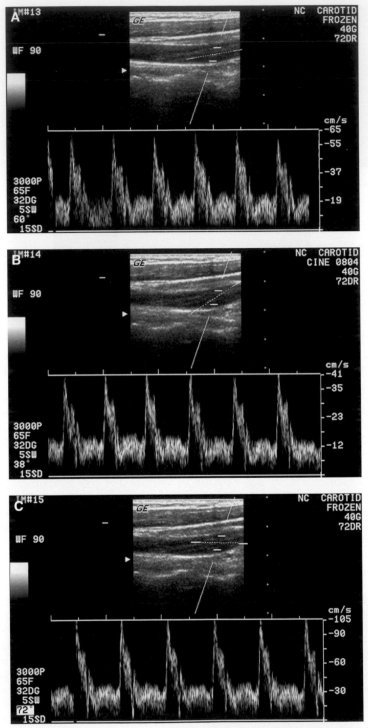

Fig. 3. Angle-corrected velocity. (*A*) Correct angle, as depicted by line through Doppler cursor, is parallel to center of lumen and yields peak systolic velocity of 65 cm/s. (*B*) Angle is too low, at 38°, which results in calculated velocity of only 41 cm/s. (*C*) Angle is only slightly off at 72° but velocity is now calculated to be 105 cm/s. Small changes in angle greater than 60° result in much larger errors than small changes below 60°.

itself. These wall echoes are large amplitude causing a loud "wall thump" on the audio Doppler output [4]. Fortunately, these signals are also low frequency. By using a threshold that cuts off these low frequency noises, a cleaner high-velocity blood-flow signal is displayed; however, if the wall filter threshold is set too high, true blood flow also is discarded from the display. Low velocity venous flow and the filter for venous Doppler should be kept at the lowest practical level, usually 50 to 100 Hz or less [**Fig. 2**] [2].

Doppler Gain

This setting controls the amplitude of the color display in color or power Doppler mode and the spectral display in pulse Doppler mode. For spectral Doppler, the tracing should be continuous and easy to visualize, without any low-level noise band above and below the baseline. Excess spectral gain in pulse wave Doppler produces noise that may be mistaken for flow [**Fig. 1**]. In arterial spectra, excess gain fills in the tracing as low velocity echoes and mimics turbulent flow [5]. For color imaging, the gain should be turned up until scattered isolated color pixels can be seen overlying the gray-scale background. Then the gain should be turned back until they disappear.

If the color gain settings are too low, flow may be present but not visualized. If the settings are too high, color or power signals may overwrite gray-scale clot. A machine setting related to gain for color and power Doppler is the color-write priority. The color-write priority determines whether a given pixel is written as a gray-scale value or as color [3]. If the gray-scale signal is above some threshold (eg, medium gray), the pixel remains gray, and if the signal is below the threshold (ie, the pixel is dark gray or black), the pixel is written as color. If the gray-scale gain is too high or the color-write priority too low, some color pixels may not be displayed.

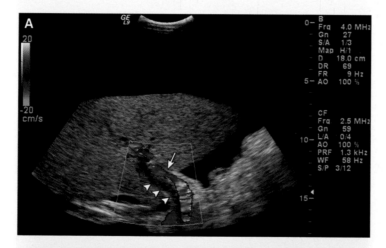

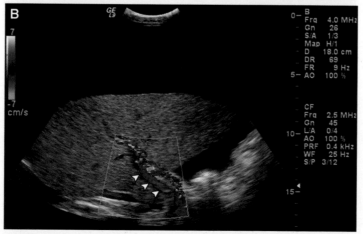

Fig. 4. Portal vein pseudoclot. (*A*) Longitudinal CDUS image in cirrhotic patient with portal hypertension. Velocity scale is set at 20 cm/s. Good flow in hepatic artery anteriorly (*arrow*) but none in adjacent portal vein (*arrowheads*). (*B*) Scale is appropriately lowered to 7 cm/s and slower flow in portal vein (*arrowheads*) can now be demonstrated.

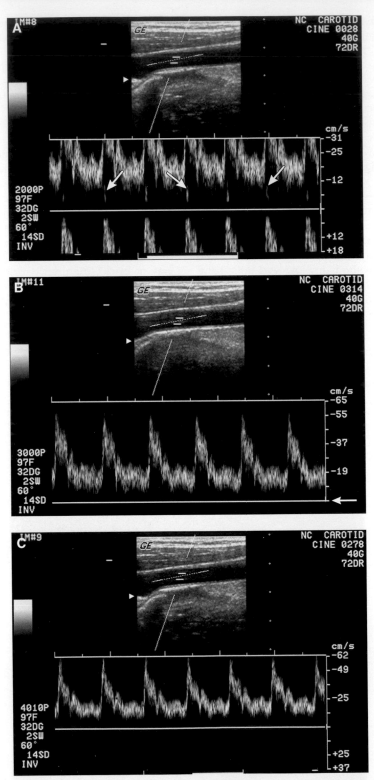

Fig. 5. Spectral aliasing. (*A*) Longitudinal spectral Doppler evaluation of common carotid artery (CCA) demonstrates spectral aliasing as higher Doppler shift frequencies "wrap around" scale and peaks (*arrows*) are written coming from opposite side of baseline. Note that peaks can actually cross baseline and overwrite existing spectral display. (*B*) Dropping baseline (*arrow*) eliminates aliasing. (*C*) Increasing scale (from 31 to 62 cm/s) eliminates aliasing.

Velocity scale

The velocity scale controls the range of frequencies displayed and is critical in color and spectral Doppler imaging. If the scale is too high (similar to a too-wide window in CT), the dynamic range is too large and low velocity signals are missed simulating an area of thrombosis [**Fig. 4**], particularly in low flow vessels, such as the portal vein. If the velocity scale is too low, the dynamic range is too small to display the high-velocity signals accurately and aliasing results (see later discussion).

Doppler artifacts

Doppler artifacts can be grouped into three broad categories [1]: (1) artifacts caused by technical limitations, including aliasing, improper Doppler angle with no flow, indeterminate Doppler angle, blooming, and partial volume artifact; (2) artifacts caused by patient anatomy, including mirror image arti-fact, flash artifact, and "pseudoflow"; and (3) artifacts caused by machine factors, including edge artifact and twinkle artifact.

Aliasing

Aliasing is an inaccurate display of color or spectral Doppler velocity and occurs when the velocity range exceeds the scale available to display it. The maximum velocity scale is limited by the number of US pulses per second that can be transmitted and received by the transducer (ie, the pulse repetition frequency [PRF]). Accurate depiction of frequency shifts requires a scale that is twice as large as the maximum shift (known as the Nyquist limit) [4]. If the scale is too small, large shifts exceed the available range and are displayed as multiples of small shifts. Practically, the display "wraps around" the scale and overwrites the existing data. For spectral Doppler flow toward the transducer, the velocity peak is cut off at the top of the scale and the

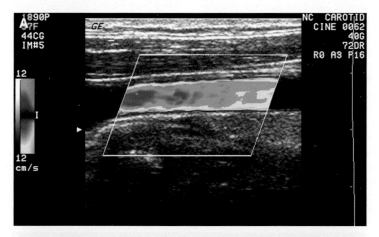

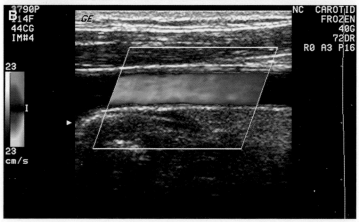

Fig. 6. Color Doppler aliasing. (*A*) Longitudinal CDUS image of CCA directed away from transducer should be red with maximum central velocity displayed as bright yellow. Instead, color scale "wraps around" and colors are displayed sequentially from red and yellow adjacent to wall to light blue and then dark blue in central lumen. Velocity scale range is 12cm/s. (*B*) At proper scale range of 23 cm/s color display no longer aliases and flow direction is depicted appropriately.

missing portion is written from the lowest portion of the scale back toward the top [**Fig. 5**]. The solutions to spectral aliasing are first to drop the baseline or increase the velocity scale (ie, the PRF) to increase the available velocity range [**Fig. 5**]. If the scale is still inadequate, decrease the Doppler frequency shift by using a lower insonating frequency or by increasing the Doppler angle [4].

For color Doppler assume a scale ranging from red (slow) to yellow (faster) toward the transducer and dark blue (slow) to light blue (faster) away. Aliasing within a vessel is displayed as adjacent colors from red to yellow to light blue to dark blue [**Fig. 6**]. Increasing the velocity scale [**Fig. 6**] or decreasing the frequency can also be diminished by color Doppler aliasing. In areas of the vessel where the flow actually reverses direction, the color palette also goes from red to dark blue but without the yellow and light blue components in between. Instead there is the black line of no flow dividing the areas in which the flow has changed direction [**Fig. 7**]. Power Doppler has no aliasing because it has no directional or velocity component.

Aliasing is disadvantageous in that high velocities may not be accurately measured; however, in day-to-day scanning, color Doppler aliasing can be useful because it quickly localizes the highest velocity region within a vessel for spectral sampling for carotid and other vascular studies [**Fig. 8**] [6]. Aliasing rapidly identifies the abnormal area in assessment of transjugular intrahepatic portal-systemic shunt TIPS [**Fig. 9**] and displays the direction of high-velocity jets for angle-corrected velocity determination. In addition, color Doppler aliasing readily identifies abnormal high-velocity vessels, which are often invisible on gray-scale. In particular, arteriovenous fis-

tulae, a common sequelae to renal or hepatic biopsy [**Fig. 10**] [7] are often undetectable on gray-scale.

Blooming artifact

In common terms this is known as "color bleed" because the color spreads out from within the vessel and "bleeds" beyond the wall into adjacent areas. Color bleed can occur because the color US image is actually two images superimposed, the color and the gray-scale; thus, depending on how the parameters are set, the color portion of the image can extend beyond the true gray-scale vessel margin. This extension usually occurs deep to the vessels and, most commonly, is caused by abnormally high gain settings [**Fig. 11**] [8]. The unwanted result, however, is that the information within the vessel (ie, partial thrombus) can be "written over" and obscured. Color blooming artifact can also be seen with US contrast agents and occurs soon after the bolus injection, at the time the increase in signal strength is the highest [9]. B-flow, an alternative US-based blood flow detection method, does not use Doppler and is acquired as part of the gray-scale image; thus, the "flow" cannot overwrite the gray-scale anatomy. This type of imaging may be useful when color imaging is problematic [10].

Directional ambiguity

Directional ambiguity or indeterminate flow direction refers to a spectral Doppler tracing in which the waveform is displayed with nearly equal amplitude above and below the baseline in a mirror image pattern. This pattern results when the interrogating beam intercepts the vessel at a 90° angle [5] and is most common in small vessels, especially those that may be traveling in and out of the imaging plane

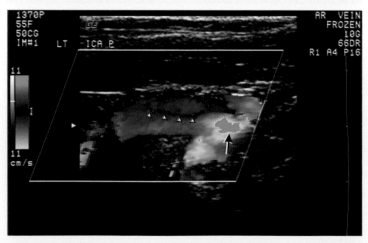

Fig. 7. Color Doppler aliasing and flow reversal. Longitudinal CDUS image of left CCA bifurcation demonstrates focal aliasing centrally (*arrow*). True flow reversal (*arrowheads*) in ICA bulb is recognized by thin black line that separates blue reversed flow near wall from adjacent red forward flow in central lumen. (*From* Zynda-Weiss A, Carson NL. Carotid arterial and vertebral Doppler ultrasound. In: Dogra V, Rubens DJ, editors. Ultrasound secrets. New York: Elsevier; 2004; with permission.)

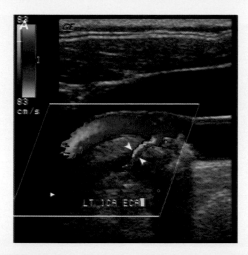

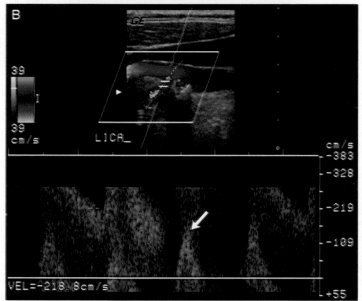

Fig. 8. Color Doppler aliasing. (*A*) Longitudinal CDUS image of left common carotid artery bifurcation demonstrates focal aliasing within ICA (*arrowheads*) indicating high-velocity jet caused by stenosis. (*B*) Spectral Doppler obtained at this region also demonstrates aliasing, even with maximized scale settings. Despite this, if peak (*arrow*) is added to portion written above baseline, velocity can be calculated at 275 + 219 = 494 cm/s, which indicates a severe stenosis. (*From* Zynda-Weiss A, Carson NL. Carotid arterial and vertebral Doppler ultrasound. In: Dogra V, Rubens DJ, editors. Ultrasound secrets. New York: Elsevier; 2004; with permission.)

[Fig. 12]. In a study by Ratanakorn and colleagues [11], this artifact adversely effected measured transcranial Doppler blood-flow velocities.

Directional ambiguity should not be confused with true bidirectional flow. In the latter case, blood actually flows in two directions, such as in the neck of a pseudo-aneurysm [Fig. 13]. The clue here is that the flow is first in one direction, then in the opposite, all within a single cardiac cycle. Another type of bidirectional flow occurs in the setting of high resistance organ flow (eg, torsion, venous thrombosis, or other causes of parenchymal edema) and is represented as diastolic flow reversal

[Fig. 14] [12]. The difference between true bidirectional flow and an indeterminate direction spectral tracing is that bidirectional flow is never simultaneously symmetric above and below the baseline. The flow direction varies within the cardiac cycle. True bidirectional flow is not an artifact. In the visceral arteries it is always abnormal and must be recognized to make the correct diagnosis.

Partial volume artifact

Partial volume artifact results from a slice thickness that is not infinitely thin. Echoes and Doppler signals can be acquired from objects that may be partly

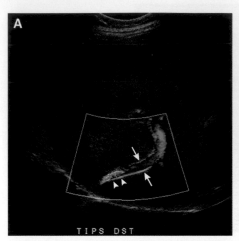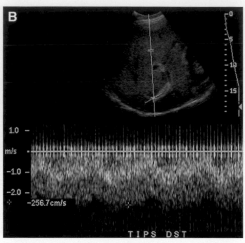

Fig. 9. Color Doppler aliasing in transjugular intrahepatic portal-systemic shunt (TIPS). (*A*) Longitudinal CDUS image of TIPS (*arrows*) demonstrates aliasing (*arrowheads*) in hepatic end of shunt suggesting focally elevated velocity. (*B*) Corresponding Doppler spectrum confirms shunt stenosis with angle- corrected flow velocity measuring 256.7 cm/s (normal velocity is <200 cm/s). (*From* Zynda-Weiss A, Carson NL. Carotid arterial and vertebral Doppler ultrasound. In: Dogra V, Rubens DJ, editors. Ultrasound secrets. New York: Elsevier; 2004; with permission.)

within the slice and partly outside of it, similar to slicing partly through a cherry in a piece of fruit cake. If viewed from one side, the slice seems to have a cherry. If viewed from the other side, no cherry seems visible. Because the signals in the US slice are summed together, the echoes produced are attributed to structures in the assumed "thin" scan plane [13]; thus, echoes can appear within anechoic structures and Doppler signals are acquired in an area in which no vessels are perceived on gray-scale [3]. For example, on a longitudinal gray-scale image, echoes from gas in the duodenum may appear within the gallbladder and mimic stones or polyps; however, if you rotate the transducer and image from the transverse plane, the gas is clearly adjacent to the gallbladder and not within it. On color flow imaging, an example of partial volume artifact is visualization of a portion of the iliac artery within the ovary giving the impression of abnormal cyst wall flow. Spectral analysis of this vessel shows the high resistance waveform typical of an iliac artery [Fig. 15] and imaging from the 90° plane clearly shows the vessel separate from the ovary. Partial volume artifact may be produced by grating lobes or side lobes, which generate information outside the expected path of the main beam. These off-axis lobes are located peripheral to the main beam axis [Fig. 16] [14]. Side lobes occur close to the primary beam whereas grating lobes can be far removed from the central beam [15]. These off-axis lobes can interrogate vessels that are separate from the primary sample volume. The lobes may appear on the spectral tracing as a flowing vessel where none is expected or display bidirectional flow as a result of interrogating the vessel from multiple angles

[Fig. 12]. These transducer related artifacts are seen mainly with the high frequency, tightly curved, convex, linear arrays used in endocavitary probes, and depend on the crystal element size and the spacing of the array elements [5].

Pseudoflow

Pseudoflow is defined as presence of flow of a fluid other than blood [7]. Pseudoflow can mimic real blood flow with color or power Doppler US, but no true vessel containing the fluid exists [Fig. 17]. The color or power Doppler signal appears as long as the fluid motion continues. These artifacts may be misinterpreted as flow unless Doppler spectral analysis is used. The spectral Doppler tracing does not exhibit a normal arterial or venous waveform [1]. Spontaneous examples of pseudoflow include ascites [Fig. 18], amniotic fluid, and urine (bladder jets). Bladder jets identify the ureteral orifice and are useful to exclude complete obstruction or to denote asymmetric ureteral emptying in the case of partial obstruction [Fig. 19] [16]. Bladder jets are not completely reliable, however, because 30% of obstructed patients may display normal jets [17]. Conversely, normal patients in the 2nd and 3rd trimester of pregnancy may have asymmetric or absent jets partly caused by uterine pressure. These jets can mostly be restored by scanning in the decubitus position, however, because the asymmetry may be physiologic and not necessarily abnormal, using diminished jets to diagnose obstruction in pregnancy still remains problematic [18].

Flash artifact

Flash artifact is a sudden burst of random color that fills the frame, obscuring the gray-scale image.

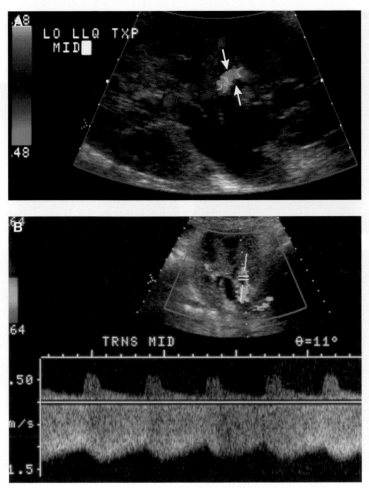

Fig. 10. Aliasing identifies an arteriovenous fistula (AVF). (*A*) Longitudinal CDUS image detects area of focal aliasing (*arrows*) indicating high-velocity flow in renal hilum, and suggests arteriovenous fistula. (*B*) Doppler spectrum demonstrates low resistance arterial waveform directed above baseline and high-velocity arterialized venous waveform below baseline, diagnostic of AVF.

This artifact may be caused by object motion or transducer motion [**Figs. 20 and 21**] [7]. Flash artifact may occur anywhere but is most commonly seen in the left lobe of the liver (as a result of cardiac pulsation) and in hypoechoic areas, such as cysts or fluid collections [**Fig. 22**] [5]. Flash artifact can be used to denote the fluid nature of solid-appearing material [**Fig. 23**] [1]. Power Doppler is more susceptible to flash artifact than color flow Doppler because of the longer time required to build the image (in general, more frames are averaged to create the image than with standard color Doppler) [19].

Although generally disruptive, motion artifacts can be extremely useful diagnostically. The so-called "perivascular artifact" or "color bruit" is a tissue motion artifact whereby the motion is generated within an organ, rather than involving an entire organ or image. This artifact appears as a random color mosaic in the soft tissues (as opposed to a single homogeneous color), occurs adjacent to vessels with turbulent flow, and is believed to be caused by actual vascular tissue vibration [20]. This artifact is the imaging equivalent to an auditory bruit or palpable thrill; varies with the cardiac cycle; is most prominent in systole; is absent or less prominent in diastole; is seen particularly in association with anastomotic sites, stenotic arteries, or arteriovenous fistulae [**Fig. 24**]; and can be extremely useful to detect their presence.

Mirror-image artifact

The mirror image artifact displays objects on both sides of a strong reflector, though they are located only on one side of it [21,22]. The reflector (eg, the diaphragm, pleural surface, or aortic wall) directs some of the echoes to a second reflector before it returns them to the transducer, resulting in a multipath reflection [**Fig. 25**] [14]. The machine "straightens out" the multipath echoes assuming

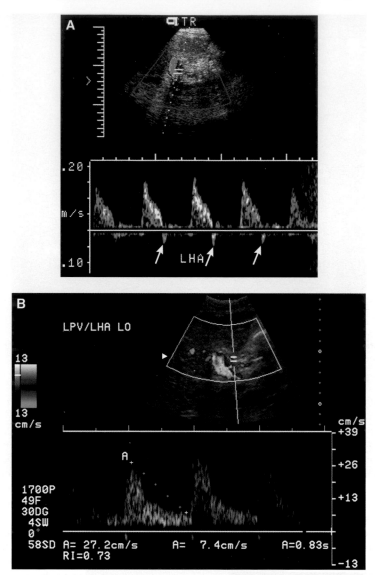

Fig. 14. Diastolic flow reversal (*A*) Spectral tracing in left hepatic artery 2 days after liver transplantation shows diastolic flow reversal (*arrows*) indicating high resistance to arterial flow. Resistive index (RI) is 1.0 (*B*) 1 day later normal continuous forward diastolic flow has been re-established and RI is normal at 0.7.

range [25]. These artifacts are more frequent at low PRF or velocity scale as a result of the increased sensitivity of the system but may also be caused by a low wall filter setting [26].

Twinkling artifact

In 1996, "twinkling artifact" was described by Rahmouni and colleagues [25] as color Doppler signals that imitate motion or flow behind a stationary strongly reflecting interface. The twinkling artifact can be seen behind any granular (irregular or rough) reflecting surface but is commonly caused by renal calculi, bladder calcification, and cholesterol crystals in the gallbladder [**Fig. 29**]. The twin-

kling Doppler is a mosaic of rapidly changing colors located deep to an echogenic reflector. With power Doppler, the signal location is the same, but the color is uniform [**Fig. 30**].

Twinkling artifact is believed to be caused by a narrow band of intrinsic machine noise called phase (or clock) jitter [27]. On a flat surface, system noise generates a narrow band of Doppler shift as a result of tiny clock errors. This tiny shift is usually excluded by the wall filter and, therefore, is not displayed as color. Rough surfaces increase the delays in measuring signal and amplify the errors, increasing the spectral bandwidth of this noise above the level of the wall filter. The spectrum is

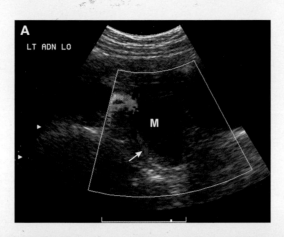

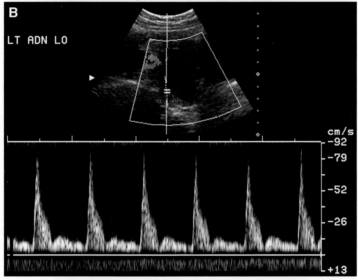

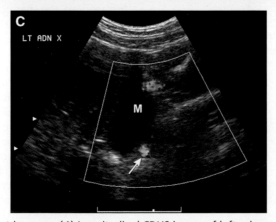

Fig. 15. Partial volume artifact in ovary. (*A*) Longitudinal CDUS image of left adnexa demonstrates vessel (*arrow*) along margin of ovarian cystic mass (M), creating concern that mass is vascular. (*B*) Doppler spectrum of this vessel reveals high resistance arterial waveform. (*C*) Axial image shows vessel (*arrows*) is actually adjacent to ovary and separate from it, not within cyst wall. (*D*) Doppler spectral waveform is identical to that in B, and is typical of internal iliac artery.

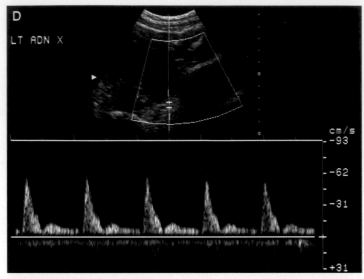

D

LT ADN X

cm/s
--93

--62

--31

-+31

Fig. 15 (continued).

typical of noise, with multiple closely applied spikes that are written equally above and below the baseline [Fig. 30].

Detection of the twinkling signal depends on the color-write priority and, in some instances, on gray-scale gain. As color-write priority decreases, more gray-scale is displayed, and the amount of twinkling artifact decreases behind the stone [27]. At high color-write priorities, the gray-scale has less effect. These settings vary from machine to machine and the relationships between the settings also vary

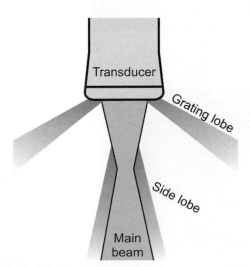

Fig. 16. Sidelobes. Diagram displays origins of side lobes and grating lobes and their relationship to main beam. Echoes returning from either of these additional lobe sources is displayed as though they originated from main beam.

with manufacturer. To consistently obtain a twinkling artifact, a high color-write priority should be selected and gray-scale gain kept to a minimum.

Why produce an artifact? Unlike many artifacts that are problematic, the twinkling artifact can be extremely useful. Similar to gray-scale shadowing, twinkling artifact also may be useful to identify stones. Small stones that may not generate a strong echo or cast an acoustic shadow still can produce a twinkling artifact, leading to their identification [Fig. 31] [1]. Similar to an acoustic shadow, twinkling does not occur 100% of the time. In a study of 32 patients by Lee and colleagues[28], only 86% of urinary calculi demonstrated a twinkling artifact; furthermore, the chemical composition of stones is related to the production of the artifact. Chelfouh and colleagues [29] reported that calcium oxalate dihydrate and calcium phosphate calculi always produced a twinkling artifact, whereas stones composed of calcium oxalate monohydrate and urate lacked a twinkling artifact. Besides renal calculi, a twinkling artifact may be seen behind material with an irregularly reflective, granular surface, such as iron filings, emery paper, ground chalk, wire mesh, an aneurysm coil during transcranial Doppler sonography [30], gall bladder adenomyomatosis [31], or, recently, encrusted stents [32]. Although the twinkling artifact cannot be generated 100% of the time, it can be extremely useful in the detection of renal calculi and some foreign bodies. The key to the twinkling artifact is that the color produced *behind* the calcification and the concomitant Doppler spectral tracing shows noise, not flow; thus, a calcified carotid plaque with twinkling can be

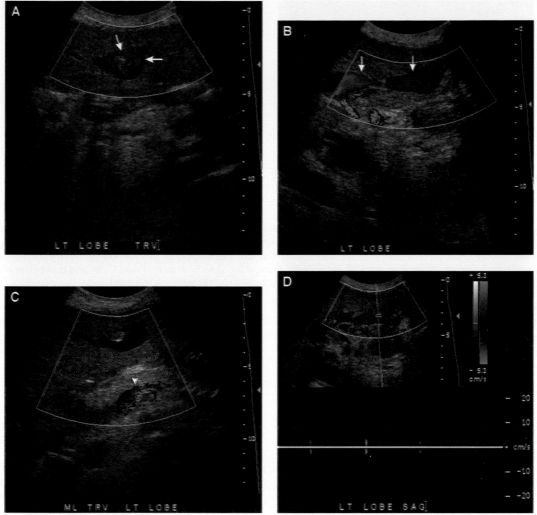

Fig. 17. Pseudoflow caused by fluid in ligamentum teres. (*A*) Transverse CDUS color flow image of liver demonstrates simulated vessel (*arrows*) coursing along falciform ligament. (*B*) Longitudinal CDUS image of same simulated vessel. (*C*) Axial image at another time point shows flow in posteriorly located splenic vein (*arrowhead*) but no flow around falciform. (*D*) Spectral Doppler tracing displays noise and no true flow. (*From* Campbell SC, Cullinan JA, Rubens DJ. Slow flow or no flow? Color and power Doppler US pitfalls in the abdomen and pelvis. Radiographics 2004;24:497–506; with permission.)

differentiated from a potentially ulcerated plaque with flow in the ulcer cavities [**Fig. 32**].

Day-to day Doppler: too much flow versus too little flow

The artifacts described in the section "Doppler Artifacts" primarily relate to the generation of Doppler signals by nonvascular structures or fluids. The key to their recognition is (1) knowing that they can occur, (2) knowing the common locations and causes for their generation, and (3) identification of the nonvascular Doppler spectrum they generate, which clinches the diagnosis. In day-to-day clinical practice, the more common problems are too much

flow, which may obscure thrombi, or too little flow, giving the false diagnosis of thrombosis.

Too much flow usually can be recognized by seeing color bleed [**Fig. 11**], or seeing aliasing in a vessel that normally does not have it [**Fig. 33**]. This problem can be corrected by increasing the scale or decreasing the gain. Another common imaging problem occurs when uninterrupted flow is imaged from a segment of a vessel and flow is assumed the same throughout the rest of the lumen. This problem usually occurrs in longitudinal vascular imaging whereby a partial thrombus or atheromatous plaque may not be imaged if it is not centered in the imaging plane [**Fig. 34**]. The fail-safe if inappropriate settings are not recognized is

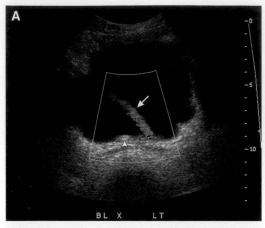
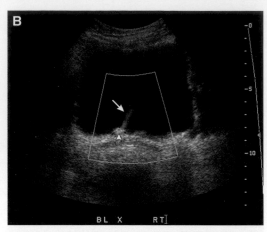

Fig. 18. Bladder jet. (*A*) Patient who presents with right renal colic. Transverse CDUS image through bladder shows normal jet (*arrow*) from asymptomatic side. Note right ureteral calculus (*arrowhead*). (*B*) Transverse CDUS image shows smaller right ureteral jet (*arrow*) indicating partial, but not complete, obstruction secondary to ureteral calculus (*arrowhead*). (*From* Campbell SC, Cullinan JA, Rubens DJ. Slow flow or no flow? Color and power Doppler US pitfalls in the abdomen and pelvis. Radiographics 2004;24:497–506; with permission.)

always to *image in two planes*; thus, even if the color-write priority is too high or the imaging plane is not centered and the thrombus is overwritten in the long axis of the vessel, the clot can be recognized in the short axis plane [**Fig. 34**].

The more common problem is too little flow, which mimics thrombosis. First, Doppler angle should be as small as possible. Obtaining signals for flow at 90° to the probe is always difficult [**Fig. 2**]. The scale should be set appropriately for the vessel you being interrogated. Too high a scale eliminates slow flow within the vessels [**Fig. 35**]. The frequency should be appropriate: low frequency for deep structures [**Fig. 36**] and high frequency for superficial ones [**Fig. 1**]. The frequency to demonstrate color flow Doppler is generally lower than the frequency needed for gray-scale imaging, so the Doppler frequency may need to be decreased if it does not default to the correct frequency. Frequency filters and other algorithms designed to decrease color tissue noise can eliminate display of slow flowing blood if they are set too high [**Fig. 2**]. In general, reducing the size of the color box reduces the sample size and increases the frame rate, leading to better overall sensitivity and resolution of the color image. Lastly, the color-write priority may be set automatically or manually. With a high color-write priority the sensitivity for color

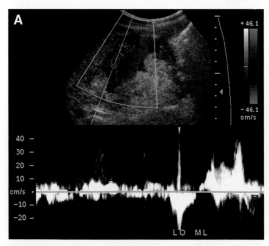
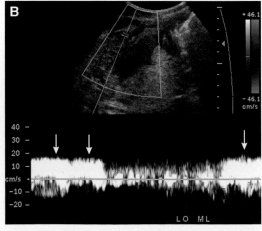

Fig. 19. Pseudoflow in ascites. (*A*) Longitudinal CDUS image in mid-abdomen in cirrhotic patient with ascites. Two linear flowing streams exist. More caudal stream (with Doppler cursor) has spectral Doppler waveform, which has random flow above and below baseline unrelated to any visceral vascular pattern. Motion in ascites occurs. (*B*) Cranial stream is continuous, unidirectional, and monophasic (*arrows*), typical of portal vein, representing patent umbilical collateral vessel. (*From* Campbell SC, Cullinan JA, Rubens DJ. Slow flow or no flow? Color and power Doppler US pitfalls in the abdomen and pelvis. Radiographics 2004;24:497–506; with permission.)

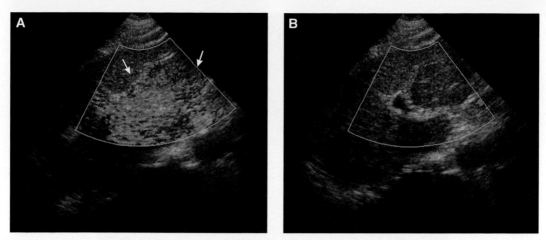

Fig. 20. Flash artifact: patient motion. (*A*) Longitudinal CDUS through the left lobe of liver with flash artifact (*arrows*) produced by respiratory motion. (*B*) Longitudinal CDUS with no motion shows normal vascular flow with no artifact.

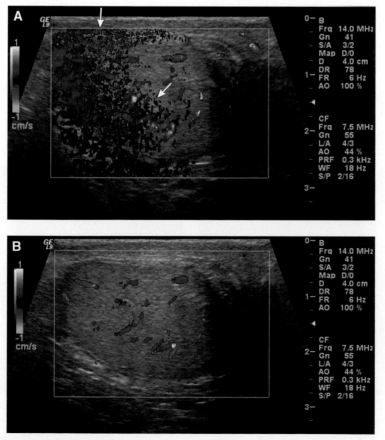

Fig. 21. Flash artifact: transducer motion. (*A*) Longitudinal CDUS of the left testis with flash artifact (*arrows*) caused by transducer motion. (*B*) Without motion, normal testicular vessels are easily identified.

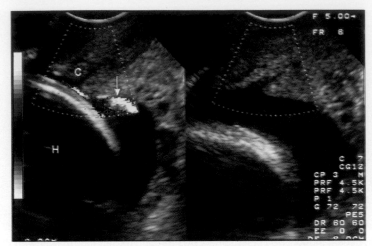

Fig. 22. Flash artifact in amniotic fluid caused by motion of fetal head. CDUS image (*left*) of lower uterine segment showing fetal head (H) and cervix (C). Flash of color (*arrow*) appears across internal os caused by application of fundal pressure while scanning, and simulates vasa previa. On corresponding CDUS image with no fundal pressure applied (*right*), no color is detected. (*From* Campbell SC, Cullinan JA, Rubens DJ. Slow flow or no flow? Color and power Doppler US pitfalls in the abdomen and pelvis. Radiographics 2004;24:497–506; with permission.)

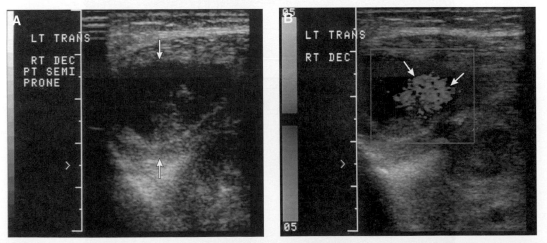

Fig. 23. Flash artifact to identify fluid for aspiration. (*A*) Transverse CDUS image in left thigh of immunocompromised patient presenting with left leg pain, originally evaluated for venous thrombosis with negative examination. Imaging in area of tenderness showed hypoechoic mass (*arrows*) with some internal echoes. (*B*) With compression applied to mass, anterior portion fills with color (*arrows*) indicating liquid, not solid mass. The apparent "mass" was aspirated and was an abscess.

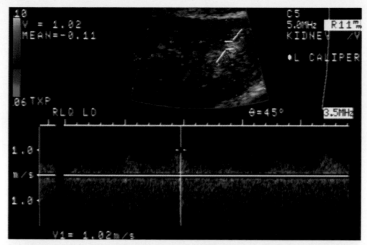

Fig. 24. Color Doppler bruit sampling in region of color Doppler bruit (mosaic of colors) shows typical spectrum of arteriovenous fistula with high-velocity arterial flow (1 m/s) and even higher venous flow (below baseline).

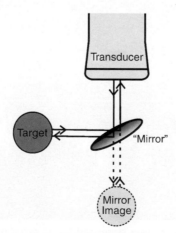

Fig. 25. Multipath reflection diagram of US wave path required to produce mirror image artifact. Pulse begins at transducer, is deflected by "mirror" (usually diaphragm or pleura) and hits target. Reflected echo returns to mirror and then to transducer, requiring much longer transit time than if pulse had interacted with object directly; thus, "mirror" image is displayed deeper in field of view.

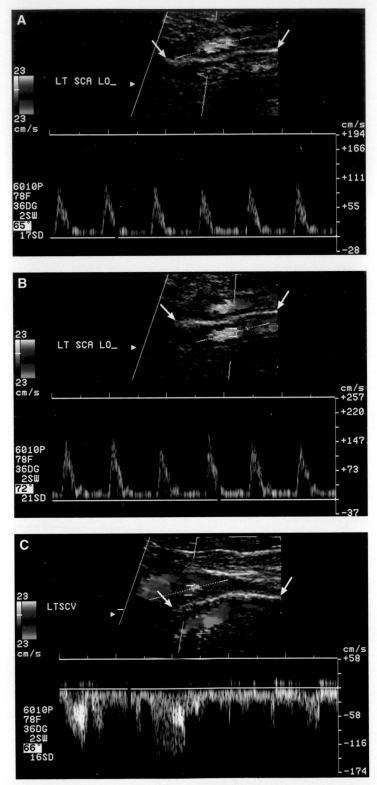

Fig. 26. Mirror-image artifact. (*A*) Anterior true vessel and (*B*) posterior mirror image of subclavian artery show identical spectra. Mirror in case is pleura (*arrows*). (*C*) Similar situation is noted with subclavian vein anteriorly and (*D*) its mirror image posteriorly with pleura (*arrows*) between them. Mirror-image vein should not be mistaken for collateral vessel.

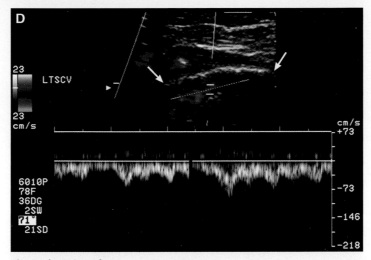

Fig. 26 (*continued*).

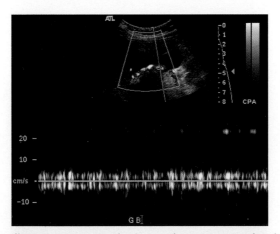

Fig. 27. Edge artifact from gallstone. Power Doppler image demonstrates color signal along rim of gallstone simulating a gallbladder mass. Spectral tracing is typical of noise, with nonvascular pattern displayed equally above and below baseline. (*From* Campbell SC, Cullinan JA, Rubens DJ. Slow flow or no flow? Color and power Doppler US pitfalls in the abdomen and pelvis. Radiographics 2004;24:497–506; with permission.)

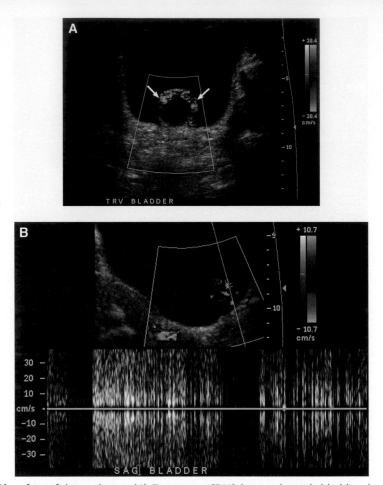

Fig. 28. Edge artifact from foley catheter. (*A*) Transverse CDUS image through bladder shows spherical mass centrally with marked Doppler signal around its margins (*arrows*). (*B*) Spectral Doppler confirms high amplitude continuous noise, equal and symmetric above and below baseline.

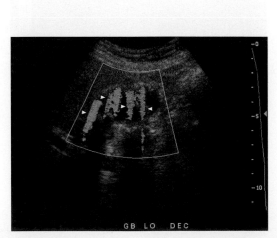

Fig. 29. Twinkling artifact longitudinal CDUS in patient with cholesterol crystals in gallbladder. Crystals generate twinkling artifact (*arrowheads*) posteriorly.

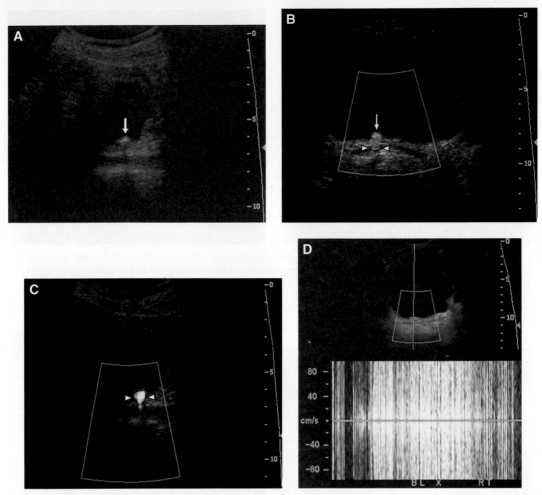

Fig. 30. Twinkling artifact. (*A*) Longitudinal image of bladder shows typical ureterovesical junction stone (*arrow*) with posterior shadow. (*B*) Transverse CDUS image of bladder shows right ureteral calculus (*arrow*) and twinkling artifact generated posteriorly (*arrowheads*). (*C*) Power Doppler also generates signal (*arrowheads*) posterior to stone. (*D*) Corresponding Doppler spectrum through twinkling color shows equal amplitude noise above and below baseline. Same spectral tracing is generated whether color or power Doppler images "twinkle." (*From* Campbell Campbell SC, Cullinan JA, Rubens DJ. Slow flow or no flow? Color and power Doppler US pitfalls in the abdomen and pelvis. Radiographics 2004;24:497–506; with permission.)

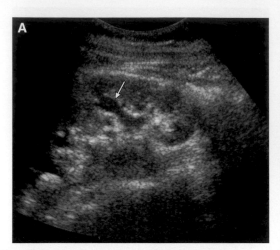
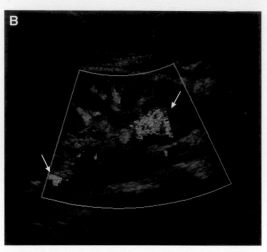

Fig. 31. Small renal stones with twinkling artifact. (*A*) Longitudinal US image through kidney shows minimal hydronephrosis (*arrow*) but no stones. (*B*) CDUS image in same position shows marked twinkling artifacts (*arrows*) at upper and lower poles, identifying stones, which do not cast an acoustic shadow.

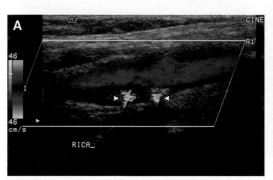
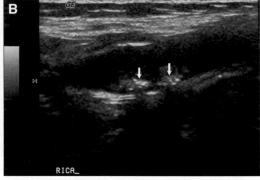

Fig. 32. Twinkling artifact in carotid. (*A*) Twinkling artifact (*arrowheads*) occurs behind calcifications (*arrows*) in atherosclerotic plaque, not to be mistaken for ulceration and disturbed flow. (*B*) Calcifications (*arrows*) are better visualized on gray-scale image. (*From* Campbell SC, Cullinan JA, Rubens DJ. Slow flow or no flow? Color and power Doppler US pitfalls in the abdomen and pelvis. Radiographics 2004;24:497–506; with permission.)

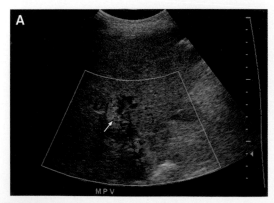
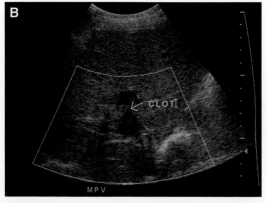

Fig. 33. Portal vein clot obscured. (*A*) Initial transverse CDUS image through portal vein shows color filling lumen; however, aliasing is occurring (*arrow*) and scale is too low at 23. (*B*) Repeat imaging with scale increased to 38 with other factors remaining constant permits detection of clot (*arrow*), which is isoechoic to liver.

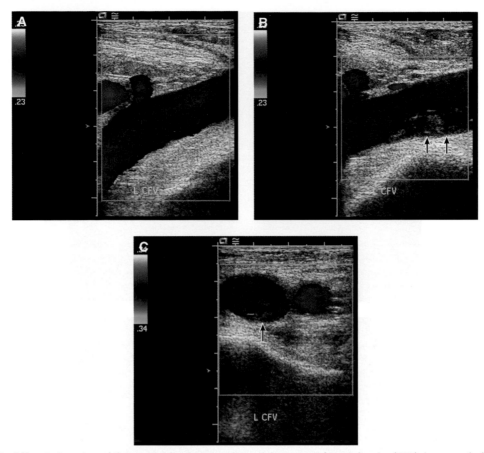

Fig. 34. Off axis imaging. (*A*) Longitudinal CDUS through common femoral vein (CFV) is normal. (*B*) With slight repositioning of transducer, large partial thrombus is identified posteriorly (*arrows*). (*C*) Transverse imaging shows partial thrombus centered in vein. Imaging in sagittal plane angled either side of thrombus creates false negative diagnosis.

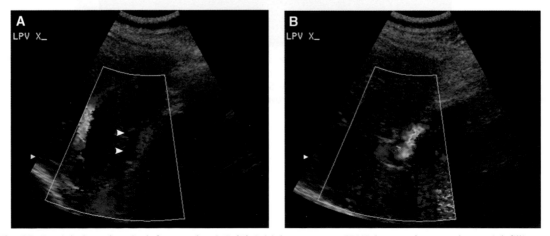

Fig. 35. Partial thrombus in left portal vein? (*A*) Initial transverse CDUS image shows only partial filling of left portal vein, simulating a thrombus (*arrowheads*) on right wall. Mean velocity scale is 17cm/s, too high for slow-flowing portal vein. (*B*) Repeat transverse image with scale at 10 cm/s shows normal filling of vein and no thrombus.

tients who had 70% to 99% internal carotid artery stenosis [3,4]. The Asymptomatic Carotid Atherosclerosis Study evaluated the efficacy of endarterectomy in patients who were asymptomatic and had carotid artery stenosis greater than 60% and showed that these patients had a reduced risk for subsequent stroke [5]. Before and after these impor-

tant studies, much effort has been directed at accurately detecting variable levels of stenosis with ultrasound, using measurements such as peak systolic velocity and various spectral Doppler ratios [6]. A multidisciplinary Society of Radiologists in Ultrasound consensus conference met recently to develop some general guidelines for carotid ultra-

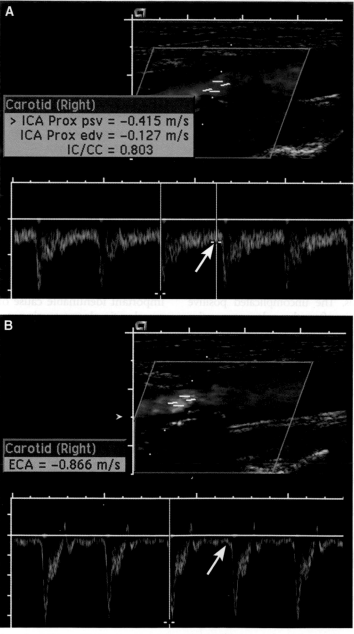

Fig. 1. Normal carotid study. (*A*) Longitudinal spectral Doppler of ICA has normal low-resistance flow with higher EDV (*arrow*) than the ECA or CCA. Prox, proximal. (*B*) Normal high-resistance spectral waveform is present in the ECA. EDV (*arrow*) is lower than in the ICA or CCA. (*C*) CCA spectrum shows low-resistance flow with no spectral broadening. The EDV (*arrow*) is between that of the ICA and the ECA. (*D*) Spectral Doppler of vertebral artery shows low-resistance waveform with moderate EDV (*arrow*).

sound for use in laboratories that do not have their own internally validated criteria [7]. Although it is optimal to perform an analysis of one's own laboratory ultrasound findings with respect to angiographic findings, it can be a difficult exercise. Generally, few angiograms are performed to corroborate sonographic findings, and exact determination of the percent diameter stenosis at surgery is not usually performed, making correlation difficult.

Using defined internal laboratory standards or standards derived from a multidisciplinary consensus panel does not guarantee a high-quality ultrasound examination. The examinations need to be performed by appropriately trained personnel, with national credentials such as Registered Diagnostic Medical Sonographer (RDMS), Registered Vascular Technologist (RVT), or the American Registry of Radiologic Technologists, Vascular Sonography, R.T. (R) (VS) (ARRT). Laboratory accreditation is essential in demonstrating a commitment to excellence and adherence to standards, as defined by the American College of Radiology, American Institute of Ultra-

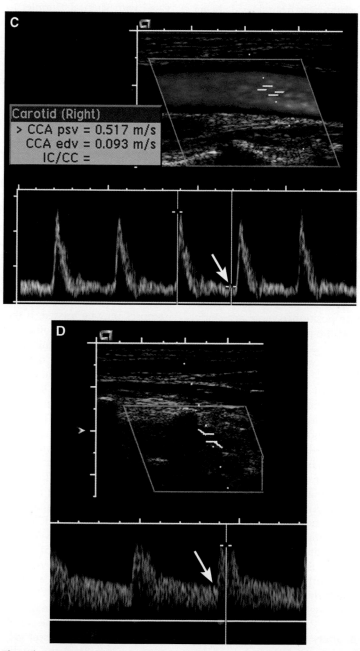

Fig. 1 (*continued*).

sound in Medicine, or the Intersocietal Commission for the Accreditation of Vascular Laboratories.

Carotid ultrasound examination

Scanning technique

General

The patient should be examined in the supine position with arms by the sides. The shoulders should be lowered to increase access to the neck if needed. It is often helpful to tell the patient to reach for the feet if they have a short or thick neck. The head should be turned slightly away from the side being examined. In general, the patient is not scanned with a pillow under the head. If adequate access to the neck is still difficult, a pillow under the shoulders may help hyperextend the neck. Sonographer position is variable, with some sonographers preferring to sit at the top of the patient's head and table, scanning facing downward from the patient's head to his shoulders. Others prefer to scan from the patient's side, facing upward toward the head.

A 5-MHz or higher linear transducer should be used, with images optimized to examine the carotid in the near field. A higher frequency linear transducer is encouraged to optimize gray-scale imaging if technically possible. Particular attention should be paid to placing the focal zone at the level of the carotid so that the gray-scale images show the finest detail possible. The transducer should be placed slightly posterolaterally on the neck, using the sternocleidomastoid muscle as an acoustic window. The transducer can be positioned more anteriorly, along with changes in the patient's neck position, if necessary.

B-mode (gray-scale)

It is important to get an overall impression of the amount of atherosclerotic disease in the carotid artery and the location of the branches before focusing on a particular arterial segment. The transverse plane is used in this initial analysis, scanning from the proximal common carotid artery (CCA) through the bifurcation, and then to the internal and external carotid arteries (ICA and ECA, respectively). The probable positions of the ICA and ECA can be determined and verified later with spectral Doppler. The ECA is usually a smaller artery oriented more medially and anteriorly than the ICA, as it supplies the face. The ICA tends to be slightly larger than the ECA, with angulation posteriorly and laterally with respect to the ECA, although anatomic variability can occur.

Next, the carotid artery is scanned longitudinally from the origin of the CCA through the bifur-

cation. The transducer is angled slightly anteriorly toward the face to image the ECA. The ICA is found using slight angulation of the transducer posteriorly and laterally in most patients. A complete gray-scale evaluation includes a general assessment of soft and hard plaque and the documentation of less-common findings, such as plaque ulceration or dissection.

Color/power Doppler

Color Doppler can be useful in detecting areas of flow abnormality that need to be further investigated with spectral Doppler to assess their significance. Optimizing color Doppler in an individual vessel segment is important, as it can speed up the task of finding stenoses. As is the case with spectral Doppler, the angle of the color box should be 60° or less. Modern ultrasound scanners have preprogrammed scanner settings individualized for different vessels, such as the carotid artery. The sophisticated sonographer should feel comfortable with the many aspects that are controllable in the image, and change them as necessary to optimize the information displayed.

One of the first things that should be addressed when imaging a vessel is the color Doppler gain. It should be increased until color speckles are seen outside of the lumen, then turned down until the color is displayed only within the vessel lumen. If the color Doppler gain is set too high, color pixels may be placed outside of the true lumen of the artery, termed an artificial color "bleed" outside of the vessel lumen. If this event occurs, plaque and stenoses may be missed. If the color Doppler gain is set too low, the amount of flow in a vessel can be underestimated significantly and an occlusion could be erroneously diagnosed. Power Doppler should be used when occlusion or a trickle of flow is suspected, as it is a more sensitive low-flow, angle-independent technique [8].

The color velocity scale is another parameter that should be individually optimized for each vessel segment. The color velocity scale should be adjusted so that color is seen within the lumen and the direction of flow in the vessel is clear. If the velocity scale is set too low, aliasing will occur and important information regarding areas of flow disturbance and flow jets from stenoses could potentially be overlooked. The velocity filter controls the amount of flow seen within the vessel depending on its velocity characteristics, and should be set as low as possible if an occlusion is suspected.

The color Doppler image is based on the average Doppler shift within the vessel, not the peak Doppler shift within the vessel [9]. Color Doppler will give an estimate of the qualitative amount of the stenosis. Spectral Doppler is a necessary component of the carotid ultrasound examination to quantitate the degree of stenosis.

Spectral Doppler

After the gray-scale and color Doppler images have been optimized, accurate measurement of the spectral Doppler signal is arguably the most important portion of the examination. The angle of spectral Doppler insonation should be 60° or less for reproducible and accurate velocity measurement. There is some debate as to the correct placement of the angle correction cursor. The normal default position should be parallel to the posterior carotid wall segment. The exception to this rule occurs when there is a color jet seen, usually extending distally

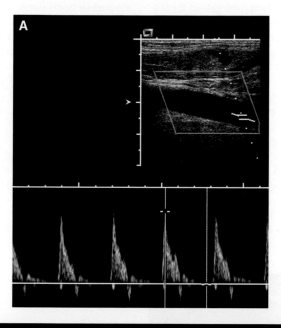

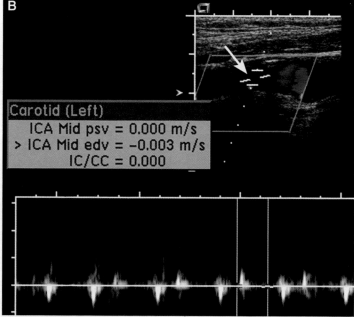

Fig. 2. High-resistance CCA. (*A*) Longitudinal spectral Doppler shows unilateral high-resistance flow (with no diastolic flow) in the CCA, suggesting ICA stenosis versus occlusion. (*B*) No flow is identified in the mid-distal ICA on color and spectral Doppler (*arrow*).

or downstream from a stenosis. In this instance, the angle should be placed parallel to the direction of the jet and not the posterior carotid wall.

It is important to not only assess the angle, but also the sample gate width when performing reproducible accurate spectral Doppler. A small sample gate width should be used, between 1.5 and 2.5 mm wide. Even in normal laminar flow, the range of velocities present in the bloodstream ranges from highest in the middle of the vessel to lower near the vessel wall. The range gate is meant to depict the representative flow in the vessel, not all the spectral velocities that exist in the vessel. Therefore, a small sample gate should be used at the center of the vessel or in the center of a jet distal to a stenosis. If too large a spectral gate is used, a widened spectral Doppler tracing (spectral broadening) could lead to the erroneous diagnosis of disturbed or turbulent flow.

Disturbed flow patterns indicate that the movement of blood is less orderly than in laminar flow, and can be found in vessel kinks, curves, areas of arterial branching, and areas of mild stenosis. Turbulent flow is defined as areas of flow reversal, and usually occurs at areas of severe stenosis when a jet of blood with high velocity encounters a normal or increased lumen diameter beyond the stenosis [9]. Flow reversal normally occurs within the carotid bulb, but is abnormal in any other location. Spectral broadening can also be erroneously depicted on the spectral tracing when the Doppler gain is set too high, causing a spurious filling in of the spectral waveform. Likewise, if the Doppler gain is set too low, not all of the clinically important velocities may be displayed.

Because the accurate diagnosis of the degree of carotid stenosis depends on velocity measurement, the peak velocity needs to be properly displayed. The pulse repetition frequency must be set high enough to be able to accurately measure the arterial signal, encompassing the entire signal within the velocity scale chosen. The spectral waveform needs be appropriately scaled so that the waveform is not too small, but not so large as to have aliasing.

Imaging protocol

After all of the imaging parameters are optimized, standard images should be obtained according to laboratory and accreditation standards. Transverse gray-scale images of at least the proximal and distal CCA, bulb, bifurcation, and proximal ICA and ECA should be obtained with detailed labeling. Longi-

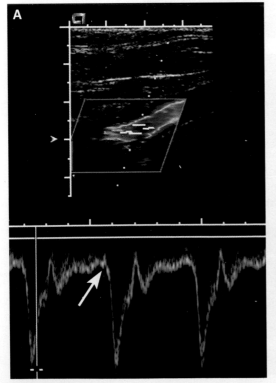
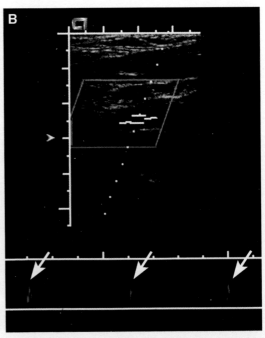

Fig. 3. Low-resistance "internalization" of ECA flow. (*A*) Longitudinal spectral Doppler of the ECA shows low-resistance flow with prominent diastolic component (*arrow*). (*B*) Spectral Doppler of the ICA has brief high-resistance flow (*arrows*), consistent with a high-grade stenosis or occlusion of the ICA.

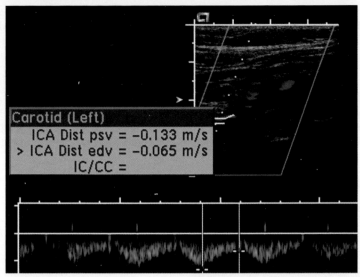

Fig. 4. Low-resistance, low PSV flow distal to CCA stenosis. Longitudinal spectral Doppler of the ICA shows a typical poststenotic "parvus-tardus" arterial waveform with delayed upstroke and low peak velocity of 13 cm/s. Dist, distal.

tudinal gray-scale images of at least the proximal and distal CCA, bulb to CCA, proximal ECA extending into the CCA, and proximal ICA extending into the CCA should be obtained. It is not necessary to record gray-scale images of the vertebral artery without spectral Doppler, as only a limited portion of the vertebral artery can be seen between the vertebral segments.

After the gray-scale images are obtained, optimized color Doppler images with their accompanying spectral waveforms are recorded. Longitudinal color Doppler and spectral waveforms are obtained in the proximal and distal CCA; proximal ECA; proximal, mid, and distal ICA; and the vertebral artery. The peak systolic velocity (PSV) and end diastolic velocity (EDV) are measured for each segment. The location of the distal CCA PSV measurement is important, as CCA PSVs decrease distally from the heart [10,11]. Accordingly, the location at which the distal CCA waveform is measured within the CCA is standardized at 2 cm proximal to the bulb. If any stenoses are found, spectral waveforms should be obtained at and distal to the stenosis, with corresponding PSV and EDV measurements.

Waveform analysis

Normal carotid ultrasound waveform pattern analysis

The brain requires oxygen and nutrients throughout systole and diastole of the cardiac cycle. Thus, the internal carotid artery has a low-resistance waveform pattern. There is a tall and sharp upstroke in systole with a moderate amount of diastolic flow. The entire waveform shows antegrade flow throughout the cardiac cycle [**Fig. 1A**].

In contradistinction, the muscles of the face do not require blood flow in diastole. Therefore, the flow in the external carotid artery is high-resistance flow. There is a tall and sharp upstroke in systole, but the waveform quickly returns to near baseline, with little flow during diastole [**Fig. 1B**]. A small amount of diastolic flow in the ECA may normally be seen.

The normal CCA waveform is a combination of the distal high-resistance waveform pattern of the ECA and the lower-resistance waveform pattern of the ICA [**Fig. 1C**]. It is critical to begin with the CCA waveform in the carotid ultrasound analysis because the CCA is a combination of the downstream ECA and ICA hemodynamics.

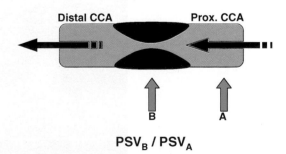

$$PSV_B / PSV_A$$

Fig. 5. CCA stenosis. The PSV ratio is used to characterize the severity of the stenosis in this region. PSV_B is at the CCA stenosis and PSV_A is 2 cm proximal to the stenosis. Prox, proximal.

The last artery to be analyzed in the carotid artery ultrasound is the vertebral artery. Like the ICA, the vertebral artery has a sharp upstroke and moderate low-resistance flow throughout all of diastole [**Fig. 1D**].

Abnormal carotid ultrasound waveform pattern analysis

After a high-quality accurate carotid ultrasound has been performed using the techniques detailed earlier,

the next steps in interpretation are equally critical. Following is a summary of the diagnostic possibilities, pearls, and pitfalls that should be considered when interpreting a carotid ultrasound examination.

Common carotid artery

The first thing that should be assessed when interpreting a carotid ultrasound is the CCA waveform, because the CCA waveform is a combination of the ECA and ICA waveforms, and should have a mod-

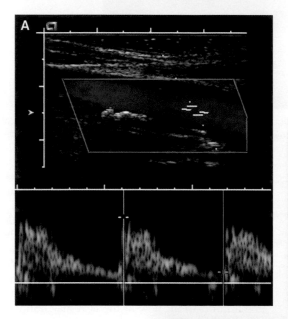

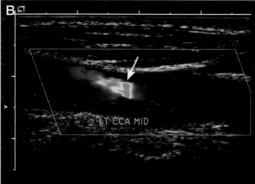

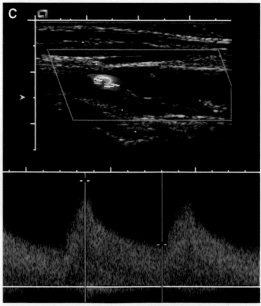

Fig. 6. CCA stenosis. (*A*) Longitudinal spectral Doppler of proximal CCA has mildly elevated resistance. (*B*) Color Doppler in the CCA demonstrates visible luminal narrowing with color aliasing (*arrow*). LT, left. (*C*) Spectral Doppler at the same location has high-velocity flow (PSV 627 cm/s) with severe turbulence. (*D*) Delayed systolic acceleration (*arrow*) and low PSV of 43 cm/s (tardus-parvus waveform) are present in the ICA.

erate amount of diastolic flow. If this waveform is abnormal, downstream or upstream stenoses or occlusions are likely. Thus, the more distal (or proximal) waveforms can be assessed with a high degree of suspicion for abnormality. The usual waveform abnormalities of the CCA encountered include an abnormally high-resistance waveform, an abnormally low-resistance waveform, and either low or high PSVs. These are considered individually later.

The classic cause of a high-resistance waveform pattern in the CCA is a high-grade ICA stenosis or occlusion, termed *externalization of the CCA*. If a high-resistance waveform is seen in the CCA, the diagnosis of severe ICA stenosis or occlusion is suggested, and the distal waveforms should be assessed to determine whether they support the diagnosis [**Fig. 2**]. However, there is an exception to this rule. If the process is bilateral and the peak PSVs are low, this waveform pattern could indicate aortic stenosis or severe cardiac failure, discussed later.

A pitfall occurs when the ECA is providing collateral flow to adjacent arteries, typically occurring with long-standing internal carotid artery occlusion. When collaterals are fed from the ECA, the waveform becomes a lower-resistance waveform with some diastolic flow. In this instance, there may be an ICA occlusion present, but the CCA waveform is not such a noticeably high-resistance pattern because of the low-resistance contribution of the collateralized ECA [**Fig. 3**]. When there is an occlusion of one artery, and differentiation of ICA versus ECA is not clear, the temporal tap can be a helpful maneuver, as detailed later.

A normal CCA PSV should be in the range of approximately 0.6 to 1.0 m/s [12]. If the CCA PSV is lower than this range, the contralateral CCA waveform should be examined. If the PSVs are symmetric, the cause of the low PSV is likely secondary to a low cardiac output, such as that seen with congestive heart failure. If the contralateral PSV appears more normal, the CCA with the low PSV is usually abnormal and needs to be investigated further.

Potential causes for a unilateral low PSV in the CCA include a proximal or distal high-grade stenosis or occlusion. The first step in differentiating between these two causes can be made by determining whether the waveform is high-resistance or low-resistance. A high-grade stenosis can occur in either proximal CCA. On the right side, the stenosis or occlusion can also occur in the innominate artery (brachiocephalic artery), typically at its origin off the aortic arch. A high-grade proximal CCA stenosis will be evidenced by a downstream low-resistance waveform. Poststenotic turbulence may be demonstrated if sampled close to the stenosis, and sometimes a tardus parvus waveform can be seen [**Fig. 4**]. Occasionally the waveforms look normal, and the only way a proximal CCA stenosis can be suspected is by noting the asymmetry in the PSVs. A high-grade stenosis distal to the point of sampling in the CCA, such as higher in the neck or in the carotid siphon, will be reflected in a high-resistance waveform.

If a focal stenosis in the CCA is seen, a ratio needs to be calculated to determine the degree of stenosis.

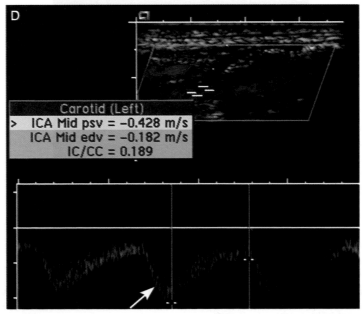

Fig. 6 (*continued*).

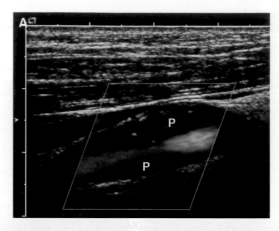

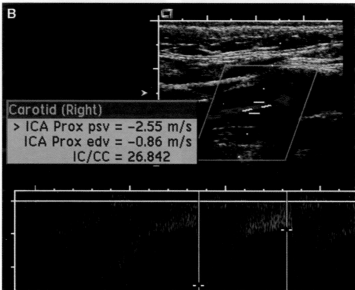

Fig. 11. ICA stenosis of 70% to near occlusion. (*A*) Longitudinal power Doppler of carotid bulb demonstrates only a narrow stream of flow through a large region of soft plaque (P). (*B*) Narrow lumen is confirmed with spectral Doppler PSV elevation of 255 cm/s. Prox, proximal.

ICA to the skull base [**Fig. 12**A]. Usually the ICA stenosis is localized, extending from the bulb only for a few centimeters [**Fig. 12**B]. The appearance of a "string sign," or narrow column of flow in the distal ICA on the angiogram, is because the heavier radiographic contrast does not fill the carotid lumen distally. The narrow lumen seen on the angiogram is not because there is a high-grade stenosis throughout the entire ICA. Ultrasound has limitations in its ability to differentiate occlusion [**Fig. 13**] from a trickle of flow.

The ICA should always be compared with the ECA waveform. An uncommon pitfall occurs in the scenario of an occluded ICA. It is possible to overlook an occluded ICA and think that the bifurcation into the ECA and ICA occurs at the first visible branch of the ECA. This situation can be diagnosed by realizing that the ICA and ECA waveforms are identical. Noticing that identical ICA and ECA waveforms are present should be a key toward making this provisional diagnosis. The sonographer then needs to re-examine that site for the diagnostic possibility of ICA occlusion. When this mistake occurs, the sonographer will frequently remark that the bifurcation looked unusual or that the examination was difficult. Occasionally this scenario will be seen in a patient who has an extremely low carotid bifurcation and no ICA occlusion [**Fig. 14**].

External carotid artery

A normal ECA waveform has a high-resistance waveform pattern because the muscles of the face

Table 1: Doppler criteria for internal carotid artery diameter stenosis detection developed by the Society of Radiologists in Ultrasound consensus conference

	ICA PSV cm/s	Plaque/diameter	ICA/CCA ratio = PSV_{ICA}/PSV_{CCA}	ICA EDV cm/s
Normal	<125	None	<2	<40
<50%	<125	<50%	<2	<40
50%–69%	125–230	≥50%	2–4	40–100
≥70 to near occlusion	>230	≥50%	>4	>100
Near occlusion	High, low, or undetectable	Visible	Variable	Variable
Total occlusion	Undetectable	Visible, no detectable lumen	N/A	N/A

Abbreviation: N/A, not applicable.

do not need blood flow throughout diastole. In general, little evaluation of the ECA distal to its origin from the CCA needs to be performed. The two major reasons the ECA needs to be evaluated are to differentiate the ECA from the ICA and to identify the source of an audible bruit other than the ICA. The temporal tap maneuver is useful for accurate differentiation when it is not immediately obvious which vessel is the ECA versus the ICA.

The temporal artery is a branch of the ECA located several finger breadths anterior to the ear

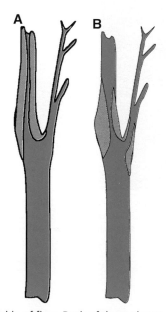

Fig. 12. Trickle of flow. Both of these plaque configurations correlate with the "string sign" on angiography. (*A*) Severe concentric atherosclerotic plaque extends all the way up the ICA into the distal ICA. (*B*) Marked atherosclerotic plaque at the bulb extends for a short distance into the ICA, causing severe narrowing of the proximal ICA. Note the more distal ICA is relatively stenosis free.

on the patient's cheek. Tapping in this location will transmit pressure waveforms through the temporal artery to the ECA [**Fig. 15**]. If there is no significant stenosis of either the ECA or the ICA, the temporal tap may be seen in both arteries. It is debatable whether or not the temporal tap needs to be performed if no significant stenosis is seen in either the ICA or ECA. However, most feel that it should be included in every examination.

In the scenario of a significant stenosis in one vessel off of the bifurcation, there are two choices for the stenotic vessel—either the ICA or ECA. The temporal tap can be useful in differentiating the ICA from the ECA [Table 2]. In scenario 1, ECA stenosis, if there is a significant stenosis in the ECA, the temporal tap will not be transmitted to the ICA from the ECA because of the significant ECA stenosis. In this scenario, an alteration in the waveform caused by the temporal tap will be appreciable in the ECA waveform and not in the ICA. In the second scenario, ICA stenosis, if there is a significant stenosis in the ICA, the temporal tap waveforms will not be transmitted to the ICA from the ECA because of the significant ICA stenosis. As in the first scenario, the temporal tap will only be appreciated in the ECA waveform. This maneuver thus allows the definitive differentiation of the ECA from the ICA once the hemodynamics behind the technique are understood [16].

Vertebral artery

Evaluation of the vertebral artery is performed bilaterally as a routine part of the carotid artery ultrasound. Spectral waveforms and direction of flow are assessed. Reversal of flow in the left vertebral artery is more common than the right and indicates a proximal subclavian artery stenosis or occlusion, usually at the origin from the aortic arch. Flow reversal in the right vertebral artery indicates either a proximal subclavian artery stenosis or occlusion, or a significant brachiocephalic artery stenosis or occlusion. If the flow reversal occurs

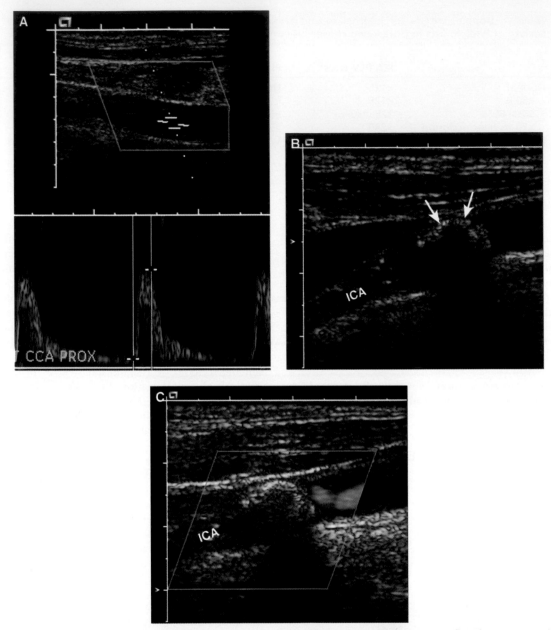

Fig. 13. Occlusion versus trickle of flow. (*A*) Spectral Doppler of CCA shows high-resistance flow but no stenosis. Prox, proximal. (*B*) Gray-scale image of the ICA and bulb shows severe plaque (*arrows*) with shadowing. (*C*) Color Doppler of the proximal ICA beyond the plaque shows no definite flow. A trickle of flow cannot be excluded by conventional ultrasound.

in the right vertebral artery, a small footprint transducer should be used to attempt to visualize the proximal right subclavian artery and a portion of the brachiocephalic artery, which occasionally can be well visualized. Lesser degrees of subclavian or brachiocephalic stenosis result in transient systolic flow reversal in the vertebral artery [17]. There are progressive degrees of midsystolic deceleration patterns that ultimately completely reverse and correlate to the degree of proximal stenosis. Kliewer and colleagues [17] developed an excellent grading scheme for abnormal vertebral artery waveforms that are not completely reversed, which is also covered in the subsequent article.

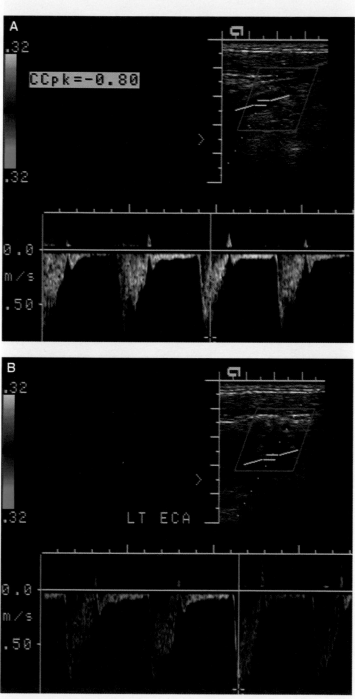

Fig. 14. Severe ICA stenosis and low carotid bifurcation with first ECA branch mistaken for carotid bulb. (*A–C*) Longitudinal spectral Doppler images that were initially labeled CCA, ECA, and ICA, and interpreted as no stenosis, have identical waveforms, suggesting that all are part of the ECA system. LT, left. (*D*) Further investigation demonstrates a very low bifurcation of the CCA and a focal ICA stenosis is confirmed on spectral Doppler (PSV 219 cm/s). CCpk, common carotid peak systolic velocity.

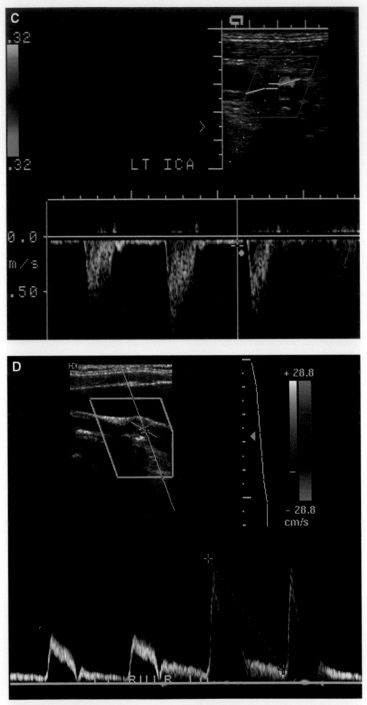

Fig. 14 (continued).

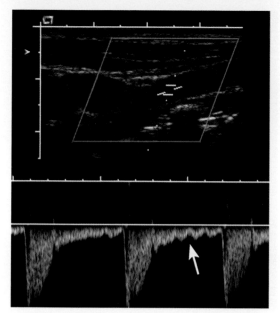

Fig. 15. Temporal tap for ECA identification. Repeated jagged reverberations (*arrow*) are transmitted from the temporal artery to the ECA and are displayed in the spectral waveform.

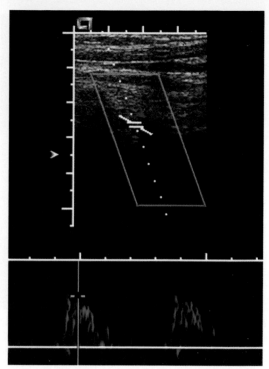

Fig. 16. Abnormal vertebral artery high-resistance flow. Spectral Doppler of a left vertebral artery in a patient who has distal vertebral artery stenosis versus occlusion shows abnormal high-resistance flow with absence of any diastolic component.

A high-resistance waveform in the vertebral artery is consistent with a distal stenosis, occlusion, or a hypoplastic artery [**Fig. 16**]. Differentiation between these causes is important, as some centers are performing vertebral artery angioplasty and stent placement for significant vertebral artery stenosis. A potential vertebral artery stenosis by ultrasound should always be correlated with the patient's clinical symptomatology. Dizziness and unsteady walking can be signs of vertebral basilar insufficiency or impending stroke from vertebral artery stenosis. If the vertebral artery cannot be detected, the differential diagnosis is vertebral artery occlusion versus a small or congenitally absent vertebral artery.

A low-resistance, low PSV waveform in the vertebral artery may indicate a more proximal stenosis [18]. Although the left vertebral artery origin is difficult to see with ultrasound because of overlying lung, the right proximal vertebral artery origin off of the subclavian artery can often be seen with a small footprint transducer to identify an area of stenosis [**Fig. 17**].

Summary

A high-quality ultrasound examination can be readily achieved using the techniques and principles discussed above. Once the hemodynamics of the carotid system are understood, the arterial waveforms encountered become understandable and predictable. A pattern recognition approach to waveform analysis makes accurate interpretation

Table 2: **Temporal tap: internal and external carotid artery findings**

	ICA temporal tap	ECA temporal tap
Normal	+/−	+
Sig. ICA stenosis	−	+
Sig. ECA stenosis	−	+

+, present; −, not present; +/−, possibly present.

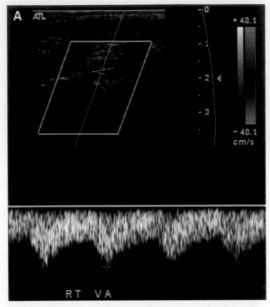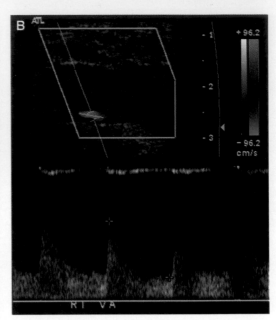

Fig. 17. Vertebral artery stenosis. (*A*) Longitudinal spectral Doppler of right vertebral artery demonstrates low-resistance "parvus-tardus" waveforms. RT, right. (*B*) Further investigation discovered a focal stenosis of the vertebral artery origin with elevated PSV of 272 cm/s. RT, right; VA, vertebral artery.

more likely, with a greater chance of avoiding the various pitfalls commonly encountered.

References

[1] Consensus Group. Consensus statement on the management of patients with asymptomatic atherosclerotic carotid bifurcation lesions. Int Angiol 1995;14:5–17.

[2] Timsit SG. Early clinical differentiation of cerebral infarction from severe atherosclerotic stenosis and cardioembolism. Stroke 1992;23:486–91.

[3] North American Symptomatic Carotid Endarterectomy Trial (NASCET) Steering Committee. North American Symptomatic Carotid Endarterectomy Trial: methods, patient characteristics, and progress. Stroke 1991;22:711–20.

[4] North American Symptomatic Carotid Endarterectomy Trial Collaborators. Beneficial effect of carotid endarterectomy in symptomatic patients with high grade carotid stenosis. N Engl J Med 1991;325(7):445–53.

[5] Executive Committee for the Asymptomatic Carotid Atherosclerosis Study. Endarterectomy for asymptomatic carotid artery stenosis. JAMA 1995;273(18):1421–8.

[6] Moneta GL, Edwards JM, Papanicolaou G, et al. Screening for asymptomatic internal carotid artery stenosis: duplex criteria for discriminating 60% to 99% stenosis. J Vasc Surg 1995;21(6):989–94.

[7] Grant EG, Benson CB, Moneta GL, et al. Carotid artery stenosis: gray-scale and Doppler US diagnosis—Society of Radiologists in Ultrasound Consensus Conference. Radiology 2003;229(2):340–6.

[8] Robbin ML. The utility of contrast in the extracranial carotid ultrasound examination. In: Goldberg BB, Raichlen JS, Forsbert F, editors. Ultrasound contrast agents: basic principles and clinical applications. 2nd edition. London: Martin Dunitz Publishers; 2001. p. 239–51.

[9] Zwiebel WJ, Pellerito JS. Basic concepts of Doppler frequency spectrum analysis and ultrasound blood flow imaging. In: Zwiebel WJ, Pellerito JS, editors. Introduction to vascular ultrasonography. 5th edition. Philadelphia: Elsevier Saunders; 2005. p. 61–89.

[10] Meyer JI, Khalil RM, Obuchowski NA, et al. Common carotid artery: variability of Doppler US velocity measurements. Radiology 1997;204(2):339–41.

[11] Lee VS, Hertzberg BS, Workman MJ, et al. Variability of Doppler US measurements along the common carotid artery: effects on estimates of internal carotid arterial stenosis in patients with angiographically proved disease. Radiology 2000;214(2):387–92.

[12] Zwiebel WJ. Normal findings and technical aspects of carotid sonography. In: Zwiebel WJ, Pellerito JS, editors. Introduction to vascular ultrasonography. 5th edition. Philadelphia: Elsevier Saunders; 2005. p. 143–54.

[13] Kallman CE, Gosink BB, Gardner DJ. Carotid duplex sonography: bisferious pulse contour in patients with aortic valvular disease. AJR Am J Roentgenol 1991;157(2):403–7.

[14] Bluth EI, Stavros AT, Marich KW, et al. Carotid duplex sonography: a multicenter recommenda-

tion for standardized imaging and Doppler criteria. Radiographics 1988;8(3):487–506.

[15] Abou-Zamzam Jr AM, Moneta GL, Edwards JM, et al. Is a single preoperative duplex scan sufficient for planning bilateral carotid endarterectomy. J Vasc Surg 2000;31(2):282–8.

[16] Budorick NE, Rojratanakiat W, O'Boyle MK, et al. Digital tapping of the superficial temporal ar-

tery: significance in carotid duplex sonography. J Ultrasound Med 1996;15(6):459–64.

[17] Kliewer MA, Hertzberg BS, Kim DH, et al. Vertebral artery Doppler waveform changes indicating subclavian steal physiology. AJR Am J Roentgenol 2000;174(3):815–9.

[18] Sidhu PS. Ultrasound of the carotid and vertebral arteries. Br Med Bull 2000;56(2):346–66.

ULTRASOUND
CLINICS

Ultrasound Clin 1 (2006) 133–159

Waveform Analysis of the Carotid Arteries

Leslie M. Scoutt[a],*, Felix L. Lin, MD[b], Mark Kliewer, MD[c]

- Changes in systolic contour
- Alteration in diastolic flow patterns
- Abnormal waveforms effecting the entire cardiac cycle
- Summary
- References

Stroke is the third leading cause of death in the United States and a leading cause of severe long-term disability. It is estimated that 700,000 strokes occur yearly in the United States with an associated mortality of 162,672 and an estimated health care cost of $56.8 billion [1]. It is believed that up to 20% to 30% of strokes are the result of disease at the carotid bifurcation, with the mechanism of injury most likely emboli from friable plaque dislodged by the high-velocity turbulent jet occurring at the site of the atherosclerotic stenosis [2,3]. Several recently published prospective, multicenter, randomized, double-blind trials demonstrate convincingly that carotid endarterectomy significantly reduces the risk of stroke and death in comparison to medical therapy in patients who have hemodynamically significant stenosis ($\geq$60%–70%) of the internal carotid artery (ICA) [4–7]. Hence, when performing a carotid ultrasound (US) examination, pulse Doppler waveforms are used primarily to measure peak systolic velocity (PSV) or PSV ratio (PSVR = PSV in ICA ÷ PSV in distal common carotid artery [CCA]) in order to quantitate the degree of stenosis. More careful analysis of the shape and contour of the pulse Doppler waveform, however, can provide physiologic information regarding the distal circulation/vascular bed and the proximal vessels, areas that cannot be interrogated or visualized directly on US examination. The purpose of this review article is to discuss how changes in the shape of the Doppler waveform tracing can provide clues as to proximal or distal cardiovascular disease and identify more unusual regional disease in the carotid and vertebral vessels, including iatrogenic conditions involving the carotid arteries.

Careful attention to technique of the US examination is required to reduce inherent error in Doppler measurements of PSV and to ensure reproducibility of the Doppler examination. Pulse Doppler tracings should be obtained from longitudinal images with the sample volume placed centrally within the vessel or at the brightest spot in an area of color aliasing. The sample volume should be of adequate size to encompass the stenotic jet or central parabolic flow but should not extend to the vessel wall itself. The Doppler angle should be kept between 45° and 60° and should be calculated in relation to the direction of blood flow in the jet or

[a] Diagnostic Radiology, Chief Section of Ultrasound, Yale University School of Medicine, 333 Cedar Street, New Haven, CT 06520, USA
[b] Diagnostic Radiology, Yale University School of Medicine, 333 Cedar Street, New Haven, CT 06520, USA
[c] Diagnostic Radiology, University of Wisconsin Medical School, 600 Highland Avenue, Madison, WI 53792, USA
* Corresponding author. Yale University School of Medicine, Department of Diagnostic Radiology, 333 Cedar Street, New Haven, CT 06520.
E-mail address: scoutt@biomed.med.yale.edu (L.M. Scoutt).

1556-858X/06/$ – see front matter © 2005 Elsevier Inc. All rights reserved.
ultrasound.theclinics.com

doi:10.1016/j.cult.2005.09.012

the vessel lumen rather than to the vessel wall. The wall filter should be kept as low as possible and the pulse repetition frequency or scale should be set to maximize the size of the spectral training without allowing aliasing.

Allowing for slight variability from patient to patient, the internal, external, common carotid, and vertebral arteries demonstrate characteristic pulse Doppler waveform patterns reflecting the nature (oxygen consumption) of the vascular bed supplied. The ICA, which supplies the low-resistance vascular bed of the brain, typically demonstrates a low-resistance waveform pattern characterized by continuous forward diastolic flow reflecting the low impedence and high oxygen consumption of the intracranial circulation. The systolic upstroke

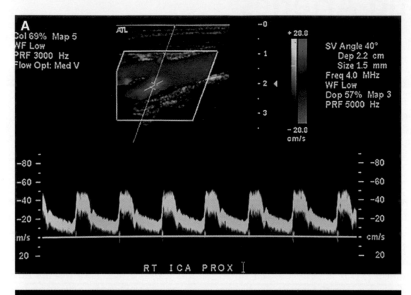

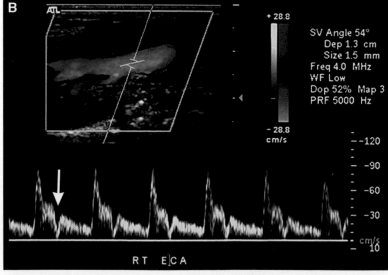

Fig. 1. Normal Doppler waveforms of the carotid and vertebral arteries. (*A*) ICA: the systolic upstroke is sharp with a thin spectral envelope. The systolic peak is blunted slightly and there is gradual tapering of velocity from end systole through diastole with continuous forward diastolic flow. (*B*) ECA: the systolic upstroke is sharp and the spectral envelope is thin. Note characteristic early diastolic notch (*arrow*) and reduced diastolic flow in comparison to the ICA. (*C*) ECA: this patient has no diastolic flow in the ECA. The amount of diastolic flow in the ECA is variable but should be equal in the right and left ECA in a given patient. Transient reversal of flow in early diastole can be a normal finding in the ECA. (*D*) CCA: note intermediate amount of diastolic flow and sharp systolic upstroke. (*E*) Vertebral artery: note sharp systolic upstroke and continuous forward diastolic flow. Widening of the spectral envelope and fill in of the spectral window may be observed, most often the result of poor visualization and, hence, poor angle of insonation.

should be sharp and the spectral envelope thin, although slightly thicker in diastole than in systole [**Fig. 1A**]. The systolic peak may be slightly blunter than the systolic peak of the external carotid artery (ECA). The ECA, which supplies the higher impedance muscular bed of the face, neck, and scalp, has a higher resistance waveform pattern, characterized by an early diastolic notch and little to no diastolic flow [see **Fig. 1B,C**]. There can be considerable variability in the amount of diastolic flow in the ECA from patient to patient. The amount of diastolic flow in the ECA, however, should be symmetric in the right and left ECA in a given patient. The systolic upstroke of the ECA should be sharp

and the spectral envelope quite thin. The waveform of the CCA is a combination of these two patterns, characterized by an intermediate amount of continuous, forward diastolic flow, a sharp systolic upstroke, and thin spectral envelope [see **Fig. 1D**]. Flow below the baseline or filling in of the spectral window normally should not be seen in the extracranial carotid arteries. Where the carotid bulb widens, however, peripheral reversal of flow or a helical flow pattern may be observed normally, reflecting a phenomenon, termed boundary layer separation. The vertebral artery usually is visualized incompletely but should demonstrate a sharp systolic upstroke and an intermediate

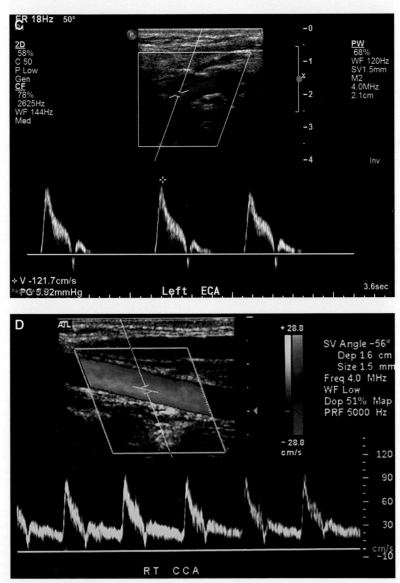

Fig. 1 (continued).

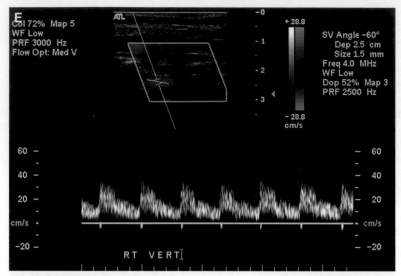

Fig. 1 (*continued*).

amount of continuous forward diastolic flow [see **Fig. 1E**].

Changes in systolic contour

PSV and end-diastolic velocity increase at the site of a carotid stenosis in the 50% to 96% diameter reduction range. In addition, the waveform pattern changes, demonstrating broadening of the spectral envelope, fill-in of the spectral window, and turbulent flow (ie, flow above and below the baseline). The rate of systolic upstroke remains brisk. Once the degree of stenosis exceeds an approximately 96% diameter reduction, however, PSV begins to fall although spectral broadening and turbulence persists [8].

The pulsus tardus (delayed) and pulsus parvus (diminished) waveform most commonly is observed distal to a severe proximal stenosis [9,10]. The tardus parvus waveform develops because of a delay in systolic acceleration. Initially, loss of the normal sharp systole upstroke with prolongation of the acceleration time (length of time from the onset of systole to the early peak systolic complex) is observed. The slope of systolic upstroke becomes more horizontal or flattened rather than sharply vertical. When pronounced, the tardus parvus wave-form is characterized by a round, widened systolic peak of diminished absolute PSV [**Fig. 2**] [9]. The tardus parvus waveform phenomenon becomes more exaggerated the farther away from the stenosis that the vessel is sampled. Hence, if the stenosis is in the CCA or at the carotid bifurcation, the waveform in the distal ICA is more abnormal than in the proximal ICA. Thus, if the carotid bifurcation cannot be seen well because of shadowing from calcified plaque, for example, it is important to sample the distal ICA as high (cephelad) as possible to look for this indirect, but important, sign of a more proximal stenosis. If the stenosis is unilateral, there is marked asymmetry in the systolic contour of the waveforms of the right and the left ICAs. If the stenosis is central, such as with aortic stenosis, the waveforms are affected bilaterally. Thus, the level of the proximal stenosis often can be identified by the pattern of distribution of the tardus parvus waveform phenomenon [11]. For example, a tardus parvus waveform is noted in both CCAs, ICAs, ECAs, and both vertebral arteries in patients who have aortic stenosis [**Fig. 3**]. If the right inominate artery is stenosed, however, the tardus parvus waveform is observed only in the right CCA, ICA, ECA, and vertebral artery and the waveforms in the left carotid and vertebral arteries

Fig. 2. Tardus parvus waveform. (*A*) Note delay (tardus) in systolic acceleration indicated by rounding and widening of the systolic peak and diminished (parvus) PSV in the distal right CCA. PSV is diminished. Identification of a tardus parvus waveform contour is indicative of a high-grade proximal stenosis in 91% of cases. The stenosis may be found anywhere from the level of the aortic valve to the carotid bifurcation. This patient had a severe right inominate stenosis. In comparison, note that the PSV is normal and that the systolic upstroke is sharp in the left CCA (*B*). This patient also has reversed flow in the right vertebral artery (*C*).

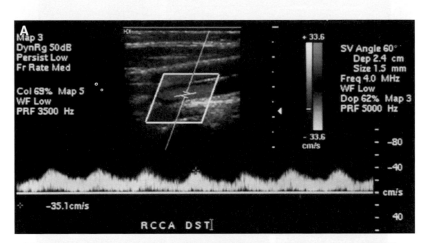

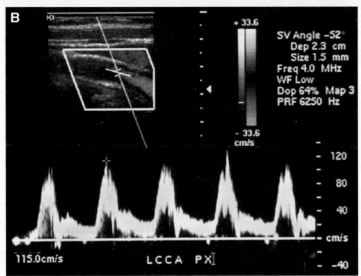

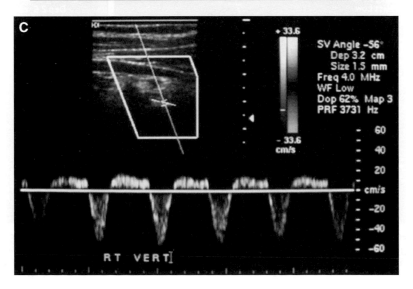

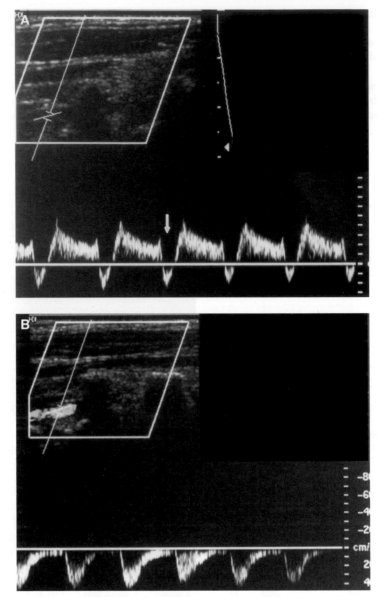

Fig. 8. Subclavian steal: conversion of a presteal waveform to a complete steal following provocative maneuvers. (*A*) Waveform of the left vertebral artery at rest in an 83-year-old woman who has a known left subclavian stenosis demonstrates a prominent midsystolic reversal of flow (*arrow*). (*B*) After inflation of a blood pressure cuff on the left arm and rapid deflation, there is conversion of the presteal waveform to a complete steal, with reversal of direction of blood flow throughout the cardiac cycle. The blood pressure cuff maneuver induces reactive hyperermia in the distal arm and increases blood flow across the subclavian stenosis, resulting in a complementary pressure drop and change in direction of blood flow in the ipsilateral vertebral artery towards the now lower-pressure subclavian origin. (*From* the Rohren EM, Kliewer MA, Carroll BA, et al. A spectrum of Doppler waveforms in the carotid and vertebral arteries. AJR Am J Roentgenol 2003;181:1695–704; with permission.)

sion/stenosis or cause of increased peripheral vascular resistance that the vessel is sampled. There is a spectrum of waveform patterns progressing from reversal of early diastolic flow to absence of diastolic flow, which reflects the severity of the distal disease and the proximity to the obstructing lesion.

Ultimately, PSV drops just proximal to a vascular occlusion, resulting in a "blip" of extremely low velocity systolic flow with completely absent or reversed early diastolic flow. It is possible to distinguish a carotid dissection from atherosclerotic occlusive disease as a cause of such a waveform

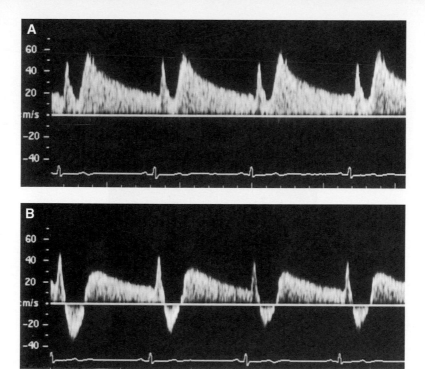

Fig. 9. Vertebral artery waveform changes induced by provocative maneuver (reactive hyperemia maneuver). (*A*) Doppler tracing of the vertebral artery obtained at rest in a 67-year-old woman status post stroke. Note "bunny profile" characteristic of a type 2 waveform pattern. Although there is continuous antegrade flow throughout the cardiac cycle, there is a prominent midsystolic notch. The velocity at the trough of the notch is slightly below end-diastolic velocity. The first systolic peak is sharp and narrow; the midsystolic decrease in velocity is abrupt and rapid; and the second systolic peak is broader and slightly rounded. Note synchronously obtained EKG below Doppler tracing. (*B*) After inflation of a blood pressure cuff to greater than systolic arterial pressure on the ipsilateral arm for 3 to 5 minutes and rapid deflation of the cuff, a repeat tracing from the vertebral artery demonstrates conversion of the type 2 waveform to a type 4 waveform. Note transient reversal of flow (below the baseline). (*From* Kliewer MA, Hertzberg BS, Kim DH, et al. Vertebral artery Doppler waveform changes indicating subclavian steal physiology. AJR Am J Roentgenol 2000;174;815–9; with permission).

by identification of the echogenic intraluminal dissection flap on gray-scale imaging or by the observation that in patients who have carotid dissections, the vessel is narrowed and the waveform is abnormal over a relatively long segment of the ICA and little atherosclerotic plaque is observed. Increased intracranial pressure, diffuse vasospasm, or bilateral severe atherosclerosis can cause a similar pattern bilaterally in the carotid arteries [**Fig. 15**].

Abnormal waveforms effecting the entire cardiac cycle

Complex abnormal flow patterns affecting systole and diastole also can be observed. Such diffusely abnormal waveforms often are the result of iatrogenic or traumatic conditions, such as intra-aortic

balloon pumps, pseudoaneurysms (PSAs), arteriovenous fistulae (AVF), or carotid dissections.

In patients who have an intra-aortic balloon pump, inflation of the balloon during systole causes a second peak of forward flow. Deflation of the balloon results in a transient decrease of flow at end diastole [**Fig. 16**]. The intra-aortic balloon pump may not be inflated during every cardiac cycle (a 1:1 ratio). If it is set at a 1:2 ratio, it inflates with every other systole and the second systole peak is observed every second cardiac cycle with an intervening normal systolic peak complex. Although placement of an intra-aortic balloon pump results in an increase in total volume of forward blood flow during systole, PSV typically is decreased, which makes grading of carotid stenosis using only PSV criteria unreliable.

Carotid PSAs occur most commonly after inadvertent needle sticks to the carotid artery but also

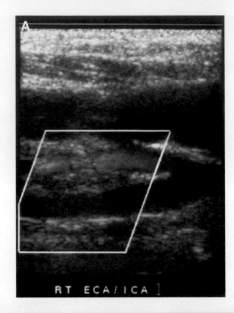

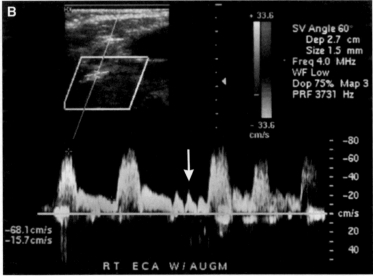

Fig. 10. "Internalization" of the ECA waveformresulting from complete occlusion of the ipsilateral ICA. (A) Color Doppler image demonstrates a single patent vessel above the carotid bifurcation. Is this the ECA or the ICA? (B) Pulse Doppler waveform demonstrates a moderate to large amount of continuous forward diastolic flow (ie a typical ICA waveform). Temporal tapping (arrow) confirms, however, that the patent vessel is the ECA and the ICA is occluded.

may occur after other types of penetrating or blunt trauma, carotid endarterectomy, carotid graft placement, or invasion of the carotid artery by a malignant mass. If the lumen of the neck of the PSA is narrow, Doppler interrogation of the neck reveals a to-and-fro pattern characterized by flow heading towards the PSA during systole and reversed flow heading towards the carotid artery during diastole [Fig. 17]. If the neck is wide, this to-and-fro flow pattern may not be observed and the waveform is randomly irregular and turbulent. PSAs are recognized easily on gray-scale imaging as an outpouching arising from the carotid artery, which fills in with color on color flow imaging. A variable amount of intraluminal thrombus may be noted.

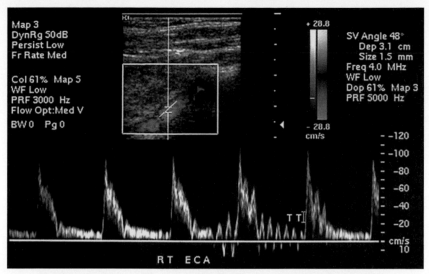

Fig. 11. Temporal tapping in the ECA. Note small regular deflections (TT). The frequency corresponds to the rate of temporal tapping. The deflections are seen best during diastole.

AVF most often are congenital or traumatic in origin and more rarely can occur secondary to malignant invasion. As in AVFs or arteriovenous malformations elsewhere, the feeding arterial vessel demonstrates a low-resistance waveform pattern characterized by increased PSV and increased continuous forward diastolic flow. The arterial waveform distal to the AVF, however, has a normal waveform pattern. The draining vein should demonstrate a pulsatile arterialized waveform with a normal venous flow pattern noted in the proximal vein. A soft tissue color bruit also may be observed as a result of tissue reverberation from the high-velocity flow [Fig. 18].

Dissections of the ICA occur most often in the setting of trauma, especially seat belt injury or repetitive trauma. The trauma can be minor but still compress the ICA significantly on the spine. Occasionally, dissections may occur spontaneously and isolated to the carotid arteries in patients who have predisposing conditions, such as Marfan syndrome, Ehlers-Danlos syndrome, fibromuscular dysplasia, cystic medial necrosis, hypertension, or drug abuse [28]. CCA dissections also may develop from direct extension of an aortic dissection. Acute onset of headache or Horner's syndrome is the most common presenting symptom. Although rare, dissection of the ICA is the most common cause of stroke in young patients [28]. Most ICA dissections occur at the level of the carotid bifurcation. The echogenic intraluminal flap may be visualized on longitudinal or transverse images [Fig. 19A], and color flow imaging may reveal flow in both lumens. The Doppler waveform pattern is highly variable, dependent on whether or not the true or false lumen is sampled, the diameter of the lumen, the length of the dissection, and involvement of the proximal aorta. Often the waveform pattern is extremely bizarre in configuration: low PSV velocity with a highly irregular waveform contour with many spikes or fluttering with reversed or bidirectional of flow, such that it may be difficult to distinguish systole from diastole [Fig. 20] [26–29]. Sometimes, however, a carotid dissection results in an intramural hematoma, causing a long-segment tapering of the ICA without a break in the intima and creation of a false lumen [see Fig. 19B]. The residual lumen may be narrowed markedly, creating a "string sign." Thrombosis of the false lumen creates a similar US appearance on gray-scale or color flow imaging. In such cases, a very pulsatile, sometimes dampened, waveform with little or no diastolic flow is noted on pulse Doppler examination, particularly if sampling is just proximal to a long-segment stenosis [27,28]. The waveform may be indistinguishable from a stenosis except that typically it extends over a much longer segment and often no plaque is visualized. Trauma also is the leading cause of vertebral artery dissections [27]. Vertebral artery dissections tend to occur higher in the neck at the level of the craniocerebral junction, however,

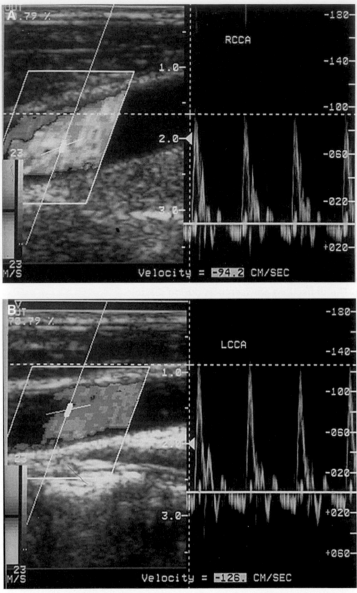

Fig. 12. Water hammer pulse. Note symmetrically reversed early and end-diastolic flow in the right (*A*) and left (*B*) CCAs, indicating a widened pulse pressure. PSV is elevated and systolic upstroke is sharp with a rapid deceleration in this patient who has severe aortic regurgitation.

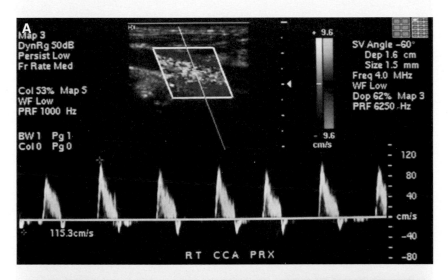

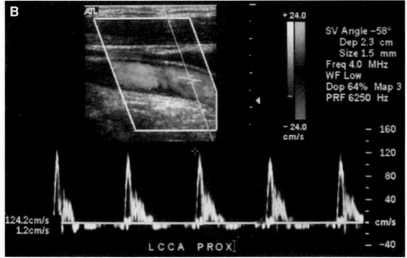

Fig. 13. Aortic regurgitation. Reversed diastolic flow is noted in the right (*A*) and left (*B*) CCAs in this 63-year-old patient who has moderate aortic regurgitation. Diastolic flow is normal in the more distal right (*C*) and left (*D*) ICAs, however. Note midsystolic retraction (*arrow*), the bisferiens phenomenon, also likely a result of the aortic regurgitation.

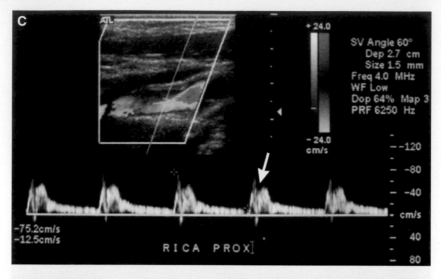

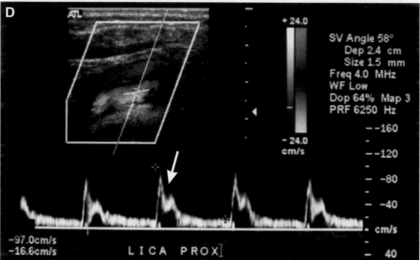

Fig. 13 (continued).

Fig. 14. Knocking waveform. (A) Doppler tracing from the right CCA demonstrates a high-resistance waveform pattern with no end-diastolic flow. This observation should raise suspicion for a distal occlusion or high-grade stenosis. (B) PSV is diminished markedly with reversed/absent diastolic flow, a knocking waveform pattern in the right ICA immediately proximal to the level of the high-grade ICA stenosis. (C) Note near occlusion of the ICA with distal string sign on this sagittal power Doppler image.

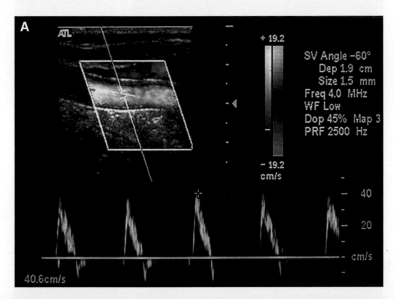

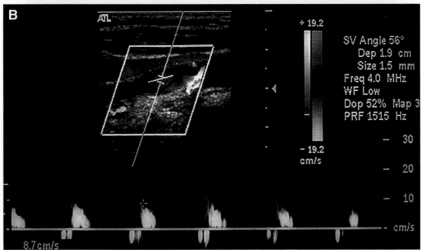

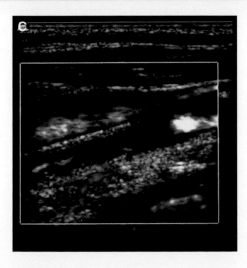

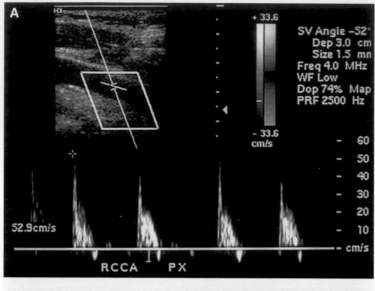

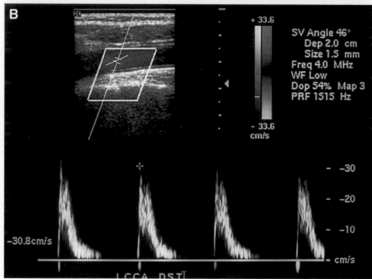

Fig. 15. A high-resistance waveform pattern is noted bilaterally in both CCAs (*A,B*) and right ICA (*C*) in this patient who has increased intracranial pressure resulting from a massive stroke. Note evidence of early herniation (*arrow*) on CT scan of the brain (*D*).

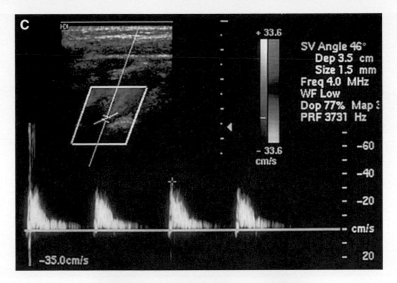

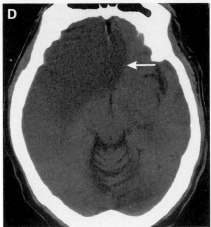

Fig. 15 (*continued*).

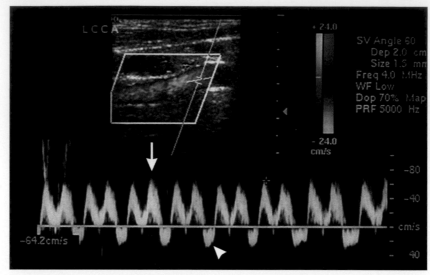

Fig. 16. Intra-aortic balloon pump. Note second systolic peak of forward flow (*arrow*) resulting from inflation of the intra-aortic balloon pump in this 58-year-old man who has severe ischemic cardiomyopathy. Deflation of the balloon results in a transient reversal of flow (*arrowhead*) at the end of diastole.

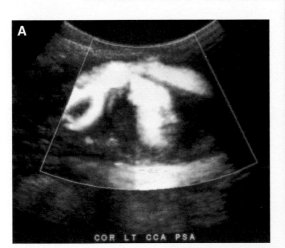

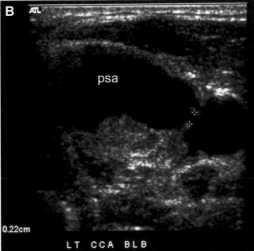

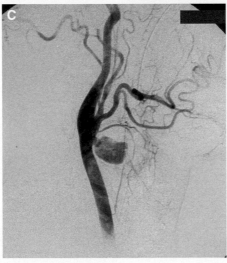

Fig. 17. Carotid PSA. (*A*) Sagittal power Doppler image demonstrates a large PSA arising from the CCA just below the bifurcation. (*B*) Transverse gray-scale image demonstrates a narrow neck (calipers) pseudoaneurysm (psa). (*C*) Angiogram demonstrating carotid PSA. (*D*) Doppler waveform demonstrating to-and- fro flow with an ir- regular contour in the neck of the PSA.

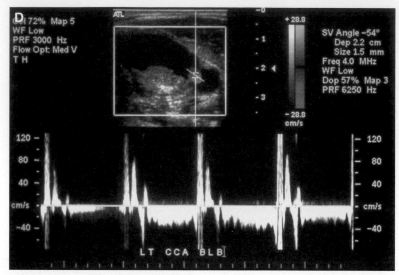

Fig. 17 (continued).

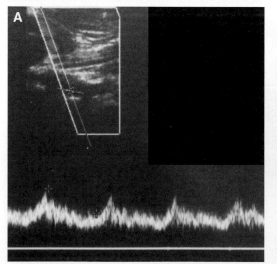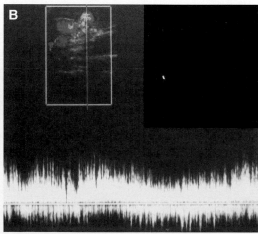

Fig. 18. Carotid AVF. (*A*) Color Doppler image reveals a vertebrojugular AVF in a 19-year-old male status post gunshot wound to the neck. (*B*) Waveform of the right vertebral artery demonstrates increased systolic and diastolic velocities. Pulsatile, high-velocity flow is noted in the draining vein. (*From* Rohren EM, Kliewer MA, Carroll BA, Hertzberg BS. A spectrum of doppler waveforms in the carotid and vertebral arteries. AJR Am J Roentgenol 2003;181;1695–704; with permission.)

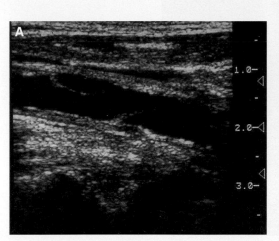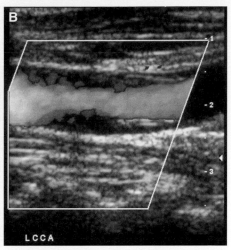

Fig. 19. Carotid dissection. (*A*) Note thin echogenic intraluminal flap on sagittal gray-scale image in this patient who has a carotid dissection. (*B*) This 22-year-old patient presented with a left neck hematoma and pain after a motor vehicle accident. Color Doppler image demonstrates marked hypoechoic circumferential "thickening" of the wall of the CCA consistent with an intramural hematoma/dissection. Note that the vessel wall is quite narrowed over a long segment.

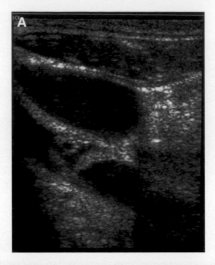

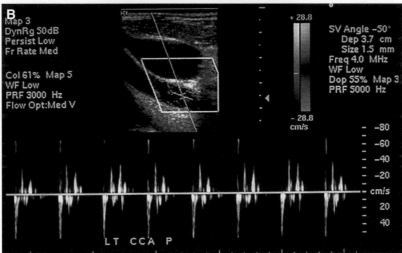

Fig. 20. Carotid dissection. (*A*) Gray-scale image reveals a thick echogenic flap in this 40-year-old patient who has a carotid dissection. (*B*) Pulse Doppler image demonstrates a markedly irregular waveform.

and are, therefore, more difficult to diagnose by US examination.

Summary

The normal Doppler waveform patterns of the carotid and vertebral arteries reflect the nature of oxygen consumption of the vascular bed that they supply. Careful attention to changes in the arterial waveforms can provide important clues regarding associated pathology, such as proximal cardiac or great vessel pathology, distal intracranial disease, and nonatherosclerotic carotid disease. Careful analysis and judicious use of provocative maneuvers also can help to distinguish accurately between the ICA and ECA when only one vessel is seen above the carotid bifurcation and to identify a subclavian stenosis by converting a presteal to a complete vertebral steal. In addition, certain iatrogenic conditions can be recognized by their characteristic Doppler waveforms and gray-scale features. Lastly, it is extremely important to recognize the effect of such conditions, especially proximal and distal disease, which cannot be visualized on direct US examination, on the Doppler waveform to avoid pitfalls in grading carotid stenosis using Doppler velocity criteria.

References

[1] American Heart Association. Heart disease and stroke statistics—2005 update. Dallas (TX): American Heart Association; 2005.
[2] Timsit SG, Sacco RL, Mohr JP, et al. Early clinical differentiation of cerebral infarction from severe

atherosclerotic stenosis and cardioembolism. Stroke 1992;23:486–91.

[3] Hademenos GJ, Massoud TF. Biophysical mechanisms or stroke. Stroke 1997;28:2067–77.

[4] North American Symptomatic Carotid Endartectomy Trial Collaborators. Beneficial effect of carotid endarterectomy in symptomatic patients with high grade stenosis. N Engl J Med 1991;325: 445–53.

[5] Barnett H, Taylor D, Eliasaw M, et al. Benefit of carotid endarterectomy in patients with symptomatic moderate or severe stenosis. N Engl J Med 1998;339:1415–25.

[6] Executive Committee for Asymptomatic Carotid Atherosclerosis Study. Endarterectomy for asymptomatic carotid artery stenosis. JAMA 1995;273: 1421–8.

[7] European Carotid Surgery Trialists' Collaborative Group. MRC European Carotid Surgery Trial: interim results for symptomatic patients with severe (70–99%) or with mild (0–29%) carotid stenosis. Lancet 1991;337:1235–43.

[8] Spencer MP, Reid JM. Quantitation of carotid stenosis with continuous wave (CW) Doppler ultrasound. Stroke 1979;10:326–30.

[9] Kotval PS. Doppler waveform parvus and tardus: a sign of proximal flow obstruction. J Ultrasound Med 1989;8:435–40.

[10] Bude RO, Rubin JM, Platt JF, et al. Pulsus tardus: its cause and potential limitations in detection or arterial stenosis. Radiology 1994;190:779–84.

[11] Horrow MM, Stassi J. Sonography of the vertebral arteries: a window to disease of the proximal great vessels. AJR Am J Roentgenol 2001; 177:53–9.

[12] O'Boyle MK, Vibhakar N, Chung J, et al. Duplex sonography of the carotid arteries in patients with isolated aortic stenosis; imaging findings and relation to severity of stenosis. AJR Am J Roentgenol 1996;166:197–202.

[13] Kallman CE, Gosink BB, Gardner DJ. Carotid duplex sonography: bisferious pulse contour in patients with aortic valvular disease. AJR Am J Roentgenol 1991;157:403–7.

[14] Rohren EM, Kliewer MA, Carroll BA, et al. A spectrum of Doppler waveforms in the carotid and vertebral arteries. AJR Am J Roentgenol 2003; 181:1695–704.

[15] Cohn KE, Sandler H, Hancock EW. Mechanisms of pulsus alternans. Circulation 1967;36:372–80.

[16] Gosselin G, Walker PM. Subclavian steal syndrome; existence, clinical features, diagnosis and management. Semin Vasc Surg 1996;9:93–7.

[17] Kliewer MA, Hertzberg BS, Kim DH, et al. Vertebral artery Doppler waveform changes indicating subclavian steal physiology. AJR Am J Roentgenol 2000;174:815–9.

[18] Horrow MM, Stassi J. Sonography of the vertebral arteries: a window to disease of the proximal great vessels. AJR Am J Roentgenol 2001; 177:53–9.

[19] Grant EG, Elsaden S, Modrazo B, et al. Inominate artery occlusive disease: sonographic findings. AJR Am J Roentgenol, in press.

[20] Delaney CP, Couse NF, Mehigan D, et al. Investigation and management of subclavian steal syndrome. Br J Surg 1994;81:1093–5.

[21] AbuRahma AF, Pollack JA, Robinson PA, et al. The reliability of color duplex ultrasound in diagnosing total carotid artery occlusion. Am J Surg 1997;174:185–7.

[22] Verbeeck NY, Vazquez Rodriguez C. Patent internal and external carotid arteries beyond an occluded common carotid artery: report a case diagnosed by color Doppler. JBR-BTR 1999;82: 219–21.

[23] Macchi C, Catini C. The anatomy and clinical significance of the collateral circulation between the internal and external carotid arteries through the ophthalmic artery. Ital J Anat Embryol 1993; 98:23–9.

[24] Kliewer MA, Freed KS, Hertzberg BS, et al. Temporal artery tap: usefulness and limitations in carotid sonography. Radiology 1996;201:481–4.

[25] Budorick NE, Rojratanakiat W, O'Boyel MK, et al. Digital tapping of the superficial temporal artery: Significance ion carotid duplex sonography. J Ultrasound Med 1996;15:459–64.

[26] Hennerici M, Neuerburg-Heusler D, editors. Vascular diagnosis with ultrasound. Stuttgart (Germany): Georg Thieme Verlag; 1998. p. 72–3.

[27] Hennerici M, Steinke W, Rautonberg W. High-resistance Doppler flow pattern in extracranial carotid dissection. Arch Neurol 1989;46:670–2.

[28] Khaw KT, Griffiths PD. Non-invasive imaging of the cervical carotis and vertebral arteries. Imaging 2001;13:376–90.

[29] Gardner DJ, Gosink BB, Kallman CE. Internal carotid artery dissections: Duplex US imaging. J Ultrasound Med 1991;10:607–14.

ELSEVIER
SAUNDERS

ULTRASOUND
CLINICS

Ultrasound Clin 1 (2006) 161–181

Ultrasound of the Intracranial Arteries

Susan L. Voci, MD*, Nancy Carson, MBA, RDMS, RVT

In 1954, Leksell introduced echoencephalography to evaluate the midline and paramedian structures [1]. In 1982, transcranial Doppler sonography was developed by Aaslid and colleagues [2]. Using a 2 MHz Doppler device, they measured blood mean flow velocities of the arteries of the circle of Willis, which was a major advance to detect and monitor noninvasively vasospasm related to subarachnoid hemorrhage. In 1990, transcranial color-coded duplex sonography (TCCS) provided clinical-imaging capability in addition to transcranial Doppler (TCD). TCCS combines B-mode imaging with color flow Doppler, permitting direct visualization of the basal cerebral arteries in addition to their flow direction so angle-corrected veloci-

ties can be obtained. Ultrasound contrast agents and other techniques, such as three-dimensional ultrasound, power Doppler, and harmonic imaging are used with TCCS for more diagnostic accuracy [3]. This article discusses the technique for performing TCD and TCCS and clinical applications and new developments for intracranial vascular ultrasound.

Indications for TCD and TCCS include but are not limited to (1) detection of intracranial stenosis and occlusion, (2) the course of vasospasm in patients who develop subarachnoid hemorrhage, (3) the detection of cerebral emboli, (4) prediction of stroke associated with sickle cell disease, (5) evaluation of the vertebrobasilar system, (6) assessment of collateral pathways, (7) evaluation for

Department of Radiology, University of Rochester Medical Center, 601 Elmwood Avenue, Rochester, NY 14642, USA
* Corresponding author.
E-mail address: susan_voci@urmc.rochester.edu (S.L. Voci).

1556-858X/06/$ – see front matter © 2005 Elsevier Inc. All rights reserved.
ultrasound.theclinics.com

doi:10.1016/j.cult.2005.09.007

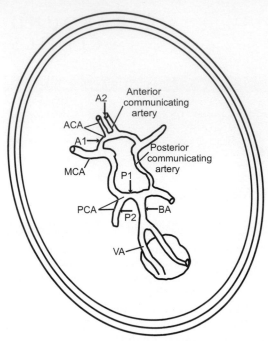

Fig. 1. Intracraninal arteries axial view at level of circle of Willis: MCA, ACA, PCA, BA, and VA. (*From* Carson NL, Voci SL. Transcranial Doppler. In: Dogra V, Rubens DJ, editors. Ultrasound secrets. Philadelphia: Hanley & Belfus; 2004; with permission.)

brain death, and (8) detection of possible emboli from a patent foramen ovale. Examination protocols and the vessels interrogated vary based on the indication for the examination.

Transcranial Doppler and transcranial color-coded duplex sonography equipment

Transcranial imaging equipment must have an excellent signal-to-noise ratio because most of the examination is performed through the highly reflective skull. The machines specifically designed for TCD have a lower bandwidth, which results in a larger and less-defined sample volume [4]. The TCD examination is performed with a 2-MHz, focused, bidirectional pulsed Doppler transducer that displays only a spectral waveform. The TCCS examination uses a duplex ultrasound machine with a low frequency (ie, 1.8–2.6 MHz) phased array sector transducer. The image consists of a gray-scale picture with the vessels displayed as an overlay of color (or power) Doppler. In addition to inherent machine settings, such as adjustable Doppler gate size and depth, the ultrasound beam must be able to focus at a depth of 40 to 60 mm. The display should be configured so the peak systolic, end diastolic, and time-averaged velocities can be displayed in real-time [4].

The transcranial Doppler examination

The complete TCD examination obtains spectral Doppler signals from the following arteries; middle cerebral artery (MCA), anterior cerebral artery (ACA), posterior cerebral artery (PCA), distal internal cerebral artery (dICA), basilar artery (BA), vertebral artery (VA), extracranial internal carotid artery (eICA), and for some indications, the ophthalmic artery (OA) and carotid siphon [Fig. 1]. These arteries are known collectively as the basal cerebral arteries of the circle of Willis [5]. To obtain the Doppler information from the entire set of vessels, the examiner must use four different windows: the transtemporal window, the transorbital window, the suboccipital window, and the submandibular window [Fig. 2]. Vessel identification during the TCD examination depends on several factors: the depth of focus; window used (ie, submandibular, occipital, and so forth); the direction of the reflected Doppler signal (toward or away from the transducer); flow velocity (peak systolic velocity [PSV], mean velocity); the traceability of the vessel, and the direction of probe angulation (ie, anterior, posterior, caudal) [5].

Transtemporal window

The transtemporal window location varies with each patient and the ability to penetrate the temporal bone varies with age, sex, and ethnicity. The

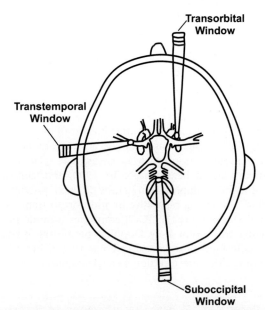

Fig. 2. Acoustic windows for TCD. (*From* Carson NL, Voci SL. Transcranial Doppler. In: Dogra V, Rubens DJ, editors. Ultrasound secrets. Philadelphia: Hanley & Belfus; 2004; with permission.)

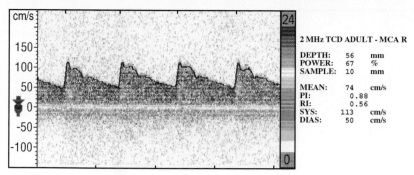

Fig. 3. Normal MCA. Using transtemporal window, depth is 56 mm, and mean velocity is 74 cm/s. Flow is toward transducer. (*From* Carson NL, Voci SL. Transcranial Doppler. In: Dogra V, Rubens DJ, editors. Ultrasound secrets. Philadelphia: Hanley & Belfus; 2004; with permission.)

thinnest part of the bone tends to be above the zygomatic arch. Rotating the transducer in a circular manner above the arch is helpful in finding the best window. Once the window is located, small adjustments in angulation are necessary to optimize the signal as the vessels are followed. The vessels interrogated through the transtemporal window include the MCA, the ACA, the PCA, and the dICA. Several factors need to be checked if difficulty occurs in finding the vessels through this window. First, the power should be set at maximum and the Doppler frequency chosen must be the lowest available. Other factors and actions to consider include: increasing the scale (or PRF), opening the Doppler gate, increasing the gain, and increasing the amplitude if possible.

The MCA can be found at a depth as shallow as 40 to 52 mm and can be followed in to a depth of approximately 56 to 62 mm until it joins with the ACA at the level of the dICA bifurcation. The M1 segment, which is the most distal segment closest to the outer skull, is found at approximately 38 to 42 mm, depending on diameter of the head. Flow in the MCA is toward the transducer, thus displayed

above the baseline [Fig. 3]. At the level of the bifurcation of the dICA (54–64 mm), MCA flow is above the baseline and ACA flow is depicted below the baseline signifying flow away from the transducer [Fig. 4]. From the bifurcation at 54 to 64 mm, the ACA can be followed anteriorly. Flow continues to be away from the transducer; it is often necessary to angle the transducer slightly superiorly or anteriorly to follow the ACA. The ACA may be traced to depths of approximately 68 to 78 mm. The examiner may notice the MCA signal disappearing from above the baseline as the ACA is followed distally [Fig. 5].

Doppler signals are obtained from the dICA by returning to the level of the bifurcation, 54 to 64 mm. Here, the transducer should be angled slightly inferiorly; the signal from the dICA is toward the transducer and lower in amplitude than that of the MCA or ACA. The dICA can be tortuous, thus the Doppler signal may be displayed on both sides of the baseline [Fig. 6].

The PCA is found by returning the sample volume to the level of the bifurcation then angling posterior. Flow in the PCA is displayed above the

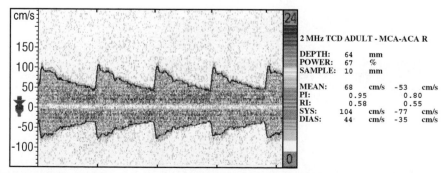

Fig. 4. Normal bifurcation of ICA at depth of 64 mm. MCA is above baseline, and ACA is below baseline. Mean velocity of MCA is 68 cm/s and flow is toward transducer. ACA has mean velocity of 53 cm/s, and flow is away from transducer. (*From* Carson NL, Voci SL. Transcranial Doppler. In: Dogra V, Rubens DJ, editors. Ultrasound secrets. Philadelphia: Hanley & Belfus; 2004; with permission.)

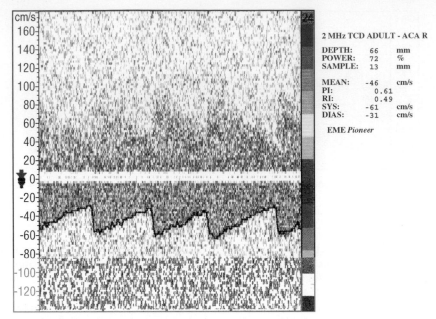

Fig. 5. Normal ACA. Depth is 66 mm, mean velocity is 46 cm/s, and flow is away from transducer.

baseline. The PCA is distinguished from the MCA (also above the baseline) by its lower velocity and its posterior location [**Fig. 7**]. The PCA is followed posteriorly 68 to 72 mm and the flow becomes bidirectional. At this point, the PCA has been traced to the top of the basilar artery (TOB), at its point of bifurcation [**Fig. 8**]. The signal below the baseline represents the contralateral PCA. While interrogating the intracranial vessels without color Doppler, only the P-1 segment of the PCA is sampled be-

cause of the sharp angle of the P-2 segment as it wraps around the midbrain.

The TCD examiner should keep in mind the normal depths and velocity relationships of the vessels. The MCA has a higher mean velocity than the ACA, and the MCA and ACA have higher mean velocities than the PCA and dICA. The examiner may need to go back and forth (shallow to deep, deep to shallow) several times to determine the identity of the vessels before recording any waveforms.

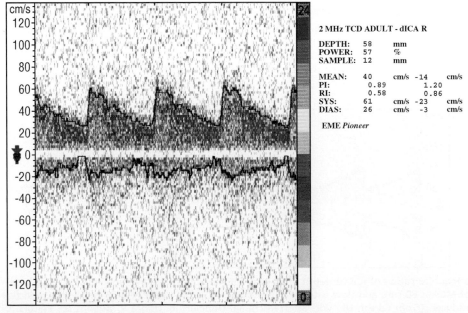

Fig. 6. Distal ICA. Flow is toward transducer, depth is 58 mm, and mean velocity is 40 cm/s.

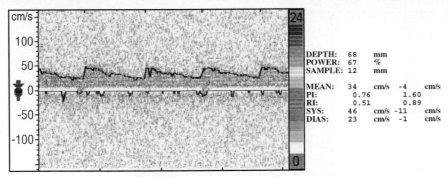

Fig. 7. Normal PCA. Transducer is angled slightly posterior, and depth is 68 mm. Flow is toward transducer and mean velocity is 34 cm/s. (*From* Carson NL, Voci SL. Transcranial Doppler. In: Dogra V, Rubens DJ, editors. Ultrasound secrets. Philadelphia: Hanley & Belfus; 2004; with permission.)

Occasionally, a patient has an adequate transtemporal window on one side and not the other. In this case, often the contralateral MCA and ACA can be interrogated by scanning from the side with the optimum window. The examiner increases the depth of the Doppler gate until the ipsilateral MCA disappears and the midline has been crossed. At this point, if the penetration is adequate, the contralateral side begins to appear. The MCA is depicted below the baseline, indicating flow away from the transducer, and the ACA is above the baseline, indicating flow toward the transducer. Using calipers and measuring the diameter of the head at the level of the zygomatic arches can be helpful to determine where the midline is.

Suboccipital window

The intracranial VAs and the BA are evaluated using the suboccipital approach. The patient is seated with the head tipped forward slightly. The transducer is placed at the nape of the neck and the foramen magnum is used as the window. If the patient cannot sit up, reclining in a sideways position is sufficient as long as the spine is kept in a horizontal plane. The chin is still tipped forward.

The VA signals are obtained at a depth of about 60 to 85 mm. The transducer must be angled slightly to the right or left of midline to follow the vessels. The net direction of flow is away from the transducer, but occasionally the signal may be

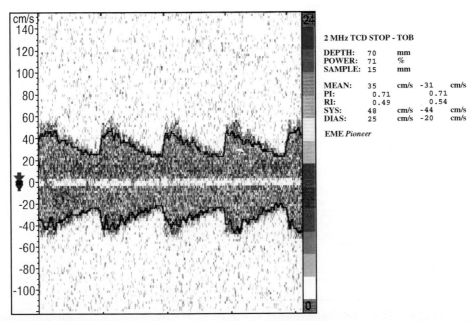

Fig. 8. PCAs at top of basilar artery (TOB). Spectral tracing above baseline represents ipsilateral PCA, tracing below baseline is contra lateral PCA.

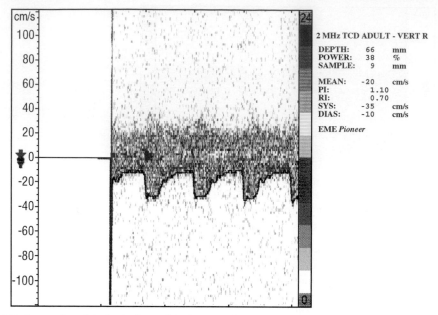

Fig. 9. Right VA from suboccipital window. Flow is away from transducer, depth is 66 mm, and mean velocity is 20 cm/s.

bidirectional as the arteries course through the foramen of the transverse spinous processes [Fig. 9]. From this window, the VAs join to form the BA. The BA is followed distally to a depth of 100 to 120 mm. The Doppler signal is below the baseline with a higher mean velocity than that of the VAs [Fig. 10]. If after several attempts, no signal is obtained from the suboccipital window the chin may be tipped too far forward. Tip the head back and angle the transducer so it is in the same plane as the bridge of the nose.

Transorbital window

Doppler signals from the OA and the carotid siphon are obtained using the transorbital approach. When using the transorbital window, the ultrasound beam travels through the eye. To minimize exposure to the eye, the acoustic power must be reduced to a low setting, 10% to 25% of maximum, and the examination time should be as short as possible. The transducer is placed directly on the closed eyelid. The depth of the sample volume should be approximately 40 to 50 mm with a slight medial angle. Normal blood flow in the OA is directed toward the transducer. The waveform may be highly pulsatile because it is supplying blood to the globe of the eye [Fig. 11].

The carotid siphon is interrogated from this window at approximately 56 to 70 mm. The angle of the transducer should be adjusted slightly as the depth is increased. The signal from the carotid siphon changes from highly pulsatile in the OA to low resistance in the carotid siphon. The direction

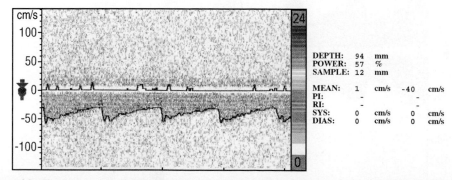

Fig. 10. Normal basilar artery. Suboccipital window at a depth of 94 mm, flow is directed away from transducer, with mean velocity of 40 cm/s. (*From* Carson NL, Voci SL. Transcranial Doppler. In: Dogra V, Rubens DJ, editors. Ultrasound secrets. Philadelphia: Hanley & Belfus; 2004; with permission.)

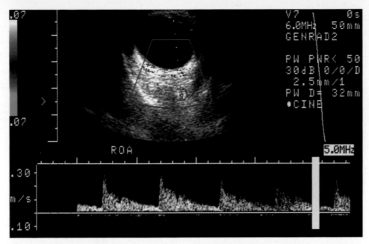

Fig. 11. OA normal. Right OA flow is towards transducer.

of the signal in the siphon depends on the location of the Doppler gate within the vessel. The carotid siphon is S-shaped and is divided into three parts, the parasellar, the genu, and the supraclinoid. The signal from the parasellar region is toward the transducer, the signal is bidirectional in the genu, and the signal is away from the transducer in the supraclinoid section [**Fig. 12**]. All three sections may not be represented for each transorbital examination.

Submandibular window

The submandibular window is used to obtain a signal from the extracranial portion of the internal carotid artery. With the head tilted slightly to the contralateral side, the transducer is placed at the angle of the mandible aiming toward the head with a slight medial angle. The depth of the sample volume is at 50 to 64 mm and the direction of flow is away from the transducer [**Fig. 13**].

Documentation

Several tracings are recorded at 2 to 4 mm intervals as the vessels are followed. The velocity measurements taken from the spectral tracings include the PSV, the end diastolic velocity, and the mean velocity. With the TCD method, all velocities are calculated by the equipment assuming a Doppler angle of 0°. In some laboratories, the pulsatility index (PI), which provides information regarding distal resistance, is recorded. In the setting of vasospasm, the ratio of the MCA to the eICA is calculated. TCD studies show a decline in flow velocities with increasing age. Several published ta-

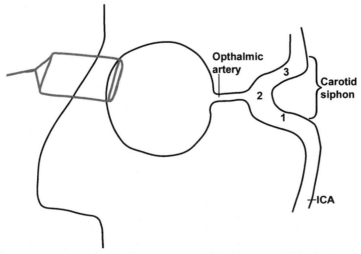

Fig. 12. Transorbital window. Transducer is placed on closed eyelid. From here, depth and angle are adjusted to insonate OA and carotid siphon. Carotid siphon is divided into three parts: (1) parasellar portion, (2) genu, and (3) supraclinoid portion.

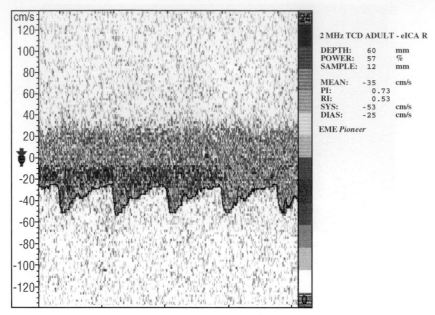

2 MHz TCD ADULT - eICA R

DEPTH:	60	mm
POWER:	57	%
SAMPLE:	12	mm
MEAN:	-35	cm/s
PI:	0.73	
RI:	0.53	
SYS:	-53	cm/s
DIAS:	-25	cm/s

EME *Pioneer*

Fig. 13. Extracranial ICA. From submandibular approach, depth is 60 mm. Flow is directed away from transducer at mean velocity of 35 cm/s.

bles are available that can be used as normal criteria [Table 1] [6,7].

TCD limitations

There are several limitations to the TCD approach. The examination is highly operator dependent. Vessel identification depends on the understanding of normal anatomic relationships and knowledge of possible variations from the norm. Approximately 50% of the population have an incomplete circle of Willis [8]. Another limitation lies in the actual spectral Doppler measurements. Doppler frequency shift depends on the velocity of sound, the velocity of flow, the insonating frequency, and the angle between the ultrasound beam and the vessel; thus, the calculated velocity and the true velocity of blood flow differ as the angle of insonation increases [8]. The reported peak, diastolic, and

mean velocities may not be accurate with TCD because the angle of the vessel is unknown. Another limitation lies in the transtemporal window itself. At least 3% to 5% of patients lack an adequate window for the TCD examination. This percentage increases in older patient populations, particularly among women [9]. Some patients simply cannot be examined.

The transcranial color-coded duplex sonography examination

The TCCS method allows the examiner to visualize the vessels with color Doppler before obtaining the spectral Doppler signals. Using the color Doppler not only makes vessel identification faster and more accurate, it allows for angle correction of the Doppler cursor and, thus, more accurate velocity

Table 1: Normal TCD velocities

Artery	Depth of sample (mm)	Mean velocity (cm/sec)	Transducer window	Direction of flow
MCA	38–62	58 ± 12	Transtemporal	Towards
ACA/MCA	54–64	–	Transtemporal	Bidirectional
ACA	60–78	50 ± 12	Transtemporal	Away
dICA	56–64	38 ± 10	Transtemporal	
PCA (P1)	60–72	40 ± 10	Transtemporal	Towards
Extracranial ICA	50–64	37 ± 9	Submandibular	Away
OA	40–58	21 ± 5	Occipital	Away
VA	60–85	37 ± 10	Suboccipital	Away
BA	80–120	40 ± 10	Subocipital	Away

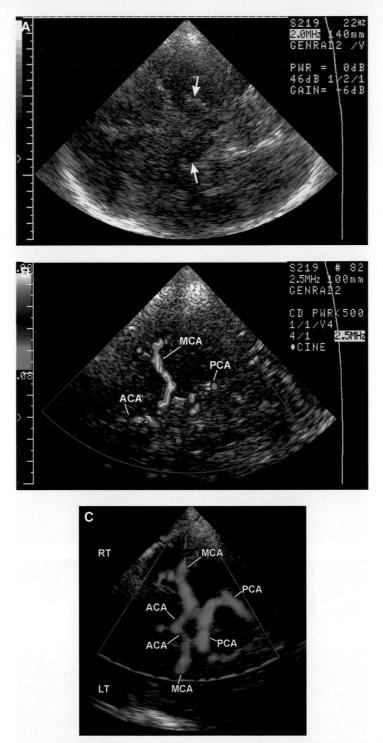

Fig. 14. Transtemporal window. (*A*) Gray-scale reference point for circle of Willis is butterfly shaped hypoechoic midbrain (*arrows*). (*B*) Color Doppler image of circle of Willis displays MCA toward transducer, ACA deep to MCA and slightly anterior, and PCA directed posterior around midbrain. (*C*) Power Doppler image shows more complete view of circle of Willis than color Doppler with bilateral MCA, ACA, and PCA displayed.

readings. Direct visualization of the vessels also decreases training time for sonographers.

The same four windows are used to perform the TCCS examination. The depths of the vessels with the TCCS approach are similar to the depths used for the TCD approach. The number of vessels interrogated also depends on the indication for the examination.

To obtain the optimum window for the transtemporal approach, the probe is placed axially along the orbitomeatal line and adjusted until the hypoechoic, butterfly-shaped midbrain is seen at the level of 6 to 8 cm [**Fig. 14A**] [4]. From this point, the color Doppler or power Doppler is turned on and the circle of Willis begins to appear [**Figs. 14B, C**]. Next, the examiner can obtain angle-corrected spectral Doppler signals from the MCA, ACA, PCA, and dICA. Angling the transducer slightly may be necessary to see all of the vessels; it is common to take the tracings from several

slightly different views. The transorbital TCCS approach is useful for vessel identification; however, the gray-scale image of the actual brain parenchyma is technically limited.

After the vessels have been interrogated from the transtemporal window, the examiner can proceed to the occipital window. The landmarks are the hypoechoic foramen magnum and the bright echo of the clivus [**Fig. 15A**] [4]. With color or power Doppler, the VAs and BA appear as a "Y" shape [**Fig. 15B**].

Despite the clear advantages of vessel identification, and angle-corrected velocities, some limitations exist with the TCCS approach. The actual shape and size of the phased array transducer that is used may make it difficult to examine patients who have small transtemporal windows. The phased array tends to be larger than the transducer used in the TCD approach; thus, TCD may

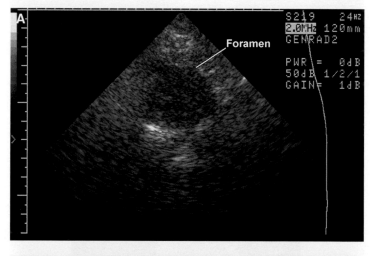

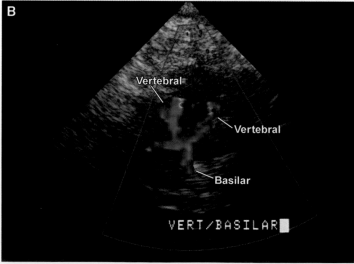

Fig. 15. Occipital window. (*A*) Reference point for VAs and BAs is hypoechoic foramen magnum. (*B*) Power Doppler shows normal VAs and BAs from occipital approach.

be better for those individuals. Another limitation with TCCS lies in the physics of color Doppler. Color Doppler, which is based on an average Doppler frequency shift of moving blood, is limited by angle dependence and aliasing. Vessels with low flow can be lost in background noise, and vessels that are at large angles with respect to the ultrasound beam may have weak or undetected signals. One solution to this is to use power Doppler as suggested by Kenton and colleagues [10] [**Fig. 14C**]. Their findings concluded power Doppler particularly helped in the visualization of the M2 portion of the MCA, the P2 portion of the PCA, and the posterior communicating artery. Another limitation is that in the presence of color Doppler, the examiner may not pay close attention to the audible Doppler signal and may miss the segment of the vessel with the highest velocity. In the TCD examination, the operator is trained to listen for the signal with the highest pitch, which correlates to the highest velocity [10].

Transcranial Doppler or transcranial color-coded duplex sonography?

When it comes to the question of true angle-corrected velocity information, TCCS clearly provides more accurate data. Several investigators have studied the differences between non–angle-corrected and angle-corrected velocities of the various intracranial arteries, and whether just using color Doppler (TCCS) without angle correction makes a difference. Neish and colleagues [11] studied a population of children with sickle cell disease and found the mean velocity measurements in the MCA, dICA, and ACA did not vary substantially between TCD and TCCS techniques. Angle correction was not used during the TCCS examination. Mean velocities discovered in the dICA, the PCA, and the BA varied substantially; these TCD velocities were higher than the non–angle-corrected TCCS velocities for the same vessels. The investigators explain that the discrepancy may be caused by the larger size of the transducer limiting the windows for interrogation of the dICA, PCA, and BA. When the examiner can see the vessels, they may not be as "tuned in" to listening for the highest pitch, which indicates the highest velocity.

Another study by Schoning and colleagues [12] compared TCD and TCCS data using an adult population. In the MCA and ACA arteries, the velocities were 10% to 15% higher using TCCS than when TCD was used. They concluded that the advantage of TCCS over TCD was more qualitative than quantitative.

Using TCCS, Krejza and colleagues studied the angle of insonation and its effect on flow velocity measurements in patients who experience MCA stenosis. Results indicated that the mean angle of insonation for a stenotic MCA M1 segment is larger than that of an unaffected normal artery. In patients who develop moderate or severe MCA stenosis, it was concluded that the angle of insonation can be substantial, thus using non–angle-corrected techniques can result in significantly underestimated peak and mean flow velocities [13].

Whether a department uses TCD or TCCS to examine the intracranial arteries often depends on the equipment available. The TCD examination requires a separate dedicated piece of equipment, an expense the laboratory may not be able to incur. The TCCS examination uses duplex equipment that already exists in the lab; however, the examination requires a transducer specifically designed for TCD applications. The TCCS approach allows for faster vessel identification but an experienced examiner can also perform the TCD examination in a timely fashion with a high level of confidence. For reporting purposes, the department must take care in choosing its reference data. The data must have been generated by the same approach (eg, nonangled TCD data or angle-corrected TCCS data).

Clinical applications

Detection and monitoring of cerebral vasospasm

One of the most serious complications of subarachnoid hemorrhage is cerebral vasospasm, which is associated with significant morbidity and mortality. Cerebral vasospasm has been reported in up to 40% of patients who present with subarachnoid hemorrhage and typically occurs 4 to 14 days following the subarachnoid hemorrhage [14]. TCD-detected vasospasm can precede clinical vasospasm by hours or days [4]. The velocity of blood flow is inversely related to the lumen of the artery. With vasospasm, the arterial lumen decreases, the blood flow velocity increases, and the condition of the vessels can be detected.

Transcranial Doppler has been shown to be a useful, noninvasive tool for the detection and evaluation of cerebral vasospasm. Flow velocity findings in the MCA correlate with clinical grade, location of blood clot, and the time course of angiographic vasospasm [15]. For the MCA, mean flow velocities greater than 200 cm/s, sharp increase in flow velocities, or a high Lindegaard ratio (mean velocity of the MCA/mean velocity of the ICA [v̄MCA/v̄ICA]) (6 ± .3) can reliably predict the presence of clinically significant MCA vasospasm [15]. Similarly, a mean flow velocity less than 120 cm/s defines no clinically significant vasospasm [Table 2]

Table 2: Sonographic criteria for vasospasm of the middle cerebral artery [6,16–20]

Mean MCA velocity (cm/s)	Vmca/ Vica	Degree of stenosis
≤80	<3.0	Normal
>80–120	<3.0	Mild
>120–160	3.0–6.0	Moderate
>160	>6.0	Severe

Side-to-side discrepancy of the MCA greater than 14% is abnormal; clinically significant vasospasm of the MCA begins at 120 cm/s.

[16–20]. A sharp increase in the flow velocity (>20cm/s/d) is associated with a poor prognosis [**Fig. 16**] [4].

Hematocrit, blood pressure, PaO2 and PCO2, collateral flow patterns, and intracranial pressure may affect blood flow velocity measurements, and therefore, should be taken into account when interpreting TCD results [15,20]. TCD velocity criteria have been found to be most reliable for detecting angiographic MCA and BA vasospasm [15]. Angiography is considered the gold standard for evaluation for cerebral vasospasm. Other modalities used include CT angiography (CTA), and magnetic resonance angiography (MRA). Obvious advantages of TCD over the other modalities are: it is noninvasive, can be performed at the bedside, can be repeated as frequently as necessary, used for continuous monitoring, does not require contrast agents, and is less expensive. Disadvantages are: it is operator dependant, an insufficient temporal or foraminal window of insonation was found in up to 20% of patients in one study [21], and vessel anatomy is variable. TCCS is also useful for evaluation of vasospasm. Because the cerebral vessels are directly visualized, angle-corrected velocities can be obtained. Studies performed to evaluate normal angle-corrected flow velocities have shown that angle-corrected velocities in adults tend to be higher than velocities obtained with TCD. TCCS may also directly visualize aneurysms, though at this time TCCS is not the screening modality of choice secondary to its low sensitivity and ready availability of CTA or MRA [1].

Detection of intracranial stenosis and occlusion

Intracranial atherosclerosis is the inciting factor in up to 10% of patients presenting with TIA or stroke [15,22]. Stenosis and occlusion of the ICA siphon, M1 segment of the MCA, intracranial VA, proximal BA, and P1 segment of the PCA can be reliably detected by TCD [15]. Sensitivity, specificity, positive predictive value, and negative predictive value of TCD are typically greater in the anterior circulation than in the vertebrobasilar circulation. This is believed to be secondary to greater variation in the vertebrobasilar anatomy and greater technical difficulties with the posterior circulation [15,3]. Fast,

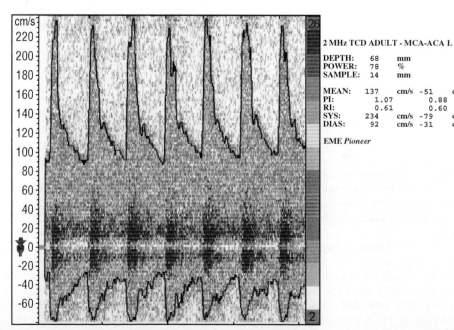

Fig. 16. Vasospasm spectral Doppler tracing is from adult status postaneurysm clipping. Mean velocity of MCA is elevated at 137 cm/s. (*From* Carson NL, Voci SL. Transcranial Doppler. In: Dogra V, Rubens DJ, editors. Ultrasound secrets. Philadelphia: Hanley & Belfus; 2004; with permission.)

noninvasive, portable, and cost effective diagnostic tools for evaluating the acute stroke patient are becoming more important because certain subgroups of patients may benefit from thrombolytic and neuroprotective treatments [23]. TCD has become extensively used in the evaluation of the acute stroke patient.

Findings on TCD for a stenosis in a major basal cerebral artery include increased flow velocity, spectral broadening of the waveform, and vibration of the perivascular soft tissues [**Fig. 17**]. Normal mean velocities for the basal cerebral arteries can be found in Table 1. Felberg and colleagues [24], looking at the accuracy of different mean flow velocity thresholds for determining the degree of stenosis,

found that using a mean velocity value of greater than or equal to 100 cm/s had a sensitivity of 100%, specificity of 97.9%, a positive predictive value of 88.8%, and a negative predictive value of 94.9% in detecting greater than or equal to 50% stenosis of the MCA [24]. TCD criteria for greater than 50% stenosis in intracranial arteries have not yet been established. Rorick and colleagues [25] found the most important confounding factor in the evaluation of velocity criteria using TCD was the presence of a greater than or equal to 75% stenosis of the eICA. Collateral flow may result leading to false positive results or a false negative result secondary to decrease in flow [25]. With TCCS, the angle-corrected PSV is used as

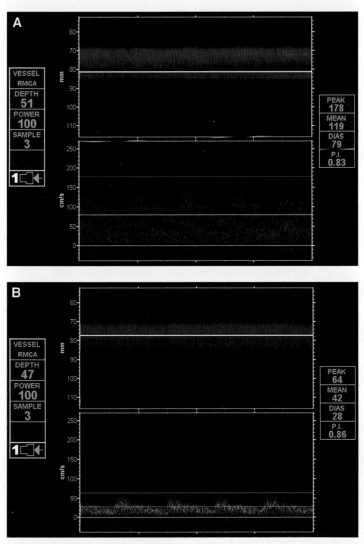

Fig. 17. Right MCA stenosis. (*A*) At the stenosis, velocities are elevated with PSV of 178 cm/s, and diastolic velocity of 79 cm/s. (*B*) Distal to stenosis, PSV in MCA decreases to 64 cm/s. (*C*) Ipsilateral ACA has increased PSV of 186 cm/s, mean of 111 cm/s, and diastolic velocity of 77 cm/s, indicating increased flow through vessel. (*D*) Corresponding angiogram shows MCA stenosis (*arrow*) and normal ACA. (*From* Carson NL, Voci SL. Transcranial Doppler. In: Dogra V, Rubens DJ, editors. Ultrasound secrets. Philadelphia: Hanley & Belfus; 2004; with permission.)

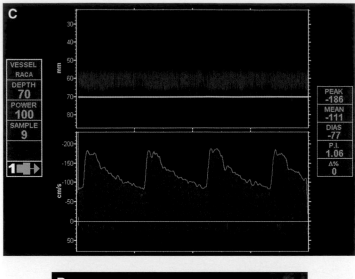

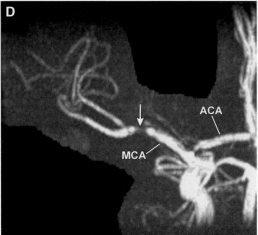

Fig. 17 (continued).

the main criteria for intracranial stenosis. Table 3 (from work by Baumgartner and colleagues [22]) gives the upper limits of normal for PSV of the intracranial arteries [4,22].

TCD can detect acute MCA occlusions with high (>90%) sensitivity, specificity, positive predictive value, and negative predictive value as compared with angiography [3,15]. TCD can also detect ICA siphon, VA and BA occlusions with good (70%–90%) sensitivity and positive predictive value and excellent specificity and negative predictive value [15]. Cerebral arterial occlusion is diagnosed on TCD by the following findings: lack of arterial signal at expected depth, presence of signals in vessels that communicate with the occluded vessel, and findings corresponding to collateral flow, such as elevated velocities in communicating arteries [4]. False positive TCD diagnoses of occlusion may occur secondary to inadequate insonation window,

displacement of arteries secondary to mass lesions, and variable anatomy of the circle of Willis [3,4].

TCCS definition of intracranial arterial occlusion is based on absence of flow. With TCCS an inadequate window of insonation is not likely to lead to a false positive. Poor Doppler angles or slow flow can limit vessel visualization with TCCS. Diagnostic confidence for intracranial arterial occlusion with TCCS is still close to 100% [4]. Ultrasound contrast agents are being used with TCCS to improve diagnostic accuracy for intracranial arterial stenoses and occlusions.

Screening for stroke prevention in children with sickle cell disease

Stroke is the most severe cerebrovascular complication in sickle cell disease. An occlusive vasculopathy results from the adhesion of abnormal cells to

Table 3: Ultrasonic detection of ≥50% intracranial stenosis (n = 31) with angiography as standard of reference

| | | Ultrasound | | | | Angiography | |
	PSV cutoff (cm/s)	Sensitivity (%)	Specificity (%)	Positive predictive value (%)	Negative predictive value (%)	No.	Mean ± SD degree (range)
ACA	≥155	100	100	100	100	4	60 ± 8 (52–71)
MCA	≥220	100	100	100	100	11	67 ± 11 (50–80)
PCA	≥145	100	100	100	91	10	63 ± 7 (50–72)
BA	≥140	100	100	100	100	3	67 ± 14 (53–85)
VA	≥120	100	100	100	100	3	69 ± 14 (55–84)

Abbreviation: SD, standard deviation.
From Baumgartner RW, Mattle HP, Schroth G. Assessment of >50% and <50% intracranial stenoses by transcranial color-coded duplex sonography. Stroke 1999;30:87–92; with permission.

the vascular endothelium and subendothelial matrix. The distal intracranial internal carotid arteries and the proximal middle cerebral arteries are most commonly involved. Eleven percent of children with homozygous (HbSS) sickle cell disease experience a stroke before the age of 20 [26–28]. The Stroke Prevention in Sickle Cell Anemia Trial (STOP) showed that children with mean flow velocities of 200cm/s or greater in the dICA or proximal MCA have a 10% risk for stroke per year. That risk is 10 to 20 times that of age-matched children who have sickle cell anemia and normal velocities [**Fig. 18**]. The STOP study also showed that this risk could be reduced to less than 1% per year with regular blood transfusions to decrease the HbSS to less than 30% of total hemoglobin. This study led to a recommendation from the National Heart Lung and Blood Institute of the National Institutes of Health that all children with HbSS sickle cell anemia between the ages of 2

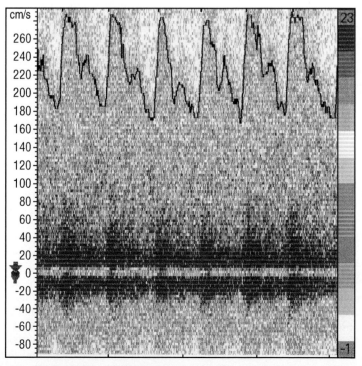

Fig. 18. Occlusive vasculopathy in sickle cell disease spectral Doppler tracing from a child with sickle cell disease shows an elevated mean velocity of MCA at 224 cm/s.

Box 1: Interpretation of the transcranial detection examination according to the Stroke Prevention in Sickle Cell Anemia Trial protocol

1. Normal: <170 cm/s (mean velocity)
2. Conditional:
   a. MCA, BIF, dICA ≥170cm/s but <200cm/s (mean velocity)
   b. PCA, TOB, BAS ≥170cm/s (mean velocity)
   c. ACA ≥170cm/s (mean velocity)
3. Abnormal: ≥200 cm/s (mean velocity)
4. Inadequate (Inadequate studies are those that cannot be interpreted. The examiner is unable to identify a minimum of information, including the M1, MCA, and BIF on temporal sides; however, if M1, MCA, BIF, or dICA is greater than or equal to 200 cm/s, then the study is interpreted as abnormal even if the other side is missing or incomplete.)

and 16 should be screened for risk for stroke [15,26–28]. The STOP trial was performed with TCD, not TCCS. The STOP protocol requires measurement of the bitemporal diameter with calipers to aid in correct identification of the ICA bifurcation. The hematocrit is also evaluated before the examination because there is an inverse relationship between hematocrit and cerebral blood flow [Box 1] [29].

Because of the results of the STOP findings, an increase in demand has occurred for TCD screening for children with HbSS. Many centers do not have access to TCD equipment but do have access to color Doppler imaging equipment; therefore, studies have been performed to compare TCD and TCCS findings in children who have sickle cell disease. Neish and colleagues [11] found that non–angle-corrected mean velocity measurements in the MCA, distal internal carotid artery, and ACA did not vary substantially between TCCS and TCD. Jones and colleagues [28] found that non–angle-corrected mean velocity measurements were lower with TCCS than TCD [27,28,30,31]. This potential difference in mean velocity measurements should be considered when screening children who develop HbSS for stroke risk with TCCS.

Vasomotor reactivity testing

Vasomotor reactivity is the ability of the vessels to undergo vasoconstriction or vasodilatation in response to various stimuli. Cerebral autoregulation is the vascular response when the stimulus is a change in perfusion pressure [32]. Transcranial Doppler can demonstrate flow velocity changes occurring over time, and therefore is an ideal test

for evaluation of autoregulation and vasomotor reactivity. Vasomotor reactivity testing is performed to evaluate the reserve mechanism of the cerebral vasculature using various stimuli. Types of stimuli include CO_2 inhalation, breath-holding, and increased or decreased systemic arterial pressure. With an intact vasomotor reserve a decrease in perfusion pressure can be offset by vasodilatation of cortical arterioles to maintain adequate cortical blood supply. In the situation where the resistance vessels are already maximally dilated they cannot respond to vasodilatory stimuli, and blood flow does not increase. This can lead to ischemic brain injury if perfusion pressure decreases further. Vasomotor reactivity testing with TCD has been used to evaluate patients who present with symptomatic or asymptomatic extracranial ICA stenosis or occlusion, cerebral small artery disease, head trauma, and subarachnoid hemorrhage [4,15]. As per the Report of the Therapeutics and Technology Assessment Subcommittee of the American Academy of Neurology, vasomotor reactivity testing was believed to be useful for detecting impaired cerebral hemodynamics in patients who present with asymptomatic severe (greater than 70%) stenosis of the eICA, symptomatic or asymptomatic eICA occlusion, and disease of the cerebral small arteries [15].

Detection of microembolic signals

Transcranial Doppler can detect microembolic signals (MES) or "high-intensity transient signals" in the intracranial arteries. Microemboli detection is based on the backscatter from the emboli. The backscatter of the ultrasound from flowing blood is less than the backscatter from solid emboli [15,33]. According to a consensus recommendation, an MES must have the following features: (1) it must be transient, lasting less than 300 ms, (2) the amplitude should be at least 3 dB greater than background signal, (3) it should be unidirectional within the Doppler velocity spectrum, and (4) the signal should be associated with a "snap," "chirp," or "moan" [**Fig. 19**] [34]. In asymptomatic patients, the identification of microembolic signals may correlate to an active embolic source, possibly identifying a subgroup of patients who are at high risk for stroke. In symptomatic patients after an acute event, identification of MES may identify those at risk for recurrent stroke. This technique may be useful in identifying the site of an embolizing lesion [33]. MES have been detected with TCD in asymptomatic and symptomatic high-grade internal carotid stenosis, prosthetic valves, myocardial infarction, atrial fibrillation, aortic arch atheroma, fat embolization, and general cerebral vascular disease. MES have also been detected during

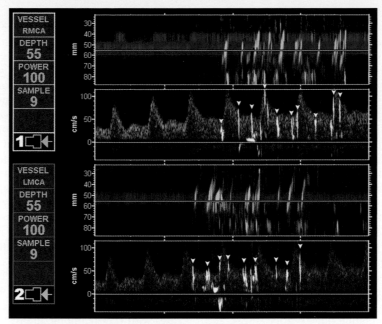

Fig. 19. Typical MES detected with TCD are bright linear high amplitude echoes (*arrowheads*).

coronary catheterization, coronary angioplasty, cardio version, cerebral angiography, carotid endarterectomy, carotid angioplasty, and cardiopulmonary bypass. TCD detection of MES has also been used to monitor antithrombotic treatment in patients who present with atherosclerotic cerebrovascular disease [15]. The introduction of new hardware and software capabilities may improve the monitoring procedure and help with discrimination from artifact [4,20].

A patent foramen ovale (PFO) is present in one third of the population and up to 50% of patients younger than 55 years of age presenting with ischemic stroke [35]. Contrast- enhanced transesophageal echocardiography (TEE) is the gold standard for detection of paradoxical emboli by way of a PFO. Data have shown a high correlation between contrast-enhanced TCD and contrast-enhanced TEE in the detection of emboli from PFO. The sensitivity and specificity of contrast-enhanced TCD can be improved with the performance of a Valsalva maneuver. The sensitivity can also be improved by increasing the volume of agitated saline used during the examination or by using a contrast agent [15,35,36].

Intraoperative monitoring

Intraoperative monitoring with TCD has been used during carotid endarterectomy and cardiac surgery with cardiopulmonary bypass. Obvious advantages of using TCD are that it is noninvasive and can

provide continuous monitoring. Most experience with TCD monitoring in the operating room has been during carotid endarterectomy where the ipsilateral MCA is monitored. Velocities and MES are evaluated. A large decrease in velocities is considered an indication for blood pressure support, shunt placement, and evaluation for shunt kinking or thrombosis. MES occur most commonly during dissection, shunting and unclamping, wound closure, and immediately postoperatively [15]. The number of MES during the dissection phase and wound closure is most predictive of postoperative stroke [4]. Greater than 50 MES/h in the early postoperative period is predictive of the development of ipsilateral focal cerebral ischemia [15]. The major cause of stroke in the postoperative period is embolism from the operative site [15].

Cerebral infarction and encephalopathy occur in up to 15% of patients undergoing coronary artery bypass surgery. Neuropsychological deficits can occur in up to 70% of patients. The degree of neuropsychological deficit correlates with the number of MES identified with intraoperative monitoring with TCD [4,15]. TCD monitoring can document changes in flow velocity and MES throughout all phases of the surgery.

Brain death

The definition of brain death is the irreversible cessation of all functions of the entire brain. Clinical criteria for brain death, such as a known cause of an unresponsive comatose state, apnea, and absence of brainstem reflexes, are usually adequate for the diagnosis of brain death. Circumstances exist where a confirmatory test is indicated. Patients treated with sedatives, patients who present with facial trauma, and ethical and legal considerations are examples of circumstances requiring a confirmatory test [37]. In addition, the increasing demand for organ donors requires prompt identification of candidates before multiorgan failure [38]. Four vessel angiography demonstrating non-filling of the cerebral arteries has been the gold standard. Angiography is invasive, expensive, and requires the patient to be transported to the angiography suite. Radioisotope studies for cerebral blood flow have also been used—this is expensive, and uses radiopharmaceutical agents. TCD is noninvasive, portable, and inexpensive. Specific intracranial arterial waveforms, which correspond to intracranial circulatory arrest, have been described with TCD. These waveforms include oscillating flow, systolic spikes, and no flow [**Fig. 20**]. To avoid false positive results, right and MCAs and the BA must be evaluated. Intracranial circulatory arrest and brain death may not occur simultaneously. A lag can occur of almost 24 hours between the TCD documentation of intracranial circulatory arrest and complete loss of brain function [38]. The sensitivity and specificity of TCD in the confirmation of brain death is 91% to 100%, and 100% respectively [37,38].

Ultrasound contrast agents

Ultrasound contrast agents in conjunction with TCCS are currently used in clinical practice in many countries, though are not yet approved by the Food and Drug Administration for use in the United States. As with TCD, a major limitation of TCCS is insufficient insonation secondary to hyperostosis of the skull, obesity, and low flow velocities [15,39]. Ultrasound contrast agents have been used to offset this limitation. Ultrasound contrast agents increase the Doppler signal intensity and increase the signal-to -noise ratio for improved transcranial insonation [15]. In a study by Zunker and colleagues [39], looking at the frequency of use, diagnostic benefit, and validity of results compared with MRA, they found that ultrasound contrast agents were indicated in 8.8% of their patients who had undergone TCD and TCCS to reliably evaluate the intracranial arteries. After ultrasound contrast use, they had a diagnostic result in 75% of cases with transtemporal and 81% during transforaminal insonation [39]. Artifacts associated with ultrasound contrast agents include the blooming effect (which occurs immediately after the bolus arrives at the image location, and can obscure vessel anatomy) and spectral bubble noise that is associated with a loud "crackling" noise, and an increase in PSV by as much as 26 cm/s plus or minus 10% [1,3,15]. Potential future applications of ultrasound contrast agents include evaluation of

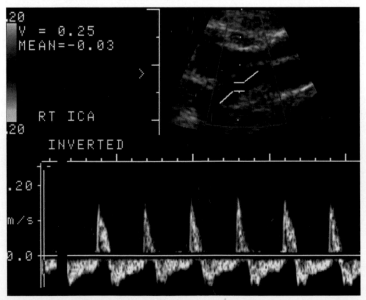

Fig. 20. Brain death characteristic to-and-fro flow is demonstrated in ICA. Flow is toward transducer in systole and away from it in diastole, with net result of no forward flow. This same waveform pattern can be demonstrated in intracranial arteries with TCD.

brain perfusion in stroke patients, and drug delivery, including delivery of thrombolytic agents [40].

New developments

Ultrasound enhanced thrombolysis

Experimental models have shown low frequency ultrasound augments the activity of fibrinolytic agents. Ultrasound enhanced thrombolysis occurs by various mechanisms, including improved drug transport, altering the fibrin structure, and increasing the binding of tissue plasminogen activator (tPA) to fibrin. Studies have been performed with ultrasound enhanced thrombolysis using KHz frequencies, as these have better penetration, but this resulted in increased risk for intracerebral hemorrhage in stroke patients [40,41]. Experimental models found that 1- to 2.2-MHz TCD also facilitated tPA infusion for clot dissolution, though tPA-enhanced thrombolysis is slower with 1 MHz than with 2 MHz frequencies [42]. At this time 2-MHz TCD is being used for diagnostic evaluation and enhancement of thrombolysis with tPA infusion. The Combined Lysis of Thrombus in Brain Ischemia Using Transcranial Ultrasound and Systemic t-PA (CLOTBUST) trial was a phase-2, multicenter, randomized clinical trial. This trial set out to determine the differences in complete recanalization and early clinical recovery rates between patients treated with tPA infusion and continuous monitoring with 2-MHz TCD compared with those treated with tPA infusion alone, and to determine the safety of continuous 2-MHz TCD monitoring of tPA infusion [43,44]. The trial concluded continuous monitoring with 2-MHz TCD did augment tPA-induced arterial recanalization in patients who experience acute ischemic stroke without an increase in bleeding. A trend toward an increase in the rate of recovery from stroke exists, though this trend was not found to be significant [41].

Summary

Since the introduction of TCD in 1982 by Aaslid and colleagues [2], TCD and TCCS have become essential tools in the diagnostic workup of cerebrovascular disorders. TCD and TCCS provide valuable information as to anatomy, hemodynamic status, and functional status, such as vasomotor reactivity and autoregulation, [Box 2].

Major advantages of TCD and TCCS over other cerebrovascular diagnostic modalities, such as angiography, CTA and MRA, are that they are noninvasive, portable, dynamic, and inexpensive. These advantages promote the use of TCD and TCCS in the operating room, emergency room, neurointensive care unit, and during thrombolysis. Exciting new developments with TCD and TCCS include ultrasound-enhanced thrombolysis and expanded United States contrast applications in cerebral vascular diagnosis and monitoring of perfusion in the stroke patient and contrast-assisted drug delivery.

Box 2: Main indications for transcranial detection and transcranial color-coded duplex sonography

- Detection and monitoring of cerebral vasospasm
- Detection of intracranial stenosis and occlusion
- Screening for stroke prevention in children with sickle cell disease
- Intra-operative monitoring
- Monitoring in the neurosurgical intensive care unit
- Evaluation for brain death
- Detection of microembolic signals
- Detection of right to left shunts
- Vasomotor reactivity testing
- Ultrasound assisted thrombolysis (new development)
- Evaluation of brain perfusion in the stroke patient (new development)

References

[1] Baumgartner R. Transcranial color duplex sonography in cerebrovascular disease: a systematic review. Cerebrovasc Dis 2003;16:4–13.

[2] Aaslid R, Markwalder TM, Norris N. Noninvasive transcranial Doppler ultrasound recording of flow velocity in basal cerebral arteries. Neurosurg 1982;57:769.

[3] Gahn G, von Kummer R. Ultrasound in acute stroke: a review. Neuroradiology 2001;43:702–11.

[4] Nabavi DG, Otis SM, Ringelstein EB. Ultrasound assessment of the intracranial arteries. In: Zwiebel WJ, Pellerito JS, editors. Introduction to vascular ultrasonography. 5th edition. Philadelphia: Elsevier Saunders; 2005. p. 225–50.

[5] Otis SM, Ringelstein EB. Transcranial Doppler sonography. In: Zwiebel WJ, editor. Introduction to vascular ultrasonography. 4th edition. Pennsylvania: W.B. Saunders Co.; 2000. p. 177–201.

[6] DeWitt LD, Rosengart A, Teal PA. Transcranial Doppler ultrasonography: normal values. In: Babikian VL, Wechsler LR, editors. Transcranial Doppler ultrasound. St. Louis (Mo): Mosby; 1993. p. 29.

[7] Fujioka KA, Douville CM. Anatomy and freehand examination techniques. In: Newell DW, Aaslid R, editors. Transcranial Doppler. New York: Raven Press, Ltd; 1992. p. 9–31.

[8] Otis SM. Pitfalls in transcranial doppler diagnosis. In: Babikian VL, Wechsler LR, editors. Transcranial Doppler sonography. St Louis (MO): Mosby-Year Book Inc.; 1993. p. 39–50.

[9] Klotzsch C, Popescu O, Berlit P. A new 1-MHz probe for transcranial Doppler sonography in patients with inadequate temporal bone windows. Ultrasound Med Biol 1998;24(1):101–3.

[10] Kenton AR, Martin PJ, Evans DH. Power Doppler: an advance over colour Doppler for transcranial imaging? Ultrasound Med Biol 1996; 22(3):313–7.

[11] Neish AS, Blews DE, Simms CA, et al. Screening for stroke in sickle cell anemia: comparison of transcranial Doppler imaging and nonimaging us techniques. Radiology 2002;222(3):709–14.

[12] Schoning M, Buchholz R, Walter J. Comparative study of color duplex sonography and transcranial Doppler sonography in adults. J Neurosurg 1993;78:776–84.

[13] Krejza J, Mariak Z, Babikian V. Importance of angle correction in the measurement of blood flow velocity with transcranial Doppler sonography. Am J Neuroradiol 2001;22:1743–7.

[14] Suarez JI, Qureshi AI, Yahia AB, et al. Symptomatic vasospasm diagnosis after subarachnoid hemorrhage: evaluation of transcranial Doppler ultrasound and cerebral angiography as related to compromised vascular distribution. Crit Care Med 2002;30(6):1348–55.

[15] Sloan MA, Alexandrov AV, Tegeler CH, et al. Assessment: transcranial Doppler ultrasonography. Neurology 2004;62:1468–81.

[16] Krejza J, Mariak Z, Lewko J. Standardization of flow velocities with respect to age and sex improves the accuracy of transcranial color Doppler sonography of the middle cerebral artery spasm. AJR Am J Roentgenol 2003;181:245–52.

[17] Proust F, Callonec F, Clavier E, et al. Usefulness of transcranial color-coded sonography in the diagnosis of cerebral vasospasm. Stroke 1999;30: 1091–8.

[18] Lindegaard KF. The role of transcranial Doppler in the management of patients with subarachnoid haemorrhage: a review. Acta Neurochir (Wien) 1999;72:59–71.

[19] Skirboll S, Newell DW. Noninvasive physiologic evaluation of the aneurysm patient. Neurosurg Clin N Am 1998;9(3):463–83.

[20] Mascia L, Fedorko L, terBrugge K, et al. The accuracy of transcranial Doppler to detect vasospasm in patients with aneurysmal subarachnoid hemorrhage. Intensive Care Med 2003;29: 1088–94.

[21] Droste DW, Kaps M, Vavabit DG, et al. Ultrasound contrast enhancing agents in neurosonology: principles, methods, future possibilities. Acta Neurol Scand 2000;102:1–10.

[22] Baumgartner RW, Mattle HP, Schroth G. Assessment of ≥50% and <50% intracranial stenoses by transcranial color-coded duplex sonography. Stroke 1999;30:87–92.

[23] Gerriets T, Goertler M, Stolz E, et al. Feasibility and validity of transcranial duplex sonography in patients with acute stroke. J Neurol Neurosurg Psychiatry 2002;73:17–20.

[24] Felberg RA, Christour I, Demchuck AM, et al. Screening for intracranial stenosis with transcranial Doppler: the accuracy of mean flow velocity thresholds. J Neuroimaging 2002;12:9–14.

[25] Rorick MB, Nichols FT, Adams RJ. Transcranial Doppler correlation with angiography in detection of intracranial stenosis. Stroke 1994;25: 1931–4.

[26] Riebel T, Betzing Kebelmann C, Gutze R, et al. Transcranial Doppler ultrasonography in neurologically asymptomatic children and young adults with sickle cell disease. Eur Radiol 2003; 13:563–70.

[27] Jones AM, Seibert JJ, Nichols FT, et al. Comparison of transcranial color Doppler imaging (TCDI) and transcranial Doppler in children with sickle cell anemia. Pediatr Radiol 2001;31: 461–9.

[28] Neish AS, Blews DE, Simms CA, et al. Screening for stroke in sickle cell anemia: comparison of transcranial Doppler imaging and nonimaging US techniques. Radiology 2002;222: 709–14.

[29] TCD in children with sickle cell disease. An intensive training course. Presented by School of Medicine, Medical College of Georgia, the Alumni Center. Augusta, January 27–30, 1998.

[30] Bulas DI, Jones A, Seibert JJ, et al. Transcranial Doppler (TCD) screening for stroke prevention in sickle cell anemia; pitfalls in technique variation. Pediatr Radiol 2000;30:733–8.

[31] Razumovsky AY. TCD methodology in children with sickle-cell anemia. Pediatr Radiol 2002;32: 690–1.

[32] Moppett IK, Mahanjan RP. Transcranial Doppler ultrasonography in anaesthesia and intensive care. British Journal of Anaesthesia 2004;93(5): 710–24.

[33] Ringelstein EB, Droste DW, Babikian VL, et al. Consensus on microembolus detection by TCD. Stroke 1998;29:275–9.

[34] Babikian VL. Basic identification criteria of Doppler microembolic signals. Stroke 1995;26:1123.

[35] Uzuner N, Horner S, Pichler G, et al. Right-to-left shunt assessed by contrast transcranial Doppler sonography. J Ultrasound Med 2004;23: 1475–82.

[36] Droste DW, Silling K, Stypmann J, et al. Contrast transcranial Doppler ultrasound in the detection of right-to-left shunts. Stroke 2000;31: 1640–5.

[37] Hadani M, Bruk B, Ram Z, et al. Application of transcranial Doppler ultrasonography for the diagnosis of brain death. Intensive Care Med 1999;25:822–8.

[38] Dosemeci L, Dora B, Yilmaz M, et al. Utility of transcranial Doppler ultrasonography for confirmatory diagnosis of brain death; two sides of the coin. Transplantation 2004;77:71–5.

[39] Zunker P, Wilms H, Brossmann J, et al. Echocontrast-enhanced transcranial ultrasound: frequency of use, diagnostic benefit, and validity

of results compared with MRA. Stroke 2002;33:
2600–3.

[40] Droste D, Metz RJ. Clinical utility of echocon-
trast agents in neurosonology. Neurol Res 2004;
26:754–9.

[41] Alexandrove AV, Wojner AW, Grotta JC, et al.
Ultrasound-enhanced thrombolysis for acute ischemic stroke. N Engl J Med 2004;351(21):2170.

[42] Alexandrove AV, Wojner AW, Grotta JC, et al.
Ultrasound-enhanced thrombolysis for acute

ischemic stroke: phase I findings of the CLOT-
BUST trial. J Neuroimaging 2004;14(21):113–7.

[43] Alexandrove AV, Molina CA, Grotta JC. CLOT-
BUST: ultrasound-enhanced systemic thrombolysis for acute ischemic stroke. J Neuroimaging
2004;14(21):108–12.

[44] Carson N, Voci SL. Transcranial Doppler ultrasound. In: Dogra V, Rubens DJ, editors. Ultrasound secrets. 1st edition. Philadelphia: Hanley &
Belfus; 2004. p. 394–402.

ELSEVIER
SAUNDERS

ULTRASOUND
CLINICS

Ultrasound Clin 1 (2006) 183–199

Ultrasound Diagnosis of Arterial Injuries and the Role of Minimally Invasive Techniques in Their Management

Nael E.A. Saad, MB, BCh*, Wael E.A. Saad, MB, Bch,
Deborah J. Rubens, MD, Patrick Fultz, MD

- ■ Natural history
- ■ Clinical features
- ■ Ultrasound imaging
- ■ Treatment
- ■ Surgery
- ■ Ultrasound-guided compression
- ■ Ultrasound-guided percutaneous thrombin injection
- ■ Endoluminal management

- ■ Arteriovenous fistulae
- ■ Natural history
- ■ Ultrasound imaging
- ■ Treatment
- ■ Surgery
- ■ Ultrasound-guided compression
- ■ Endoluminal management
- ■ Summary
- ■ References

Pseudoaneurysms (PsAs) arise from a localized disruption of the arterial wall from a variety of causes. Under high arterial pressure, blood dissects into the tissues around the damaged artery forming a perfused sac that communicates with the arterial lumen [1–3]. The wall of the PsA is formed by residual portions of the wall (the media or adventitia) or by the soft tissues surrounding the injured vessel. Modern medical imaging modalities have increased the diagnosis of PsAs [4] facilitating early detection before onset of clinical symptoms. Conventional arteriography, however, still remains the gold standard [5] for diagnosis and anatomic evaluation of PsAs. The other modalities, including ultrasonography with Doppler evaluation, magnetic resonance arteriography (MRA), and helical computed tomographic arteriography (CTA) offer noninvasive imaging options with variable results

[6,7]. As imaging guidance also improves, PsA therapy has evolved from traditional surgical management toward a less invasive, percutaneous approach. The combination of early detection and minimally invasive management has decreased dramatically the morbidity and mortality from PsAs.

Natural history

PsAs are the end result of multiple causes, including inflammation, trauma, surgical procedures [1], and other iatrogenic causes, such as percutaneous biopsy or drainage, may result in PsA formation in any artery. The high sensitivity of modern imaging modalities has made the diagnosis of PsAs more common; however, there is also a real increase in the incidence of PsAs [8] as a result of an increase in the number of vascular surgical and arteriographic

Department of Radiology, University of Rochester Medical Center, 601 Elmwood Avenue, Box 648, Rochester, NY 14642, USA
* Corresponding author.
E-mail address: nael@mindless.com (N.E.A. Saad).

1556-858X/06/$ – see front matter © 2005 Elsevier Inc. All rights reserved.
ultrasound.theclinics.com

doi:10.1016/j.cult.2005.09.008

procedures performed. Surgery causes PsAs by direct injury to the vessel or introduction of infection. Numerous procedures may induce PsAs, including those considered minimally invasive such as diagnostic angiography whereby the incidence of PsA formation is less than 1%. Therapeutic catheterization for angioplasty or stents often requires large bore sheaths, periprocedural anticoagulation, and antiplatelet therapy, which raise the incidence of PsA formation to 3.2% to 7.7% [9,10]. PsAs are also recognized complications of liver transplantation [11,12], cardiac transplantation [13], obstetric procedures (eg, dilatation, curettage, and caesarian sections [14]), and endovascular aortic stent grafts [15]. Blunt and penetrating trauma may also cause PsAs of multiple vessels, including the carotid [5], extremity [6,16], splenic [17,18], and hepatic [19] arteries. PsAs may also be caused by vascular infection or inflammation, including pancreatitis [20]. PsAs may undergo spontaneous thrombosis [7,21] or may develop complications, such as local neurovascular compression, infection, or rupture [10].

Clinical features

Asymptomatic PsAs are detected incidentally during radiologic investigation of other conditions or during surgery [22]. Symptomatic PsAs manifest with local or systemic signs and symptoms. On physical examination, a pulsatile mass, a palpable thrill, or an audible bruit may be appreciated. Local effects of a PsA are caused by mass effect on adjacent structures causing compromise of function. Ischemia of the surrounding tissues (caused by vascular com-

promise) may lead to necrosis of the overlying skin and subcutaneous tissue. Neurologic symptoms may develop secondary to nerve compression/ischemia. Compression of adjacent veins may cause edema or deep venous thrombosis. Arterial thromboembolism is also a potential complication. In addition, the PsA may rupture leading to hemorrhage with potential life threatening shock [7,10,21,23]. Rupture is the most serious cause of morbidity from PsAs; for example, rupture of splenic artery PsAs has a mortality rate approaching 100% [24]. PsAs can communicate with and rupture into the bowel, or biliary system, and the thoracic, peritoneal, pelvic, and retroperitoneal spaces [25]. Hemorrhage from these ruptures may present as a sentinel bleed, bleeding from a drain, hematemesis, melena [23], splenic rupture, or subcapsular hepatic hematoma [26].

Ultrasound imaging

Gray-scale ultrasound (US) usually demonstrates a predominantly anechoic mass adjacent to the artery [**Fig. 1**A] [8,12,14]. This mass may be spherical or irregular and may contain septations or debris [**Fig. 2**A]. The size of the PsA sac, the number of its compartments (lobes), its connection to the artery, and the length and width of the neck of the PsA can also be assessed [**Fig. 1**B] [9]. PsAs may be simple (one lobe) or complex (two or more lobes separated by a patent tract, which has a diameter smaller than the minimal dimension of the smallest lobe) [9]. In addition, a concentric hematoma within the PsA may be seen occasionally [**Fig. 3**A–C]. Gray-scale US alone is not diagnostic

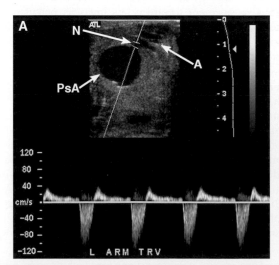
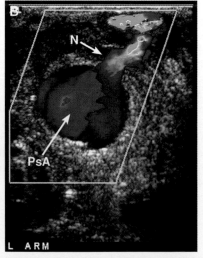

Fig. 1. (A) Gray-scale ultrasound with spectral waveform from the PsA neck depicting bidirectional flow within neck (N). The donor artery (A) supplying the PsA can also be seen. (B) Color Doppler image of same PsA with easy depiction of PsA neck (N) and the yin-yang (red-blue) Doppler appearance of the PsA sac. (*From* Saad N, Saad W, Rubens DJ. Pseudoaneurysms and the role of minimally invasive techniques in their management. Radiographics 2005;25:S173–9; with permission.)

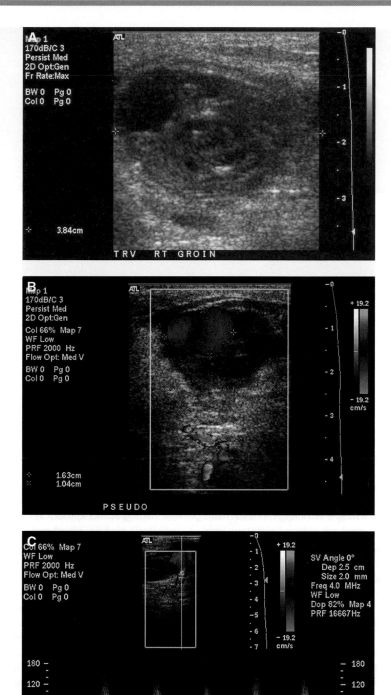

Fig. 2. (*A*) Gray-scale ultrasound image of right groin in patient who underwent catheterization demonstrates irregular mass (cursors) with mixed echogenicity. (*B*) Color Doppler image of same mass demonstrating characteristic yin-yang (red-blue) flow in sac. Area lacking flow represents thrombus within sac. (*C*) Spectral wave form from PsA neck depicting bidirectional flow within neck.

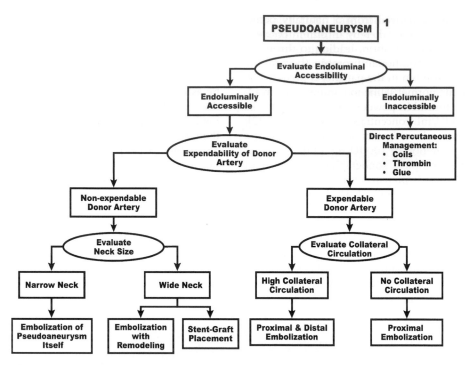

1. Superficial postcatheterization pseudoaneurysms — treat with ultrasound-guided thrombin injection (The above algorithm is not for superficial postcatheterization pseudoaneurysms).

Fig. 6. Algorithm for management of PsAs. (*From* Saad N, Saad W, Rubens DJ. Pseudoaneurysms and the role of minimally invasive techniques in their management. Radiographics 2005;25:S173–9; with permission.)

independently or in conjunction with thrombin [4,10].

Endoluminal management

These techniques serve to exclude a PsA from the circulation by placing a stent across the PsA neck or by occluding the PsA or the feeding artery. Selecting

the optimal method depends on the size of the PsA neck and the expendability of the donor artery [**Figs. 5 and 6**] [4,10]. Fig. 6 is a generalized schematic for non–catheterization-related extremity PsAs.

A PsA arising from an expendable donor artery without collaterals is treated with embolization of the afferent artery [**Fig. 7A, B**] [4]. Several visceral arteries exist that have a well-established collat-

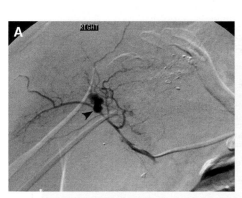
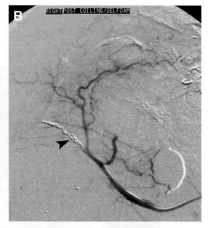

Fig. 7. (*A*) A 67-year-old man presented to emergency department after sustaining gunshot wound to right arm. Digital subtraction angiogram shows PsA (*arrow head*) of the circumflex humeral artery. (*B*) Digital subtraction angiogram showing obliterated PsA (*arrow head*). The PsA was excluded from donor artery by coil embolization. (*From* Saad N, Saad W, Rubens DJ. Pseudoaneurysms and the role of minimally invasive techniques in their management. Radiographics 2005;25:S173–9; with permission.)

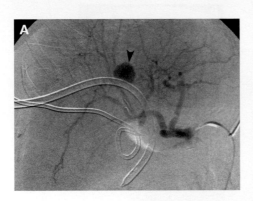

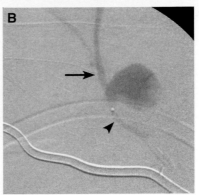

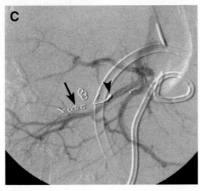

Fig. 8. (*A*) A 61-year-old woman with cholangiocarcinoma underwent Whipple procedure and multiple percutaneous transhepatic cholangiograms with biliary drainage catheter placement. Digital subtraction angiogram demonstrates PsA (*arrow head*) off branch of right hepatic artery. (*B*) Digital subtraction angiogram showing PsA with its afferent (*arrow head*) and efferent (*arrow*) hepatic artery segments. (*C*) Digital subtraction angiogram after excluding PsA by distal (*arrow*) and proximal (*arrow head*) embolization. (*From* Saad N, Saad W, Rubens DJ. Pseudoaneurysms and the role of minimally invasive techniques in their management. Radiographics 2005;25: S173–9; with permission.)

eral supply, including the gastroduodenal, hepatic, splenic, and other upper gastrointestinal arteries [4,26]. In addition, some pelvic and distal extremity arteries have a collateral supply (eg, the internal iliac artery and the profunda femoris artery respectively). When embolizing arteries with numerous collaterals, embolize proximal and distal to the PsA to exclude it completely from the circulation by preventing back flow from collateral circulation [**Fig.** 8A–C] [4].

A PsA arising from a nonexpendable donor artery must be excluded from the circulation while preserving the donor artery. A vital donor artery may be embolized in certain emergent situations (eg, rupture with active bleeding); however, this must be followed by restoration of blood flow distally by means of surgical bypass [**Fig.** 9A, B]. Most of the time, however, the PsA can be thrombosed by coils delivered into the sac or by stent-graft placement. The width of the PsA neck compared with the donor artery diameter determines which method is optimal.

If the neck is narrow, the PsA may be embolized by catheter-directed delivery of coils (the preferred em-

bolization material) into the sac itself [**Fig.** 10A, B] [4,24,25]. Coils fall under two main categories: (1) nondetachable coils and (2) detachable coils. Nondetachable coils are available in a wide array of diameters and lengths. They are linear in shape and composed of stainless steel with the addition of polyester fibers to increase their thrombogenicity. Newer coils are made of titanium, which makes them softer and allows for formation of more complex shapes (helical) and for use of fewer coils for embolization as they conform to and fill the PsA sac. Because the newer coils are softer, however, they may require initial placement of stainless steel coils to act as scaffolding. Detachable coils are held to the pusher guidewire by a mechanical connection that is released to deploy the coil, facilitating more accurate deployment and the possibility of readjusting the position of the coil before its final deployment. A disadvantage of coils as an embolization material is the potential for recanalization of the embolized sac if the coils are not packed tightly. This drawback has been overcome largely by the use of the soft helical

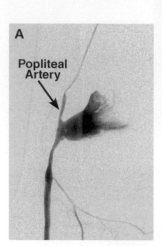
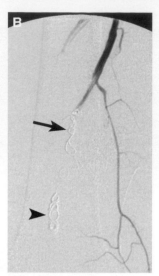

Fig. 9. (*A*) Digital subtraction angiogram showing PsA of suprageniculate popliteal artery. (*B*) Digital subtraction angiogram after successful embolization distal (*arrow head*) and proximal (*arrow*) to PsA. Patient subsequently underwent surgical bypass of occluded popliteal artery. (*From* Saad N, Saad W, Rubens DJ. Pseudoaneurysms and the role of minimally invasive techniques in their management. Radiographics 2005;25:S173–9; with permission.)

coils, which may be packed tightly in the PsA sac [48]. Other agents such as thrombin or N-butyl-2cyanoacrylate (glue) may be used alone [25,37] or in addition to coils [4].

If the neck is wide, the PsA may still be embolized by catheter-directed delivery of embolization materials; however, remodeling is required to prevent outflow of these materials into the donor artery. The goal is to ensure adequate embolization of the PsA sac while preventing distal embolization of the donor artery. A stent cage can be used in which the catheter tip is directed between the lattice before release of the coils [**Fig. 11**A, B], or the coils can be trapped by inflating a temporary occlusion balloon in the donor artery between coil deployments [10]. In cases concerning distal arterial embolization, detachable balloons may be used as the

embolic agent [9,22]. Another option if the PsA neck is wide, is stent-graft (covered stent) placement across the PsA neck to exclude it [**Fig. 12**A–C] [10]. This method is contraindicated in mycotic PsAs because of potential stent-graft infection. Stent grafts require a larger diameter catheter and a stiffer delivery system than coil embolization transcatheter delivery systems. Accordingly, the arterial anatomy and the caliber of the arteries leading to and at the PsA site should be favorable (wide and straight arteries). Currently, stent grafts are suitable for larger arteries only, because in small arteries they have a higher risk for thrombosis. Visceral PsAs are usually smaller and arise from small and tortuous donor arteries, posing a particular challenge to stent grafts.

Endovascular techniques have a lower rate of complication for the treatment of visceral PsAs when

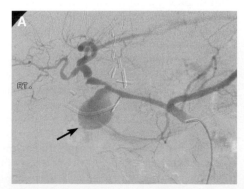
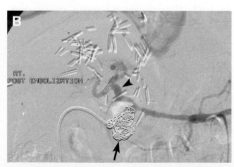

Fig. 10. (*A*) Digital subtraction angiogram showing PsA (*arrow*) off proper hepatic artery. (*B*) Digital subtraction angiogram after coil embolization of PsA itself (*arrow*) with preservation of flow in hepatic artery distally (*arrow head*). (*From* Saad N, Saad W, Rubens DJ. Pseudoaneurysms and the role of minimally invasive techniques in their management. Radiographics 2005;25:S173–9; with permission.)

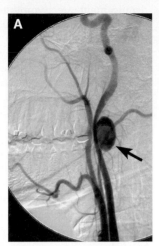
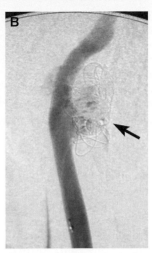

Fig. 11. (*A*) Digital subtraction angiogram of post-traumatic PsA of the common carotid artery (*arrow*). (*B*) Digital subtraction angiogram following PsA exclusion using bare-stent (uncovered stent) and coil embolization (*arrow*) of the PsA through interstices of stent. Stent acts as barrier and cages coils into PsA, excluding them from patent vital carotid artery. (*From* Saad N, Saad W, Rubens DJ. Pseudoaneurysms and the role of minimally invasive techniques in their management. Radiographics 2005;25:S173–9; with permission.)

compared with surgical management [22,25]. Complications associated with endovascular techniques include intraprocedural rupture of the PsA [24]. In addition, recanalization of the embolized vessel and reconstitution of arterial flow to the pseudoaneurysms (delayed failure of embolization) are possible, though rare [24].

Arteriovenous fistulae

An arteriovenous fistula (AVF) is an abnormal communication between an artery and a vein, and may be congenital or acquired [26,49]. Acquired AVFs may occur spontaneously as a result of rupture of arterial aneurysms into adjacent veins [50], in pa-

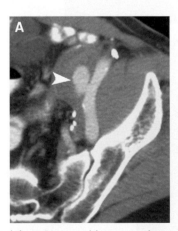
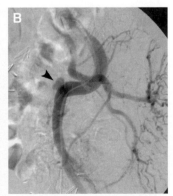
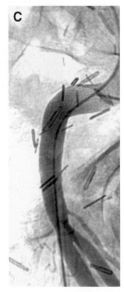

Fig. 12. (*A*) A 61-year-old man underwent prostatectomy and cystectomy with Indiana pouch creation for treatment of bladder carcinoma. A Jackson-Pratt Drain placed in surgical bed at time of surgery subsequently eroded into left external iliac artery. Contrast-enhanced CT was obtained showing PsA of left external iliac artery (*arrow head*). (*B*) Digital subtraction angiogram showing PsA (*arrow head*) before stent-graft (covered stent) placement. (*C*) Digital subtraction angiogram showing successful exclusion of PsA using stent graft. (*From* Saad N, Saad W, Rubens DJ. Pseudoaneurysms and the role of minimally invasive techniques in their management. Radiographics 2005;25:S173–9; with permission.)

tients who present with arteridities (Takayasu's arteritis or HIV-related arteritis) and connective tissue disorders (Ehlers-Danlos syndrome and Marfan syndrome), or as a result of infection or tumor [51,52]. Acquired AVFs, however, are more commonly a result of trauma (penetrating is more common than blunt) or something iatrogenic, such as surgery, catheterization, or percutaneous biopsies [52–54].

Natural history

AVFs cause left-to-right shunting of blood resulting in dilatation of the efferent veins [53]. The degree of shunting and proximity of the AVF to the heart correlates with the degree of cardiovascular derangement and clinical presentation [54]. Low-flow fistulas usually do not result in any cardiovascular derangement, are asymptomatic (incidentally diagnosed), and can spontaneously thrombose [54–56]. Moderate-flow AVFs cause venous dilatation but usually do not result in flow-overload and cardiac dilatation and often present years later [55]. Large AVFs with high flow cause early left ventricular hypertrophy and, eventually, cardiac failure [53–56]. The left-to-right shunting of arterial blood may lead to ischemia of the affected limb causing claudication [51,56] or organ failure [54]. The increased venous pressure may result in edema of the extremities [49,51]. Hemorrhage is another clinical presentation caused by rupture of the AVF [49,53,54]. Paradoxical pulmonary embolism has also been reported [50]. On physical examination an audible bruit or palpable thrill (in superficial AVFs) may be present [51,53].

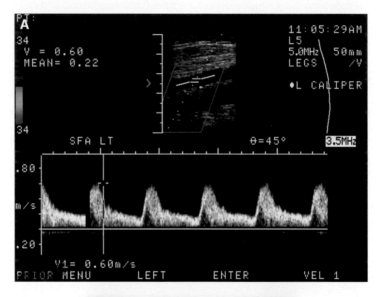

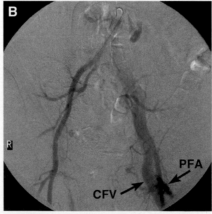

Fig. 13. (*A*) Longitudinal US image of left superficial femoral artery in patient following motorcycle accident. Spectral waveform demonstrates abnormal low resistive index, consistent with distal arteriovenous fistula. Normal extremity waveform should demonstrate high resistive index. (*B*) Digital subtraction pelvic angiogram demonstrating early filling of left common femoral vein (CFV) in arterial phase from AVF between profunda femoris artery (PFA) and CFV. Normal right common femoral vein is not seen in arterial phase imaging.

Ultrasound imaging

Gray-scale US often fails to demonstrate the connection between the artery and the vein, especially if the fistula is small; therefore, the diagnosis may be missed if color and spectral Doppler are not used [49]. In peripheral AVFs, the communication between the vessels is demonstrated as a colored jet of blood by color or power Doppler [26], often with aliasing on color Doppler caused by high velocity flow. The affected vein is often larger in caliber than the contralateral (unaffected) side [**Fig. 13**A, B]. With a high-flow AVF, poor response to a Valsalva maneuver in the involved vein occurs [26]. A normal response to the Valsalva maneuver suggests that the AVF is small with low-flow and may resolve spontaneously [26]. Spectral Doppler evaluates the flow patterns from a selected segment

of the AVF vessels [49,57]. Spectral waveforms obtained from the draining veins of the AVF demonstrate pulsatile periodic flow that varies with the cardiac cycle, and often simulate an artery [**Fig. 14**A, B]. The feeding artery shows increased diastolic blood flow resulting from the high venous outflow with low resistance [26,49]. The low resistance arterial and pulsatile venous waveforms are the spectral diagnostic criteria for a systemic AVF. In visceral AVFs (eg, arterioportal fistula), the venous pattern includes reversed flow in particular portal vein radicals, and an arterialized portal vein waveform [**Fig. 15**A–C] [58–60]. The feeding hepatic artery exhibits increased diastolic flow caused by reduced impedance, which is reflected in a reduced resistive index (peak systolic velocity − end diastolic velocity ÷ peak systolic velocity). A reduced resistive index less than 0.5 in

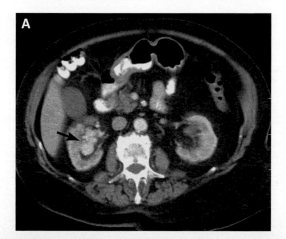

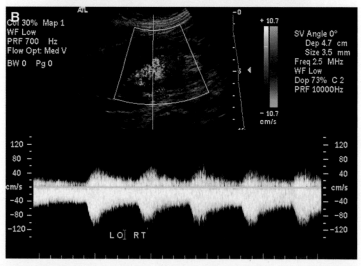

Fig. 14. (A) Axial contrast-enhanced CT image demonstrating increased attenuation in right renal hilum (*arrow*). (B) Color flow Doppler image of right renal hilum demonstrating mosaic of colors indicates aliasing and high velocity flow. Also note large volume of vessels which fill hilum. Spectral waveform shows pulsatile periodic arterial waveform on both sides of baseline. Artery flows into kidney (*above baseline*) and high velocity vein has an arterialized waveform directed below baseline as it flows out into renal hilum; diagnostic of AVF.

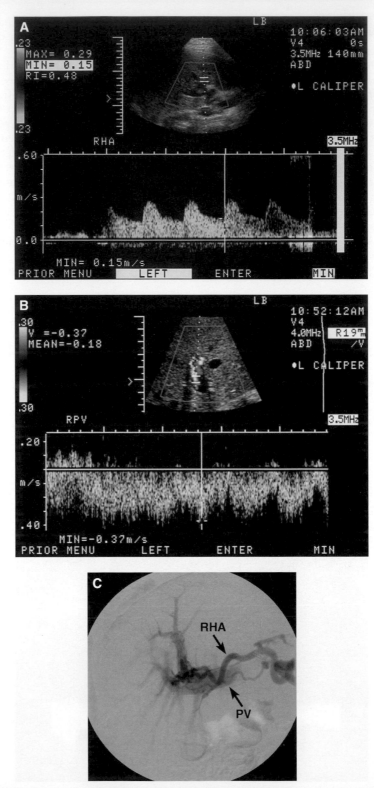

Fig. 15. (*A*) Gray-scale ultrasound with spectral waveform from right hepatic artery demonstrating low resistive index of 0.48. (*B*) Gray-scale ultrasound with spectral waveform from right portal vein demonstrating abnormally reversed flow direction, out of liver toward porta. (*C*) Digital subtraction angiogram image from selective celiac axis injection demonstrates early filling of portal venous system in hepatic arterial phase denoting an arterioportal fistula. Right hepatic artery (RHA) and portal vein (PV).

the hepatic artery is usually abnormal and is caused by ischemia or by arteriovenous shunting (tumor or AVF).

Three-dimensional US improves localization and orientation of the AVF relative to surrounding structures with results comparable with MRA [52]. Intravascular US (IVUS) provides more accurate delineation of AVFs; however, this is an invasive modality and its use is reserved for guidance of endoluminal therapy [61].

Treatment

Low-flow AVFs may be managed expectantly with close monitoring by duplex US [49,54,56]. Symptomatic AVFs should undergo definitive treatment [49,54]. As in PsAs, the traditional treatment of AVFs has been surgical repair [51]; however, over the past few years, minimally invasive therapy for AVFs has also evolved to provide an alternate to surgery [49,51]. The therapeutic options available today include observation, surgery, US-guided compression, and endoluminal management [49,51].

The goal of treatment for AVFs is to obliterate the connection between the artery and the vein [53]. The fate of the involved vessels depends on their expendability. Efforts are made to preserve continuity of vital vessels, whereas expendable vessels may be sacrificed [53].

Treatment of AVFs results in symptom relief, preservation of function, and, often, reversal of cardiomegaly [53,54].

Surgery

Surgery remains the traditional choice for therapy and, because of multiple feeding arteries and draining veins, is more often required in AVF repair than for PsA treatment. Surgical options include vascular ligation of expendable vessels [54], ligation of the AVF with preservation of vessel continuity or conduit bypass, and partial or total organ removal [49,54].

Ultrasound-guided compression

US-guided compression may be used to treat superficial postcatheterization AVFs similar to postcatheterization PsAs [26,56]; however, success rates are 30% or lower [26]. The US probe directly compresses the fistulous track between the feeding artery and the draining vein of the AVF [26]. Alternating compression cycles and concurrent continuous US monitoring are performed as they are for PsA therapy.

Endoluminal management

The same basic principles of endoluminal therapy for PsAs apply to AVFs. Expendable arteries may be embolized selectively using coils or other embolic agents [49,54,61]; however, these coils and agents carry a substantial risk for inadvertent systemic or paradoxical pulmonary embolization in large high-flow AVFs [54,61]. In such cases, a covered stent may be placed either in the artery or the vein [61]. If the stent is placed in the vein, the artery must be embolized selectively to ensure fistula closure, otherwise high pressure blood leaks around the stent and back into the vein [58]. IVUS may be helpful in the planning and deployment of stents [61]. In general, the risks of percutaneous therapy are higher and success rates lower in AVFs as compared with PsAs, often caused by multiple feeding arteries or draining veins, making it more difficult to isolate and eliminate all the abnormal vessels.

Summary

PsAs and AVFs are common vascular abnormalities. They are diagnosed more frequently as a result of increased percutaneous biopsies and procedures that cause them, and noninvasive imaging with CTA, US, and MRA, which often detect asymptomatic disease. Conventional angiography, the gold standard for diagnosis, is an invasive procedure and every effort should be made to use other noninvasive diagnostic modalities in the initial workup. The potential complications of many but not all PsAs and AVFs carry a high morbidity and mortality. Surgery has been the classic treatment of choice; however, radiology has introduced alternative minimally invasive treatment techniques that carry a lower morbidity and mortality. A complete workup of the PsA or AVF and defining the location, surrounding structures, and vascular anatomy are essential steps in the selection of the treatment technique. The therapeutic options (including observation) should be tailored to the site, rupture risk, patient comorbidities, and symptoms of the PsA or AVF in question.

References

[1] Schwartz LB, Clark ET, Gewertz BL. Anastomotic and other pseudoaneurysms. In: Rutherford RB, editor. Vascular surgery. 5th edition. Philadelphia: WB Saunders; 2000. p. 752–63.

[2] Bromley PJ, Clark T, Weir IH, et al. Radiologic diagnosis and management of uterine artery pseudoaneurysm: case report. Can Assoc Radiol J 1997;48(2):119–22.

[3] Zimon AE, Hwang JK, Principe DL, et al. Pseu-

doaneurysm of the uterine artery. Obstet Gynecol 1999;94(5 Part 2):827–30.

[4] Arata MA, Cope C. Principles used in the management of visceral aneurysms. Tech Vasc Interv Radiol 2000;3:124–9.

[5] Munera F, Soto JA, Palacio D, et al. Diagnosis of arterial injuries caused by penetrating trauma to the neck: comparison of helical CT angiography and conventional angiography. Radiology 2000; 216(2):356–62.

[6] Soto JA, Munera F, Morales C, et al. Focal arterial injuries of the proximal extremities: helical CT arteriography as the initial method of diagnosis. Radiology 2001;218(1):188–94.

[7] Ahmed A, Samuels SL, Keeffe EB, et al. Delayed fatal hemorrhage from pseudoaneurysm of the hepatic artery after percutaneous liver biopsy. Am J Gastroenterol 2001;96(1):233–7.

[8] Kresowik TF, Khoury MD, Miller BV, et al. A prospective study of the incidence and natural history of femoral vascular complications after percutaneous transluminal coronary angioplasty. J Vasc Surg 1991;13(2):328–33.

[9] Kruger K, Zahringer M, Sohngen FD, et al. Femoral pseudoaneurysms: management with percutaneous thrombin injections – success rates and effects on systemic coagulation. Radiology 2003;226(2):452–8.

[10] Morgan R, Belli A. Current treatment methods for postcatheterization pseudoaneurysms. J Vasc Interv Radiol 2003;14(6):697–710.

[11] Brancatelli G, Katyal S, Federle MP, et al. Three-dimensional multislice helical computed tomography with the volume rendering technique in the detection of vascular complications after liver transplantation. Transplantation 2002;73(2):237–42.

[12] Crossin JD, Muradali D, Wilson SR. US of liver transplants: normal and abnormal. Radiographics 2003;23(5):1093–114.

[13] Knisley BL, Mastey LA, Collins J, et al. Imaging of cardiac transplantation complications. Radiographics 1999;19(2):321–39.

[14] Kwon JH, Kim GS. Obstetric iatrogenic arterial injuries of the uterus: diagnosis with US and treatment with transcatheter arterial embolization. Radiographics 2002;22(1):35–46.

[15] Mita T, Arita T, Matsunaga N, et al. Complications of endovascular repair for thoracic and abdominal aortic aneurysm: an imaging spectrum. Radiographics 2000;20(5):1263–78.

[16] Busquets AR, Acosta JA, Colon E, et al. Helical computed tomographic angiography for the diagnosis of traumatic arterial injuries of the extremities. J Trauma 2004;56(3):625–8.

[17] Sugg SL, Gerndt SJ, Hamilton BJ, et al. Pseudoaneurysms of the intraparenchymal splenic artery after blunt abdominal trauma: a complication of nonoperative therapy and its management. J Trauma 1995;39(3):593–5.

[18] Shanmuganathan K, Mirvis SE, Boyd-Kranis R, et al. Nonsurgical management of blunt splenic injury: use of CT criteria to select patients for splenic arteriography and potential endovascular therapy. Radiology 2000;217(1):75–82.

[19] Mallek R, Mostbeck G, Gebauer A, et al. A posttraumatic pseudoaneurysm of the hepatic artery. Duplex sonographic diagnosis and follow up in spontaneous thrombosis. Radiology 1990; 30(10):484–8.

[20] Soudack M, Epelman M, Gaitini D. Spontaneous thrombosis of hepatic posttraumatic pseudoaneurysms. sonographic and computed tomographic features. Case report. J Ultrasound Med 2003;22(1):99–103.

[21] La Perna L, Olin JW, Goines D, et al. Ultrasound-guided thrombin injection for the treatment of postcatheterization pseudoaneurysms. Circulation 2000;102(19):2391–5.

[22] McDermott VG, Shlansky-Goldberg R, Cope C. Endovascular management of splenic artery aneurysms and pseudoaneurysms. Cardiovasc Intervent Radiol 1994;17(4):179–84.

[23] Okuno A, Miyazaki M, Ito H, et al. Nonsurgical management of ruptured pseudoaneurysm in patients with hepatobiliary pancreatic diseases. Am J Gastroenterol 2001;96(4):1067–71.

[24] Guillon R, Gracier JM, Abergel A, et al. Management of splenic artery aneurysms and false aneurysms with endovascular treatment in 12 patients. Cardiovasc Intervent Radiol 2003;26(3):256–60.

[25] Yamakado K, Nakatsuka A, Tanaka N, et al. Transcatheter arterial embolization of ruptured pseudoaneurysms with coils and n-butyl cyanoacrylate. J Vasc Interv Radiol 2000;11(1):66–72.

[26] Polak JF. The peripheral arteries. In: Rumack CM, Wilson SR, Charboneau JW, editors. Diagnostic ultrasound. 3rd edition. Philadelphia: Elsevier, Mosby; 2005. p. 993–1018.

[27] Tessier DJ, Stone WM, Fowl RJ, et al. Clinical features and management of splenic artery pseudoaneurysm: case series and cumulative review of literature. J Vasc Surg 2003;38(5):969–74.

[28] Katz DS, Hon M. CT angiography of the lower extremities and aortoiliac system with a multidetector row helical CT scanner: promise of new opportunities fulfilled. Radiology 2001;221(1):7–10.

[29] Katyal S, Oliver III JH, Buck DG, et al. Detection of vascular complications after liver transplantation:early experience in multislice CT angiography with volume rendering. AJR Am J Roentgenol 2000;175(6):1735–9.

[30] Ricci MA, Trevisani GT, Pilcher DB. Vascular complications of cardiac catheterization. Am J Surg 1994;167(4):375–8.

[31] Steinkamp HJ, Werk M, Felix R. Treatment of postinterventional pseudoaneurysms by ultrasound-guided compression. Invest Radiol 2000; 35(3):186–92.

[32] Friedman SG, Pellerito JS, Scher L, et al. Ultrasound-guided thrombin injection is the treatment of choice for femoral pseudoaneurysms. Arch Surg 2002;137(4):462–4.

[33] Kumins NH, Landau DS, Montalvo J, et al. Expanded indications for the treatment of postcatheterization femoral pseudoaneurysms with ultrasound-guided compression. Am J Surg 1998; 176(2):131–6.

[34] Patel JV, Weston MJ, Kessel DO, et al. Hepatic artery pseudoaneurysm after liver transplantation: treatment with percutaneous thrombin injection. Case report. Transplantation 2003; 75(10):1755–7.

[35] Lennox AF, Delis KT, Szendro G, et al. Duplex-guided thrombin injection for iatrogenic femoral artery pseudoaneurysm is effective even in anticoagulated patients. Br J Surg 2000;87(6): 796–801.

[36] Badran MF, Gould DA, Sampson C, et al. Transluminal occlusion of a pseudoaneurysm arising from a thoracic aortic graft patch using catheter delivery of thrombin. J Vasc Interv Radiol 2003; 14(9, Part 1):1201–5.

[37] Thalhammer C, Kirchherr AS, Uhlich F, et al. Postcatheterization pseudoaneurysm and arteriovenous fistulas: repair with percutaneous implantation of endovascular covered stents. Radiology 2000;214(1):127–31.

[38] Bergert H, Hinterseher I, Kersting S, et al. Management and outcome of hemorrhage due to arterial pseudoaneurysms in pancreatitis. Surg 2005;137(3):323–8.

[39] Sadiq S, Ibrahim W. Thromboembolism complicating thrombin injection of femoral artery pseudoaneurysm: management with intraarterial thrombolysis. Case report. J Vasc Interv Radiol 2001;12(5):633–6.

[40] Fellmeth BD, Roberts AC, Bookstein JJ, et al. Postangiographic femoral artery injuries: nonsurgical repair with US-guided compression. Radiology 1991;178(3):671–5.

[41] Paulson EK, Sheafor DH, Kliewer MA, et al. Treatment of iatrogenic femoral arterial pseudoaneurysms: comparison of US-guided thrombin injection with compression repair. Radiology 2000;215(2):403–8.

[42] Gale SS, Scissons RP, Jones L, et al. Femoral pseudoaneurysm thrombinjection. Am J Surg 2001; 181(4):379–83.

[43] Brophy DP, Sheiman RG, Amatulle P, et al. Iatrogenic femoral pseudoaneurysms: thrombin injection after failed US-guided compression. Radiology 2000;214(1):278–82.

[44] Cope C, Zeit R. Coagulation of aneurysms by direct percutaneous thrombin injection. AJR Am J Roentgenol 1986;147(2):383–7.

[45] Kang SS, Labropoulos N, Mansour MA, et al. Expanded indications for ultrasound-guided thrombin injection of pseudoaneurysms. J Vasc Surg 2000;31(2):289–98.

[46] Kurz DJ, Jungius K, Luscher TF. Delayed femoral vein thrombosis after ultrasound-guided thrombin injection of a postcatheterization pseudoaneurysm. Case report. J Vasc Interv Radiol 2003; 14(8):1067–70.

[47] Sheldon PJ, Oglevie SB, Kaplan LA. Prolonged generalized urticarial reaction after percutaneous thrombin injection for treatment of a femoral artery pseudoaneurysm. Case report. J Vasc Interv Radiol 2000;11(6):759–61.

[48] Krysl J, Kumpe D. Embolization agents: a review. Tech Vasc Interv Radiol 2000;3:158–61.

[49] Aziz N, Lenzi TA, Jeffrey Jr RB, et al. Postpartum uterine arteriovenous fistula. Obstet Gynecol 2004;103(5, Part 2):1076–8.

[50] Lay JP, Swainson CJ, Sukumar SA. Paradoxical pulmonary embolism secondary to aortocaval fistula: diagnosis by helical CT. Br J Radiol 1999; 72(857):507–9.

[51] Wang EA, Lee MH, Wang MC, et al. Iatrogenic left iliac-caval fistula: imaging and endovascular treatment. AJR Am J Roentgenol 2004;183(4): 1032–4.

[52] Nair R, Chetty R, Woolgar J, et al. Spontaneous arteriovenous fistula resulting from HIV arteritis. J Vasc Surg 2001;33(1):186–7.

[53] Puppinck P, Chevalier J, Ducasse E, et al. Connection between a long-standing traumatic arteriovenous fistula and development of aneurysmal disease. Ann Vasc Surg 2004;18(5):604–7.

[54] Chauvapun JP, Caty MG, Harris LM. Renal arteriovenous aneurysm in a 4-year-old patient. J Vasc Surg 2005;41(3):535–8.

[55] Hartung O, Garcia S, Alimi YS, et al. Extensive arterial aneurysm developing after surgical closure of long-standing post-traumatic popliteal arteriovenous fistula. J Vasc Surg 2004;39(4): 889–92.

[56] Ray C. Complications of percutaneous transluminal angioplasty. In: Darcy MD, Vedantham S, Kaufman JA, editors. SCVIR syllabus: peripheral vascular interventions. 2nd edition. Fairfax (VA): The Society of Cardiovascular & Interventional Radiology; 2001. p. 81–90.

[57] Rose SC, Nelson TR. Ultrasonographic modalities to assess vascular anatomy and disease [review]. J Vasc Interv Radiol 2004;15(1, Part 1):25–38.

[58] Chavan A, Harms J, Picjlmayr R, et al. Transcatheter coil occlusion of an intrahepatic arterioportal fistula in a transplanted liver. Bildgebung 1993;60:215–8.

[59] Strodel E, Eckhauser FE, Lemmer JH, et al. Presentation and perioperative management of arterioportal fistulas. Arch Surg 1987;122:563–71.

[60] Glockner JF, Forauer AR. Vascular or ischemic complications after liver transplantation: pictorial essay. AJR Am J Roentgenol 1999;173:1055–9.

[61] Sprouse II LR, Hamilton Jr IN. The endovascular treatment of a renal arteriovenous fistula: placement of a covered stent. J Vasc Surg 2002;36(5): 1066–8.

ULTRASOUND
CLINICS

Ultrasound Clin 1 (2006) 201–221

Doppler Imaging of the Uterus and Adnexae

Shweta Bhatt, MD, Vikram S. Dogra, MD*

- Normal uterine and ovarian vascular anatomy
- Sonographic technique
- Uterine pathologies
  Leiomyoma
  Color flow Doppler to assess leiomyomas
  Vascular bridging sign
  Vascular pedicle sign
  Uterine artery embolization
  Pre-embolization evaluation
  Postembolization evaluation
- Adenomyosis
  Uterine artery embolization in adenomyosis
- Endometrial polyps
- Endometrial carcinoma
- Vascular abnormalities of the endometrium
  Arteriovenous malformation
  Uterine artery aneurysm
  Uterine artery pseudoaneurysm
- Gestational trophoblastic disease
  Molar pregnancy
  Persistent trophoblastic neoplasia (invasive mole)
- Abnormal placentation
  Placenta accreta, increta, and percreta
  Vasa previa
  Retained products of conception
- Ovarian pathologies
  Torsion
  Twisted vascular pedicle/whirlpool sign
  Subtorsion of the ovary
- Massive ovarian edema
- Ectopic pregnancy
- Ovarian vein thrombosis
- Ovarian malignancy
- Summary
- References

Pelvic sonography constitutes a major proportion of the routine and the emergency ultrasound (US) examinations performed. Application of color Doppler US in addition to gray-scale imaging helps in the characterization of uterine and adnexal masses. Color flow Doppler imaging has a definitive role in the diagnosis and management of uterine leiomyomas (including arterial embolization), ovarian torsion, placental abnormalities, vascular malformations, and uterine artery aneurysms. This article describes the normal CFD features of uterine and ovarian vessels and the usefulness of color flow Doppler sonography in the evaluation of uterine and ovarian abnormalities.

Normal uterine and ovarian vascular anatomy

The uterus derives its main arterial supply from the uterine artery, a branch of the anterior division of the internal iliac artery [**Fig. 1**]. Transvaginal (TV) and transabdominal color Doppler sonography

Department of Radiology, University of Rochester School of Medicine and Dentistry, 601 Elmwood Avenue, Box 648, Rochester, NY 14642, USA
* Corresponding author.
E-mail address: Vikram_Dogra@URMC.Rochester.edu (V.S. Dogra).

1556-858X/06/$ – see front matter © 2005 Elsevier Inc. All rights reserved.
ultrasound.theclinics.com

doi:10.1016/j.cult.2005.09.010

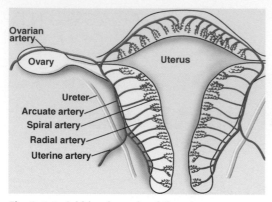

Fig. 1. Arterial blood supply of the uterus.

(CDS) can depict the origin of the uterine artery that runs medially on the levator ani to a point approximately 2 cm from the cervix where it crosses over the ureter to become medial to it [1]. The uterine artery ascends along the margin of the uterus in the broad ligament up to the uterine cornua where it courses laterally to the hilum of the ovary to join the ovarian artery. Branches arise from the main uterine arteries and penetrate the outer myometrium, forming a spoke wheel configuration of arcuate vessels [2]. Right and left uterine artery branches anastomose in the midline through the arcuate vessels, located between the outer and middle layers of the myometrium. The radial branches of the uterine artery course through the myometrium and form the basal and spiral arterioles within the endometrium [2]. The uterine plexus of veins accompanies the arcuate arteries and is larger than the associated arterial channels [1]. Doppler waveforms of uterine artery flow typically have a high-velocity, high-resistance pattern [3] with an identifiable dicrotic notch [Fig. 2]. Persistence of the dicrotic notch beyond 23 weeks of pregnancy is suggestive of intrauterine growth retar-

dation. Flow characteristics in the arcuate artery may also vary during pregnancy with lower resistive indices in placental than in nonplacental sites [4].

The ovary has a dual arterial supply through the ovarian artery and the adnexal branches of the uterine artery [Fig. 3]. Ovarian arteries arise laterally from the aorta inferior to the origin of the renal arteries. They cross the external iliac arteries and veins at the pelvic brim and course medially within the suspensory ligament of the ovary and then pass posteriorly in the meso-ovarium [1]. The right ovarian (gonadal) vein drains into the inferior vena cava (IVC), and the left ovarian vein drains into the left renal vein. Doppler waveforms of the ovarian arteries show physiologic variations within the menstrual cycle. The dormant ovary in the menstrual cycle has a low-flow (high resistive index [RI]) pattern throughout the menstrual cycle, whereas the dominant ovary demonstrates a high-flow (low RI) pattern [Fig. 4]. This pattern coincides with the luteinizing hormone surge that increases through the periovulatory period and remains at this level for 4 to 5 days after ovulation into the luteal phase of the cycle. Ovarian blood flow then gradually returns to a high-resistance pattern during the menstrual period [3,5,6].

Sonographic technique

On TV color and pulsed Doppler, the uterine artery can be sampled along the lateral aspect of the uterine body at the level of the corporocervical junction. The arcuate branches can be sampled anywhere within the myometrium [4,7].

The ovarian artery should be sampled in the infundibulopelvic ligament or from the intraovarian vessels for the best quantitative information [5]. Resistive and pulsatility indices are used to quantitate the blood flow in the ovary. RI is defined as

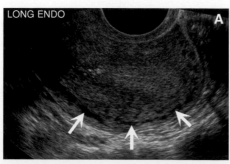
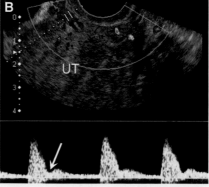

Fig. 2. Normal uterine arterial Doppler. (*A*) Longitudinal endovaginal gray-scale sonogram of uterus (UT) demonstrates normal arcuate vessels (*arrows*). (*B*) CFD image with spectral analysis of uterine artery reveals normal high-velocity, high-resistance waveform with dicrotic notch (*arrow*).

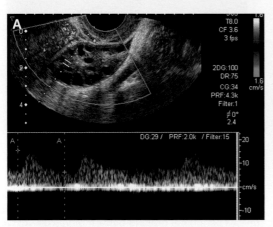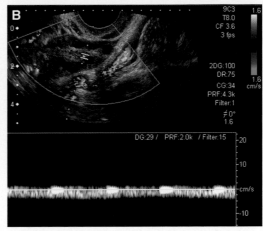

Fig. 3. Normal arterial and venous ovarian Doppler. (*A*) Normal arterial and (*B*) venous Doppler waveforms of the ovarian vessels.

(peak systolic velocity [PSV] − end diastolic velocity [EDV]) ÷ PSV and the pulsatility index (PI) is defined as (PSV − EDV) ÷ mean velocity.

Color Doppler parameters should be optimized to detect flow, to avoid a mistaken diagnosis of torsion or thrombosis. These parameters are summarized in Table 1. Power Doppler may be used for better detection of flow. Pros and cons of the use of power Doppler compared with color Doppler are listed in Box 1.

Uterine pathologies

Leiomyoma

Uterine leiomyomas, also called myomas or fibroids, are the most common gynecologic disease involving the uterus; they occur in 20% to 25% of women over 30 years of age [8,9].

Leiomyomas are classified depending on their location in the uterus. Subserosal leiomyomas are the exophytic fibroids that protrude from the outer surface of the uterus. Leiomyomas create a uterine contour abnormality and may mimic an adnexal mass. They may be pedunculated; if they are large they are prone to torsion [10]. Intramural leiomyomas, the most common type, are located within the myometrium. Submucosal leiomyomas are subendometrial and may protrude into the endometrial cavity. Most fibroids are hypoechoic, well-circumscribed masses, often with attenuation and shadowing. As they become more complex, their interfaces and, thus, their echogenicity increases.

When uterine leiomyomas increase in size, they may outgrow their blood supply and undergo various types of degeneration, such as hyaline or myxoid degeneration, calcification, cystic degeneration, and red degeneration [11]. The sonographic ap-

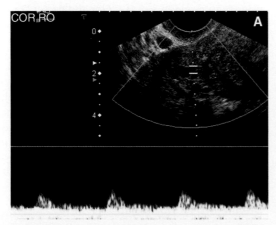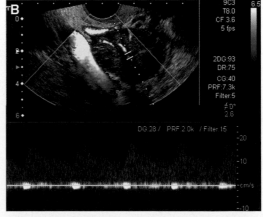

Fig. 4. Cyclical normal variation on ovarian arterial Doppler. Spectral Doppler waveform of (*A*) right ovary (dormant ovary for this menstrual cycle), demonstrates low-flow (high-resistance, RI = 0.75) pattern compared with high-flow (low-resistance, RI = 0.375) pattern seen in left ovary (*B*) (dominant ovary for this menstrual cycle).

Table 1: Optimizing color flow Doppler image

Color box	Keep color box small to improve frame rate and obtain better color resolution
Doppler gain	Set just below noise level
Color scale (PRF)	Low PRF is more sensitive to low-flow vessels but may lead to aliasing
Beam steering	Adjust to obtain satisfactory vessel angle (ie, not 90°)
Gate size (sample volume)	Set sample volume to correct size, usually two-thirds of the vessel lumen
Wall filter	High filter cuts out noise and slower flow states. Keep filter at 50–100 Hz
Focal zone	Color flow image is optimized at focal zone, so place where vessels are expected

Abbreviation: PRF, pulse repetition frequency.

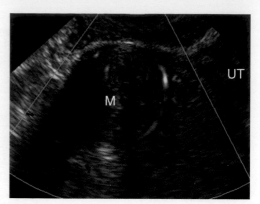

Fig. 5. Power Doppler image of uterus demonstrates leiomyoma (M) arising from the uterus (UT), which reveals peripheral draping pattern of vascularity typical of leiomyoma.

pearance of the fibroids may vary accordingly, demonstrating hypo- to anechoic areas as a result of cystic degeneration or bright hyperechoic areas with sharp acoustic shadowing in calcified leiomyomas [10].

Color flow Doppler to assess leiomyomas

Depiction of fibroid vascularity by CDS improves the delineation of the size, location, and extent of myometrial involvement [12]. Leiomyomas usually demonstrate a peripheral rim of vascularity in the pseudocapsule (covering almost three fourth circumference); this feature helps to identify isoechoic intramural myomas and aids in the diagnosis of subserosal myomas [**Fig. 5**] [2]. In addition, demonstration of a vascular bridging sign (VBS) or a vascular pedicle between the uterus and the peri-uterine mass helps to discriminate a subserosal leiomyoma from a true adnexal mass. Color flow Doppler US also has a significant role in evaluating patients for uterine artery embolization (UAE) pre- and postprocedure.

Box 1: Power Doppler versus color Doppler

1. No directional information is obtained with power Doppler.
2. Power Doppler is more susceptible to motion artifact than color Doppler.
3. Power Doppler has better sensitivity to low flows than CFD.
4. Power Doppler has less temporal resolution as a result of longer acquisition times (more frame averages).

Vascular bridging sign

A large subserosal leiomyoma may mimic a solid or heterogeneous ovarian mass, whereas the former is benign, the latter may be malignant, and the patient management is different. The presence of multiple vessels between the uterus and the presumed adnexal mass is called the VBS. The VBS is secondary to recruitment of multiple vessels feeding the exophytic uterine fibroid [**Fig. 6**] and confirms the origin of the vascular blood supply to uterine fibroids from the uterine arteries, implying that the tissue is uterine, not ovarian. Kim and colleagues [13] first demonstrated the VBS in MRI of leiomyomas whereby the bridging vessels appeared as tortuous channels with no signal connecting the uterus and the pelvic mass. In another study comparing CDS and MRI for differentiating subserosal myomas from extra-uterine tumors, the VBS was present in 39 out of 41 subserosal myomas and in 3 out of 27 extra-uterine tumors when using both modalities [14]. Color and power Doppler US alone have 100% sensitivity and 92% specificity for differentiating subserosal leiomyomas from extra-uterine tumors [14].

Vascular pedicle sign

Color flow Doppler may also demonstrate a solitary vessel originating from the uterine artery that supplies the subserosal leiomyoma, called the vascular pedicle sign [**Fig. 7**]. As with the VBS, demonstrating a common source of blood supply between the mass and the uterus implies the origin of the mass is from the uterus.

Uterine artery embolization

UAE of uterine fibroids is a minimally invasive alternative to surgical therapy (hysterectomy or myomectomy). The use of UAE in the treatment of

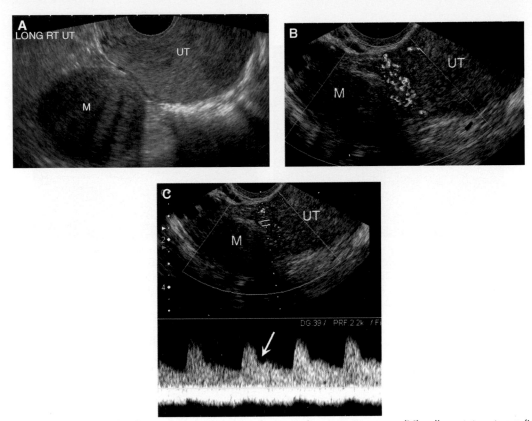

Fig. 6. VBS. (*A*) Longitudinal gray-scale sonogram of uterus demonstrates mass (M) adjacent to uterus (UT). Corresponding color (*B*) and spectral Doppler (*C*) demonstrate vascular bridge between mass and uterus, which has identical spectral waveform as uterine artery with dicrotic notch (*arrow*), suggesting common blood supply. This was confirmed to be exophytic leiomyoma.

uterine fibroids as an alternative to surgical treatment was first proposed by Ravina and colleagues [15] in 1995. Originally, UAE was used before myomectomy to reduce intraoperative bleeding and also to treat post-partum hemorrhage [16]. As a single therapeutic regimen for fibroids, UAE has been reported to be a safe and successful method to reduce fibroid-induced symptoms including bleeding, urinary frequency, and pelvic pain [17–19]. Suc-

cessful pregnancies have been reported in patients who have undergone UAE [19]; however, these pregnancies were shown to have an increased risk for preterm delivery and malpresentation [20].

Pre-embolization evaluation

Imaging parameters used to predict the effectiveness of UAE, are baseline uterine volume, baseline leiomyoma volume and location, and the number

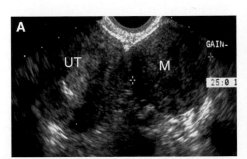
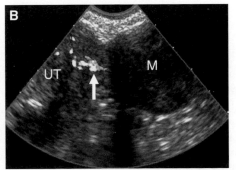

Fig. 7. Vascular pedicle sign. (*A*) Transverse gray-scale sonogram of uterus demonstrates mass (M) adjacent to uterus (UT). (*B*) Corresponding Doppler image demonstrates vascular pedicle sign (*arrow*).

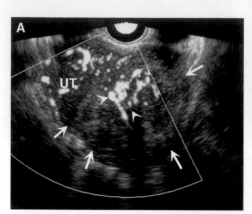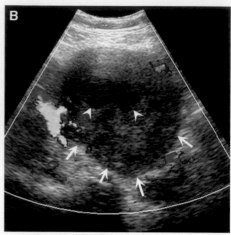

Fig. 8. UAE. (*A*) Power Doppler imaging of uterus before embolization shows fibroid (*arrows*) nearly isoechoic with uterus (UT) and has marked peripheral vascularity (*arrowheads*). (*B*) Three months after UAE, leiomyoma (*arrows*) has no vascularity and has cystic necrosis (*arrowheads*). (*From* Nicolson TA, Pelage JP, Ettles DF. Fibroid calcification after uterine artery embolization: ultrasonographic appearance and pathology. J Vasc Interv Radiol 2001;12:443–6; with permission.)

of leiomyomas. Spies [21] demonstrated that myomas with a larger baseline volume showed less symptomatic improvement and less reduction in size after UAE. The number of leiomyomas is not considered a strong predictor of efficacy of UAE; however, in Spies' study, patients who presented with two to five leiomyomas showed a better symptomatic response to therapy than patients who presented with a single leiomyoma or more than five leiomyomas [21]. The size of uterine leiomyomas remains controversial as a determining factor in the outcome of UAE; however, a size greater than 8 cm is a predictor of UAE failure. Submucosal leiomyomas have the best outcome after UAE [21]. Pedunculated and subserosal fibroids are considered unsuitable for UAE [22].

Doppler examination of overall tumor vascularity predicts therapeutic outcome. Hypervascular fibroids show more reduction in size than isovascular and hypovascular fibroids [12]. Doppler flow measurements can be used to assess UAE outcome also. McLucas and colleagues [23] reported that patients presenting with fibroids that had a PSV greater than 64 cm/s were more likely to have UAE failure, emphasizing the use of Doppler flow studies in screening for UAE.

Postembolization evaluation

MRI and color Doppler US have proven to be excellent modalities for postprocedural follow-up after UAE [24,25]. Follow-up sonographic examination is performed at 1, 3, 6, and 9 months, and 1 year after UAE [17]. Fibroid volume (size) and vascularity have been used as parameters to evaluate the therapeutic efficacy of UAE [26]. CDS depicted that along with the reduction in the fibroid volume, disappearance of the intrafibroid vessels occurred without affecting uterine vascularity [27]. Shrinkage of the fibroids continues to take place over a period of several months, peaking between 3 and 6 months after UAE, with measurable shrinkage sometimes noted for as long as 1 year [28,29]. Weintraub and colleagues [30] reported that postprocedure sonographic imaging showed decreased uterine size and echogenicity. Concomitantly, color Doppler imaging showed a marked decrease in the blood flow to the leiomyoma [**Fig. 8**]. US also may depict peripheral calcification in the fibroid after UAE, occurring as a result of aggregation of the polyvinyl alcohol particles in the peripheral tumoral arteries [31]. Gadolinium-enhanced MRI is a useful diagnostic technique to assess uterine fibroids after UAE because it can evaluate the degree of infarction in the treated tumors [32].

Adenomyosis

Adenomyosis is a benign condition of the uterus characterized by the presence of endometrial glands and stroma in the myometrium, identified on imaging by the distortion of the endometrial-myometrial junctional zone and the asymmetry of the uterus [33]. Diffuse adenomyosis appears on US as uterine enlargement with a globular configuration, heterogeneous-appearing myometrium, and subendometrial cysts [34–36]. The RI in adenomyosis is usually less than 0.7, suggesting an abnormal flow (normal RI = > 0.7) [37]. Unlike myomas, which have a peripheral blood supply, adenomyosis may be distinguished on imaging by its "rain-

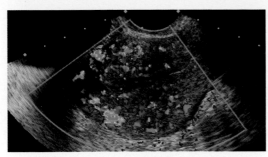

Fig. 9. Adenomyosis. Spectral Doppler evaluation of adenomyosis reveals globular configuration of uterus with increased central vascularity. RI in this patient was 0.54.

drop" appearance of blood flowing through the center of the tissue [Fig. 9]. Surrounding tissue unaffected by adenomyosis remains mostly hypovascular [23]. The PI of the arteries within or around the adenomyosis tissue is usually greater than 1.17, whereas leiomyomas have a PI of less than or equal to 1.17 [38]. The overall sensitivity and specificity of TV US for the diagnosis of adenomyosis is considered to be 80% to 86% and 50% to 96%, respectively [39].

Uterine artery embolization in adenomyosis

UAE has been proposed as an alternative to surgery for patients who present with menorrhagia as a result of adenomyosis. The success rate of UAE for controlling long-term symptoms of menorrhagia is higher (50%) in patients presenting with coexisting myomas with adenomyosis but less than in myomas alone (90%) [40]. Doppler measurement of PSV greater than 64cm/s is predictive of UAE failure in adenomyosis and leiomyomas [23]. Significant improvement of clinical symptoms following UAE correlates well with gray-scale US and CDS findings. Clinical improvement is associated with decreased uterine size, decreased vascularity, and reduced junctional zone thickness [41]. A decrease in the vascularity of normal myometrium and the adenomyosis tissue is observed during

the initial, 1-week, postembolization period, with restoration of normal myometrial vessels on the 3-month follow-up imaging [42]. Although the short-term results (3–6 months) of embolization seem to be good [43,44], the mid-term (2 years) results are not as encouraging [45]. In patients who present with pure adenomyosis, only 56% of patients demonstrated a complete resolution of adenomyosis at the 24-month follow-up after UAE as reported by Pelage and colleagues [45]. Patients who present with failed UAE in adenomyosis usually undergo hysterectomy [46].

Endometrial polyps

Endometrial polyps are intracavitatory lesions seen in peri- and postmenopausal women who present often with uterine bleeding. Polyps may be pedunculated, broad-based, or have a thin stalk. Twenty percent of these polyps are multiple. The diagnosis of an endometrial polyp is considered when hyperechoic endometrial thickening of greater than 5 mm is observed on US. Color Doppler or power Doppler imaging enable easy detection of endometrial polyps by demonstrating a single feeding artery known as the pedicle sign [Fig. 10] [47]. Observation of the feeding artery in a polyp may help to distinguish endometrial polyp from a submucosal fibroid [48]. Timmerman and colleagues [49] defined the pedicle sign as the presence of an artery within the central portion of the polyp. Using these criteria, the sensitivity of the pedicle artery sign in diagnosing an endometrial polyp on endovaginal sonography was 76%, the specificity was 95%, and the negative predictive value was 94% [49]. In more recent study comparing transvaginal color Doppler (TVCD) with sonohysterography (SHG), the sensitivity and specificity for TVCD using the pedicle artery sign for identifying endometrial polyps, was 95% and 80%, respectively. The specificity was low because of two false negative cases. Overall, TVCD has comparable efficacy to SHG in diagnosing endometrial polyps [50].

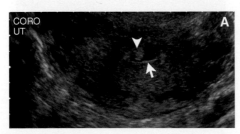
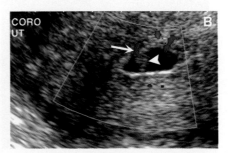

Fig. 10. Pedicle artery sign in endometrial polyp. (*A*) Coronal section of uterus on endovaginal sonography, demonstrates endometrial mass lesion (*arrowhead*) surrounded by fluid within endometrial cavity (*arrow*). Corresponding CFD image (*B*) reveals solitary vessel (*arrow*) supplying polyp (*arrowhead*).

Endometrial carcinoma

Endometrial carcinoma is the most common gynecologic malignancy in North America, occurring most commonly in postmenopausal women and manifesting as uterine bleeding, with increased incidence in women on replacement hormonal therapy. Histologically, almost all endometrial carcinomas are adenocarcinomas; typical endometrioid adenocarcinomas are the most common subtype of endometrial carcinomas followed by adenocarcinomas with squamous elements. Other less common subtypes include clear cell, serous, secretory, mucinous, and squamous carcinomas, but imaging characteristics cannot predict the histology of these cancers [51].

Sonographically, a considerable overlap exists between the morphologic characteristics of benign and malignant endometrial neoplasms. A thickened endometrium (>8 mm) in a postmenopausal woman must be considered malignant until proven otherwise. Malignancy is considered more likely when the endometrial thickening or mass is of heterogeneous echotexture with irregular borders [51,52]. Numerous studies on the use of color Doppler imaging in endometrial neoplasms have yielded variable results.

CDS depicts vessels in benign and malignant endometrial lesions. Endometrial carcinomas show an increased number of feeding vessels with moderate vascularity in the mass lesion [53–55]. Irregular and randomly dispersed vessels with complex branching in an endometrial lesion also favor malignancy [56]. Doppler indices may have a significant role in suggesting malignancy. The mean RI in the uterine artery in a normal postmenopausal woman, is 0.93 plus or minus 0.09 [57]. Low-impedance flow with a RI of less than 0.5 and a PI of less than 1, have been positively associated with the presence of malignancy [58]. Significantly lower RIs are noticed in endometrial cancers of higher histologic grade and those with lymph node metastasis [59]. An intratumoral RI of less than 0.4 has a high incidence of pelvic nodal metastasis [60,61]. A combination of transvaginal sonography and CDS can be useful in differentiating benign and malignant endometrial lesions; however, endometrial biopsy still remains the gold standard for diagnosing endometrial carcinoma.

Vascular abnormalities of the endometrium

Uterine vascular lesions are rare but may be life-threatening. They usually manifest as unexplained vaginal bleeding, occasionally massive in amount. Color Doppler US with spectral analysis is helpful in diagnosis.

Arteriovenous malformation

Uterine arteriovenous malformations (AVMs) consist of a vascular plexus of arteries and veins without an intervening capillary network. They are located in the myometrium and do not regress spontaneously with time [52,62]. AVMs may be congenital but are more commonly acquired following uterine trauma (eg, curettage, pelvic surgery,

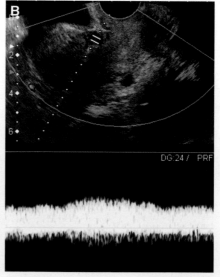
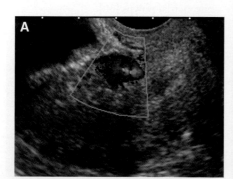

Fig. 11. (*A*) Uterine AVM. CFD image of uterus, demonstrates focal area of mosaic red and blue pattern of color signal in uterus. Corresponding spectral Doppler waveform (*B*) reveals a high velocity venous waveform suggestive of an arterio-venous malformation.

and previous treatment for gestational trophoblastic disease [GTD]). Color Doppler US in the sonographic evaluation of any unexplained cystic mass in the uterus significantly increases the detection rate of uterine AVMs [63].

The gray-scale US morphology of uterine AVM is nonspecific and may present as a hypoechoic or heterogeneous area or as multiple contiguous distinct anechoic areas in the myometrium. Color Doppler findings are more consistent and specific and include intense multidirectional turbulent flow typified by aliasing [**Fig. 11**] [52,64,65]. Spectral analysis characteristically depicts a low-resistance, high-velocity arterial flow with a low RI in the range of 0.25 to 0.55 [62]. PSV recorded within the AVM is also usually high in the range of 40 to 100 cm/s [62,65,66]. Three-dimensional power Doppler sonography provides additional use in the evaluation of uterine vascular AVMs by depicting a clearer view of the orientation of the tortuous vessels comprising the AVM. Doppler US also is used to monitor the AVMs for response or recurrence after embolization [65].

Uterine artery aneurysm

Uterine artery aneurysms are rare. A true uterine artery aneurysm is usually congenital and may manifest as uterine bleeding from rupture during pregnancy or in the puerperium [64]. On gray-scale US, a uterine artery aneurysm is a pulsating anechoic structure in the myometrium. Doppler US diagnoses the aneurysm with high sensitivity and specificity by depicting the dilatation of the uterine artery with its characteristic arterial flow pattern [64]. UAE is an effective treatment modality for uterine artery aneurysms and CDS can be used for monitoring postembolization.

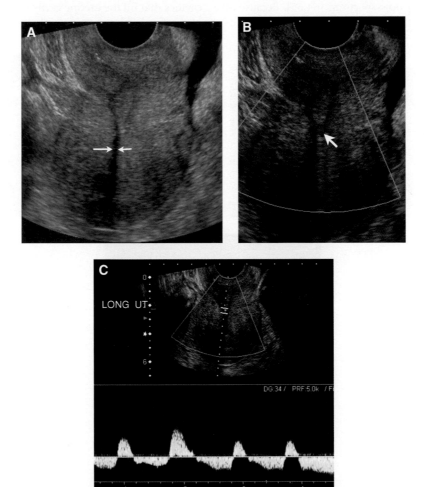

Fig. 12. Pseudoaneurysm of uterine artery. (*A*) Longitudinal section of uterus on endovaginal sonography reveals retroverted uterus with absent endometrial lining (*arrows*). Corresponding color (*B*) and spectral (*C*) Doppler images demonstrate focal area of color signal (*arrow*) in endometrium (aliasing was observed on real-time imaging) with to-and-fro spectral waveform suggestive of pseudoaneurysm resulting from thermal ablation.

Uterine artery pseudoaneurysm

A pseudoaneurysm is an extraluminal collection of blood with turbulent flow that communicates with the parent vessel through a defect in the arterial wall [67]. A pseudo-aneurysm differs from a true aneurysm because of the absence of the three layers of a vessel wall [68–70]. Uterine artery pseudoaneurysm is a rare vascular abnormality but is seen more commonly than an aneurysm. It usually arises as a complication after pelvic surgery or trauma and can be diagnosed by arteriography or, noninvasively, by CDS. CDS shows a blood-filled cystic structure with varying colors caused by the swirling movement of the arterial blood in different directions [**Fig. 12**]. Spectral analysis within the sac demonstrates turbulent multidirectional arterial flow. In the neck of the pseudoaneurysm, the blood flowing into the aneurysm in systole and out in diastole creates a characteristic bidirectional flow spectrum [64,65]. Because of the small size of the uterine artery, it may be diffi-

cult to visualize the neck of the pseudoaneurysm, and in such instances, arteriography is more useful [68].

Gestational trophoblastic disease

Molar pregnancy

GTD is a spectrum of disorders that show abnormal trophoblastic proliferation with a progressive malignant potential [71,72]. GTD includes molar pregnancy (MP) (complete and partial), invasive mole, choriocarcinoma, and placental site trophoblastic tumors (PSTT).

MP is the most common and benign form of GTD. Depending on the severity of trophoblastic proliferation and the presence or absence of fetal tissue, it may be complete or partial MP [72]. Typically, gray-scale sonography reveals abnormal hyperechoic placental tissue with cystic grapelike cavities that fill the uterine cavity [73]. Proliferation of the trophoblastic tissue with abnormal vascular

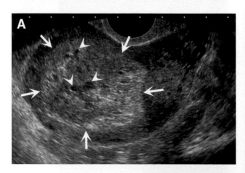
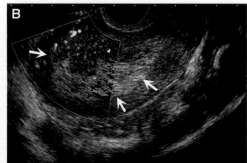
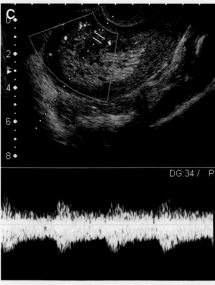

Fig. 13. Hydatiform mole. (*A*) Longitudinal gray-scale sonography of uterus demonstrates large hyperechoic mass (*arrows*) with cystic spaces (*arrowheads*) filling uterine cavity. Corresponding power (*B*) and spectral (*C*) Doppler images reveal increased vascularity with high-velocity, low-resistance waveform pattern with RI of 0.35.

shunting (or abnormal vessels) results in a high-velocity, low-impedance flow on Doppler US in the first and early second trimesters [**Fig. 13**] [71]. The RI usually measures less than 0.4 compared with 0.66 in normal pregnancy [71].

Doppler findings confirm the diagnosis combined with the elevated human chorionic gonadotropin (hCG) level and the gray-scale US findings.

Persistent trophoblastic neoplasia (invasive mole)

Persistent trophoblastic neoplasia (PTN) is a broad term that includes invasive mole (the most common), choriocarcinoma, and PSTT; it is suggested clinically by a persistent elevation of the hCG after evacuation of MP. Sonographic and Doppler findings cannot differentiate between the three entities.

The most commonly described sonographic findings in PTN are focal echogenic myometrial nodules or a bulky enlarged uterus [74–76]. Color Doppler interrogation reveals marked hypervascularity of the invasive trophoblast with extensive color aliasing within the myometrium. Spectral tracings reveal low-resistance arterial flow within the myometrium suggesting an invasion of the trophoblastic disease [77–79]. Doppler indices in PTN include a high PSV, usually greater than 50cm/s, and a low RI, often less than 0.4 (normal myometrial blood flow PSV is less than 50 cm/s with an RI of approximately 0.6–0.7) [72,77]. Doppler imaging may define the extent of invasion in an invasive mole and also its subsequent response to chemotherapy [80]. Although the trophoblastic signals on spectral Doppler are not unique to PTN, clinical correlation with an elevated hCG level and with gray-scale sonographic findings are virtually diagnostic of PTN.

Abnormal placentation

Placenta accreta, increta, and percreta

Placenta accreta is defined as a condition in which the placental tissue extends from the endometrium into the myometrium (minimal invasion). Placenta increta refers to the extension of the placenta deeper into the myometrium but confined to the myometrium. Placenta percreta is the severest form with extension of the placenta beyond the myometrium. Most of the published literature refers to these abnormalities collectively as placenta accreta [81,82]. Previous uterine surgery is a predisposing factor for these abnormal placental attachments [83]. The prenatal diagnosis of abnormal placentae is critical to avoid postpartum hemorrhage.

Color flow Doppler of placenta accreta demonstrates several placental lacunae with a highly pul-

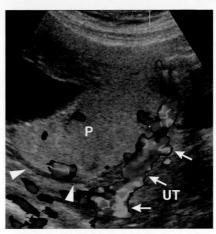

Fig. 14. Placenta accreta. Longitudinal CFD image of placenta (P) demonstrates thinning of retroplacental hypoechoic zone (*arrowheads*). CFD US demonstrates enlarged abnormal vessels (*arrows*) invading adjacent uterus (UT). (*From* Taipale P, Orden MR, Berg M, et al. Prenatal diagnosis of placenta accreta and percreta with ultrasonography, color Doppler, and magnetic resonance imaging. Obstet Gynecol 2004;104:537–40; with permission.)

satile venous flow pattern that extends from the placenta into the surrounding myometrium. Progressive thinning also occurs and disappearance of the retroplacental hypoechoic zone representing the decidua basalis [**Fig. 14**] [84–87]. Placenta accreta is found commonly in association with placenta previa [86,88]. On postpartum US, cessation of blood flow between the basal placenta and the myometrium is the sonographic hallmark of normal placental separation. Persistent blood flow demonstrated by CDS is suggestive of placenta accreta. [89]. Color Doppler has 100% sensitivity and 94% specificity to detect placenta accreta [86].

Placenta increta appears on US as an echogenic mass within the myometrium; isoechoic to the placenta. Multiple large vessels exist within the mass, which does not extend to the serosal margin of the uterus [90]. Placenta percreta is diagnosed by the interruption of the hyperechoic line between the uterine serosa and the bladder and by the presence of multiple lacunae in the myometrium. Placent percreta has the worst prognosis. A patient death caused by air embolism has been described with placenta percreta extension into the bladder [91]. Placenta percreta may more commonly result in uterine rupture [92,93].

Vasa previa

Vasa previa is defined as umbilical vessels that cross the internal os and are not supported by the placenta or the umbilical cord [**Fig. 15**]. Fail-

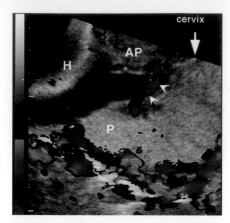

Fig. 15. Vasa previa. Sagittal CFD image of lower uterine segment demonstrates posteriorly located marginal placenta (P). Vessels (red and blue) (*arrowheads*) are seen communicating with accessory placental lobe (AP) across internal os (arrow points to cervix. H = fetal head). (*From* Taipale P, Orden MR, Berg M, et al. Prenatal diagnosis of placenta accreta and percreta with ultrasonography, color Doppler, and magnetic resonance imaging. Obstet Gynecol 2004;104: 537–40; with permission.)

ure to diagnose vas previa antenatally results in catastrophic hemorrhage following rupture of the membranes with near 100% mortality of the fetus [82]. Vasa previa is associated strongly with unusual placental findings, such as a bilobed placenta, succenturiate lobe, placenta previa, or a velamentous cord insertion [94,95]. Other risk factors include low-lying placenta in the second trimester,

multiple pregnancies, and in vitro fertilization [96–98]. Documentation of the placental cord insertion should be a part of the standard obstetric examination to identify those at risk for vasa previa [99]. Judicious use of CDS in these patients can help establish the antenatal diagnosis of vasa previa and reduce mortality by performing elective cesarean section. Transperineal sonography with Doppler evaluation may also identify vasa previa [100].

Retained products of conception

Retained products of conception (RPOC) is a well-known complication of spontaneous or induced abortion. The diagnosis usually is based on the sonographic appearance of intrauterine echogenic material. A high false-positive rate is reported from clinical and sonographic diagnosis, leading to repeated curettage of the endometrial cavity, which has immediate and long-term complications, such as perforation, bleeding, infertility and adhesions [101]. Although a focal echogenic mass in the endometrium on gray-scale US is the most useful finding to predict the presence of RPOC [102,103], such a mass may also represent a blood clot or residual decidua. Doppler US can be helpful these situations. Depiction of flow in the echogenic mass within the endometrium favors RPOC and excludes a blood clot [104]. High-velocity, low-resistance flow on color Doppler US is suspicious for RPOC [**Fig. 16**] but does not exclude GTD. The two are discriminated by clinical history of recent abortion with negative or declining beta-hCG level. A PSV

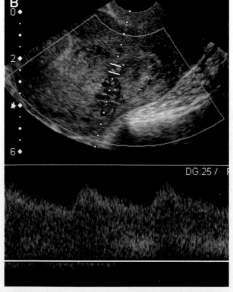

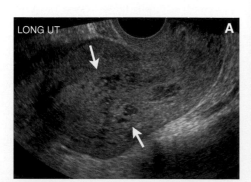

Fig. 16. Retained products of conception. (*A*) Longitudinal gray-scale US of uterus demonstrates wide endometrium with heterogeneous-appearing contents (*arrows*). (*B*) Corresponding spectral Doppler evaluation demonstrates increased vascularity in this heterogeneous area with low-resistance waveform pattern typical of trophoblastic flow.

of 21 cm/s is used as the minimum threshold for the diagnosis of residual trophoblastic tissue [105]; however, the lack of increased flow does not eliminate the possibility of RPOC. In a study by Alcazar and colleagues, abundant endometrial or myometrial flow with an RI of less than 0.45 had a sensitivity of 93% and specificity of 96% for RPOC [106]; however, low-impedance peritrophoblastic flow also can be observed after abortion even when products of conception are absent [107].

Ovarian pathologies

Torsion

Ovarian torsion accounts for about 3% of the gynecologic emergencies presenting with acute, severe, unilateral pain. Torsion most frequently involves the ovary and the fallopian tube with the broad ligament acting as the fulcrum, and is appropriately termed adnexal torsion [108]. Ovarian torsion frequently is associated with an ipsilateral benign ovarian mass but most commonly with a mature cystic teratoma [109]. Sonographic features of ovarian torsion are not sensitive and cannot lead to the diagnosis without clinical suspicion. Grayscale findings of a midline enlarged ovary plus or minus a coexistent mass, peripheral ovarian follicles (the "string of pearls" sign) [110], pelvic free fluid, and CFD findings of completely absent arterial and venous ovarian blood flow are specific for ovarian torsion [**Fig. 17**]; however, arterial and venous flow have been documented in the torsed ovary. Evidence of flow within the ovary does not exclude ovarian torsion. The presence of a dual blood supply to the ovary (through the ovarian and the adnexal branches of the uterine artery) is responsible for the variable Doppler findings in adnexal torsion. Technical errors with improper settings of the color flow parameters may result in a false positive diagnosis of adnexal torsion [111]. CFD may identify the twisted vascular pedicle sign or whirlpool sign [112].

> **Box 2: Sonographic findings in ovarian torsion**
>
> **Gray-scale US features**
> - Midline enlarged ovary superior to fundus of uterus
> - "String of pearls" sign
> - Coexistent mass within the torsed ovary
> - Free pelvic fluid
> - Extra-ovarian echogenic, target-appearing mass = twisted vascular pedicle
>
> **Color flow Doppler features**
> - Arterial and venous flow absent (diagnostic)
> - Arterial and venous flow present (does not exclude the diagnosis of torsion)
> - Arterial flow present, venous flow absent
> - Arterial flow absent, venous flow present
> - "Whirlpool sign" in the twisted vascular pedicle

Twisted vascular pedicle/whirlpool sign

A twisted vascular pedicle appears on sonography as a round, echogenic, extraovarian mass with multiple concentric, internal hypoechoic stripes, wrapping around a central axis, giving a target appearance. On CDS, these intrapedicular hypoechoic structures are identified as vessels, confirming the twisted vascular pedicle and the resultant adnexal torsion. The color Doppler "whirlpool sign" is similar to the whirlpool sign described with malrotation of the midgut with volvulus [113,114]. The presence of a whirlpool sign also indicates the potential viability of the ovary preoperatively [109,112,115]. The presence of flow should be documented in the artery and the vein in the vascular pedicle. Documentation of intraovarian central venous flow is also essential to establish the viability of the torsed ovary [116]. Intermittent absence of blood flow in the vascular pedicle can be visualized during episodes of pain brought on by intermittent episodes of incomplete torsion [115]. Flow returns when the pain is relieved. Use

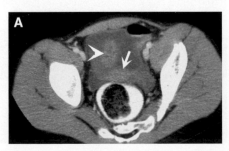
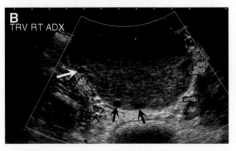

Fig. 17. Ovarian torsion. (*A*) Contrast-enhanced axial CT scan through pelvis demonstrates enlarged ovary (*arrowhead*) located in midline superior to fundus of uterus (*arrow*). CFD US (*B*) was performed because of suspicion of ovarian torsion and revealed enlarged ovary with absent blood flow and with peripherally arranged epithelial cysts (*arrows*), confirming diagnosis of ovarian torsion.

of intravenous US contrast medium improves demonstration of altered flow patterns in ischemic adnexae secondary to torsion, allowing a more confident diagnosis [117]. The sonographic findings in ovarian torsion are summarized in **Box 2**.

Subtorsion of the ovary

Subtorsion of the ovary is an early stage of torsion consequent to incomplete vessel occlusion (torsion of <360°) concomitant with a normal ovarian appearance on sonography [118]. Recognizing impending torsion of the ovary at this stage is important so that appropriate detorsion methods can be initiated to salvage the ovary before ischemia sets in. On sonography, a twisted vascular pedicle cannot be identified in subtorsion. Unilateral, congested periovarian vessels in the presence of a normal ovarian morphology and blood supply in an appropriate clinical setting, indicate subtorsion of the ovary [119].

Massive ovarian edema

Massive ovarian edema is a rare condition characterized by massive enlargement of one or both ovaries secondary to partial torsion of the ovary occluding venous and lymphatic drainage but sparing the arteries. Chronic venous and lymphatic obstruction results in marked stromal edema resulting in severe ovarian enlargement [52]. It is usually unilateral and more commonly involves the right ovary [120]. On gray-scale sonography, massive ovarian edema appears as a heterogeneous mass with cystic components [120]. Color and

pulsed Doppler demonstrate the presence of flow in the pedicle of the ovary; therefore, Doppler imaging cannot diagnose massive ovarian edema.

Ectopic pregnancy

Ectopic pregnancy (EP) is one of the most common gynecologic emergencies, presenting as vaginal bleeding and abdominal pain. Sonographically, the presence of an extra-ovarian thick-walled adnexal mass called the tubal ring is the most common feature of an EP [121,122]; however, in a pregnant patient, an exophytic corpus luteal cyst (CLC) may be mistaken for an EP [123]. The sonographer or the radiologist should identify an adnexal mass as a CLC or an EP, particularly in the absence of a sonographically visible intrauterine pregnancy so that appropriate management can be planned. EP and CLC demonstrate abundant vascularity in the periphery of the tubal ring [124] known as a "ring of fire" on color flow imaging [**Fig. 18**]. A "ring of fire" is a nonspecific sign and can also be seen around a mature ovarian follicle or a hemorrhagic cyst. Various studies have shown an overlap between the RIs of EPs and CLCs, but, in general, EPs show lower RIs [125]. In his recent study, Atri and colleagues[125] showed that low (<0.39) and high (>0.7) RIs can represent EP and were specific for an EP (100% specificity and positive predictive value). A higher RI suggests the presence of less active trophoblasts and, therefore, seems to be a predictor of spontaneous resolution of the EP [126]. Color Doppler evaluation of the endometrium may help discriminate between EP and CLC. EPs may also show endometrial blood flow but the RI is usually

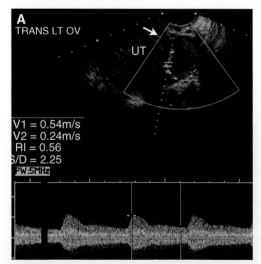
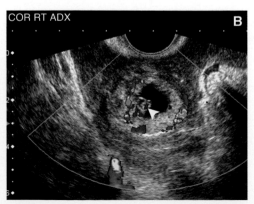

Fig. 18. Ring of fire. (A) CFD image of left adnexa in patient presenting with intrauterine pregnancy, demonstrates exophytic CLC with "ring of fire" sign. Adjacent ovarian tissue is compressed (UT, uterus). (B) CFD image of right adnexa demonstrates "ring of fire" sign in EP (live EP with cardiac pulsations visualized as red color signal, *arrowhead*).

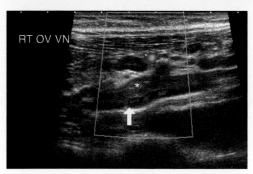

Fig. 19. Ovarian vein thrombosis. CFD image of right ovarian vein (*arrow*), demonstrates echogenic thrombus (*) which partially occludes vessel. Some flow (blue) exists adjacent to thrombus. This patient presented with right lower quadrant pain.

greater than 0.55 and the PSV is less than 15 cm/s [127,128]. Demonstration of the presence of trophoblastic tissue in the endometrium, even in the absence of a visible double decidual sac, is suggestive of an intrauterine pregnancy and excludes EP. Trophoblastic tissue is identified by the detection of a low-resistance flow in the endometrium with RI less than 0.55 and a PSV equal to or greater than 15cm/s [127]. Low resistance in the trophoblastic tissue is explained by the absence of smooth muscles in the walls of intervillous spaces.

Ovarian vein thrombosis

Ovarian vein thrombosis or thrombophlebitis, a rare condition, is seen during the postpartum period; it results from venous stasis and the spread of bacterial infection from endometritis. It commonly involves the right ovarian vein (90% cases) [52]

and mimics acute appendicitis on clinical presentation [129]. CDS is the favored initial diagnostic procedure, with CT being a supplementary tool [129]. Color Doppler imaging demonstrates the ovarian vein running cephalad and lateral to the uterus, with hypoechoic to echogenic thrombus, and absent or partially obstructed flow [Fig. 19]. The thrombus usually involves the junction of the right ovarian vein with the IVC or extends into the IVC [130]. Color Doppler imaging also can be used to follow ovarian vein thrombosis after anticoagulant therapy to demonstrate resolution of the thrombus.

Ovarian malignancy

Ovarian cancer is the fourth leading cause of cancer deaths among women in the United States and comprises 25% of gynecologic malignancies in the United States [52]. The clinician should identify whether an adnexal mass is a benign or a malignant tumor so that appropriate treatment can be planned. Ovarian masses less than 5cm in long axis are generally benign, whereas those greater than 10cm are more likely to be malignant. Imaging plays a major role in differentiating these masses, and CDS serves as the main initial modality for lesion characterization.

The two Doppler angle-independent indices, RI and PI, predominantly have been used to differentiate malignant from benign adnexal masses. Malignant masses usually have a low PI (< 1.0) and RI (<0.4) [131,132], but an overlap of these values has been noted [133]. In addition, lack of detectable flow by color Doppler US does not exclude ovarian malignancy [134].

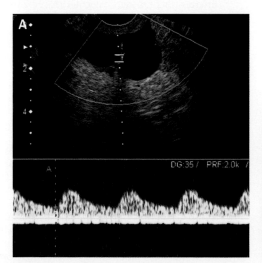

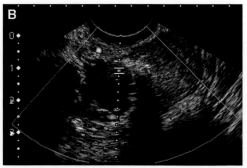

Fig. 20. Ovarian malignancy. (*A*) CFD image of right adnexa with spectral analysis, demonstrates complex ovarian mass with blood flow in septae with low-resistance waveform pattern. (*B*) Power Doppler image in another patient with ovarian malignancy demonstrates tumor vascularity in mural nodules.

> **Box 3: Sonographic findings in ovarian malignancy**
>
> - > 10 cm size
> - Increased vascularization
> - PI < 1.0, RI < 0.4
> - End diastolic velocity distribution slope of 1.90 ± 1.33
> - Shorter uptake and longer washout time of US contrast

Malignant masses are characterized typically by centrally located vessels that have low-impedance flow without a diastolic "notch" [**Fig. 20**] [135]. The decay constant of the Doppler waveform, which characterizes its decrease from systole to diastole as an exponential decay, has been recently presented as an additional measure of tumor malignancy [136]. In their study, Shaharabany and colleagues designed a new parameter characterizing the slope of the mean velocity spectrum at end-diastole (or "end diastolic velocity distribution slope" [DVD_S]). This parameter provides much better results than those obtained with previously used variables in the detection of malignancy. The mean DVD_S value for malignant tumors is 1.90 plus or minus 1.33 compared with 9.21 plus or minus 5.34 for benign masses (area under reciever operating characteristic curve = 0.983) and yields a detection rate of approximately 94% [136]. CDS and gray-scale sonography together with serum cancer antigen [CA]-125 levels still have a better sensitivity and specificity for diagnosing ovarian malignancy than CDS alone [137–140]; however, in the future, vascular analysis may be more useful because of the advent of US contrast media. Increased vessel number is a hallmark of malignant tumors. Contrast-enhanced sonography increases the accuracy to discriminate benign from malignant ovarian tumors by demonstrating a higher number of vessels in malignant lesions [141]. The kinetic properties of contrast agents, such as a shorter contrast uptake time and a longer washout time, also have the potential to diagnose malignant ovarian tumors successfully [142]. The degree, onset, and duration of Doppler signal enhancement after US contrast injection, are, therefore, supplemental to CDS for the diagnosis of malignant ovarian tumors [143]. The sonographic features of an ovarian malignancy are summarized in **Box 3**.

Summary

CFD is performed routinely in all patients who present with pelvic pain. CFD and power Doppler sonography in combination with gray-scale imaging and clinical history helps in characterization and localization of uterine and ovarian masses. CFD has a specific role in leiomyomas, in the diagnosis and the management. Subserosal leiomyomas are distinguished from adnexal masses by demonstrating a VBS or a vascular pedicle between the uterus and the peri-uterine mass. UAE is a minimally invasive therapy for leiomyomas. CFD plays an important role in pre-UAE evaluation to predict the efficacy of the procedure and also in monitoring the response post-UAE. Endometrial thickening can be categorized as an endometrial polyp or malignancy with the help of CFD by identifying the pedicle artery sign in an endometrial polyp. Diagnosis of MP, RPOC and placental abnormalities are aided by CFD findings with clinical correlation. CFD findings may be variable in some cases of ovarian torsion but clinical correlation may lead to the correct diagnosis. Other adnexal lesions, such as EP and ovarian malignancy may be diagnosed with CFD in the appropriate clinical setting. CFD of the uterus and adnexae in combination with gray- scale findings and clinical correlation leads to the correct diagnosis in most patients presenting with acute pelvic pain.

References

[1] Holt SC, Levi CS, Lyons EA. Normal anatomy of the female pelvis. In: Callen PW, editor. Ultrasonography in obstetrics and gynecology. 3rd edition. Philadelphia: WB Saunders; 1994. p. 548–68.

[2] Fleischer AC. Color Doppler sonography of uterine disorders. Ultrasound Q 2003;19:179–89.

[3] Taylor K, Burns PN, Wells PN. Ultrasound Doppler flow studies of the ovarian and uterine arteries. Br J Obstet Gynecol 1985;92:240–6.

[4] Fleischer AC, Goldstein RB, Bruner JP, et al. Doppler sonography in obstetrics and gynecology. In: Callen PW, editor. Ultrasonography in obstetrics and gynecology. 3rd edition. Philadelphia: WB Saunders; 1994. p. 503–23.

[5] Ritchie WGM. Ultrasound evaluation of normal and induced ovulation. In: Callen PW, editor. Ultrasonography in obstetrics and gynecology. 3rd edition. Philadelphia: WB Saunders; 1994. p. 569–85.

[6] Fleischer AC, Brader KR. Sonographic depiction of ovarian vascularity and flow: current improvements and future applications. J Ultrasound Med 2001;20:241–50.

[7] Pellizzari P, Esposito C, Siliotti F, et al. Colour Doppler analysis of ovarian and uterine arteries in women with hypoestrogenic amenorrhoea. Hum Reprod 2002;17:3208–12.

[8] Schwartz SM. Epidemiology of uterine leiomyomata. Clin Obstet Gynecol 2001;44:316–26.

[9] Tsuda H, Kawabata M, Nakamoto O, et al. Clinical predictors in the natural history of

uterine leiomyoma: preliminary study. J Ultrasound Med 1998;17:17–20.

[10] Kurtz AB, Middleton WD. Pelvis and uterus. In: Kurtz AB, Middleton WD, editors. Ultrasound: the requisites. New York: Taylor & Francis Inc.; 2003. p. 530–57.

[11] Murase E, Siegelman ES, Outwater EK, et al. Uterine leiomyomas: histopathologic features, MR imaging findings, differential diagnosis, and treatment. Radiographics 1999;19:1179–97.

[12] Fleischer AC, Donnelly EF, Campbell MG, et al. Three-dimensional color Doppler sonography before and after fibroid embolization. J Ultrasound Med 2000;19:701–5.

[13] Kim JC, Kim SS, Park JY. "Bridging vascular sign" in the MR diagnosis of exophytic uterine leiomyoma. J Comput Assist Tomogr 2000;24: 57–60.

[14] Kim SH, Sim JS, Seong CK. Interface vessels on color/power Doppler US and MRI: a clue to differentiate subserosal uterine myomas from extrauterine tumors. J Comput Assist Tomogr 2001;25:36–42.

[15] Ravina JH, Herbreteau D, Ciraru-Vigneron N, et al. Arterial embolisation to treat uterine myomata. Lancet 1995;346:671–2.

[16] Heaston DK, Mineau DE, Brown BJ, et al. Transcatheter arterial embolization for control of persistent massive puerperal hemorrhage after bilateral surgical hypogastric artery ligation. AJR Am J Roentgenol 1979;133:152–4.

[17] Ravina JH, Aymard A, Ciraru-Vigneron N, et al. [Uterine fibroids embolization: results about 454 cases]. Gynecol Obstet Fertil 2003;31:597–605.

[18] Brunereau L, Herbreteau D, Gallas S, et al. Uterine artery embolization in the primary treatment of uterine leiomyomas: technical features and prospective follow-up with clinical and sonographic examinations in 58 patients. AJR Am J Roentgenol 2000;175:1267–72.

[19] Pron G, Mocarski E, Bennett J. Pregnancy after uterine artery embolization for leiomyomata: the Ontario multicenter trial. Obstet Gynecol 2005;105:67–76.

[20] Goldberg J, Pereira L, Berghella V, et al. Pregnancy outcomes after treatment for fibromyomata: uterine artery embolization versus laparoscopic myomectomy. Am J Obstet Gynecol 2004;191:18–21.

[21] Spies JB, Roth AR, Jha RC, et al. Leiomyomata treated with uterine artery embolization: factors associated with successful symptom and imaging outcome. Radiology 2002;222:45–52.

[22] Walker WJ, Pelage JP, Sutton C. Fibroid embolization. Clin Radiol 2002;57:325–31.

[23] McLucas B, Perrella R, Goodwin S, et al. Role of uterine artery Doppler flow in fibroid embolization. J Ultrasound Med 2002;21:113–20.

[24] Pelage JP, Guaou NG, Jha RC, et al. Uterine fibroid tumors: long-term MR imaging outcome after embolization. Radiology 2004;230: 803–9.

[25] Pron G, Mocarski E, Bennett J, et al. Tolerance, hospital stay, and recovery after uterine artery embolization for fibroids: the Ontario Uterine Fibroid Embolization Trial. J Vasc Interv Radiol 2003;14:1243–50.

[26] Muniz CJ, Fleischer AC, Donnelly EF, et al. Three-dimensional color Doppler sonography and uterine artery arteriography of fibroids: assessment of changes in vascularity before and after embolization. J Ultrasound Med 2002;21: 129–33.

[27] Tranquart F, Brunereau L, Cottier JP, et al. Prospective sonographic assessment of uterine artery embolization for the treatment of fibroids. Ultrasound Obstet Gynecol 2002;19: 81–7.

[28] Lipman JC, Smith SJ, Spies JB, et al. IV. Uterine fibroid embolization: follow-up. Tech Vasc Interv Radiol 2002;5:44–55.

[29] Walker WJ, Pelage JP. Uterine artery embolisation for symptomatic fibroids: clinical results in 400 women with imaging follow up. BJOG 2002;109:1262–72.

[30] Weintraub JL, Romano WJ, Kirsch MJ, et al. Uterine artery embolization: sonographic imaging findings. J Ultrasound Med 2002;21: 633–7.

[31] Nicholson TA, Pelage JP, Ettles DF. Fibroid calcification after uterine artery embolization: ultrasonographic appearance and pathology. J Vasc Interv Radiol 2001;12:443–6.

[32] Katsumori T, Nakajima K, Tokuhiro M. Gadolinium-enhanced MR imaging in the evaluation of uterine fibroids treated with uterine artery embolization. AJR Am J Roentgenol 2001;177: 303–7.

[33] Azziz R. Adenomyosis: current perspectives. Obstet Gynecol Clin North Am 1989;16:221–35.

[34] Bohlman ME, Ensor RE, Sanders RC. Sonographic findings in adenomyosis of the uterus. AJR Am J Roentgenol 1987;148:765–6.

[35] Reinhold C, Atri M, Mehio A, et al. Diffuse uterine adenomyosis: morphologic criteria and diagnostic accuracy of endovaginal sonography. Radiology 1995;197:609–14.

[36] Reinhold C, McCarthy S, Bret PM, et al. Diffuse adenomyosis: comparison of endovaginal US and MR imaging with histopathologic correlation. Radiology 1996;199:151–8.

[37] Hata T, Hata K, Senoh D, et al. Doppler ultrasound assessment of tumor vascularity in gynecologic disorders. J Ultrasound Med 1989;8: 309–14.

[38] Chiang CH, Chang MY, Hsu JJ, et al. Tumor vascular pattern and blood flow impedance in the differential diagnosis of leiomyoma and adenomyosis by color Doppler sonography. J Assist Reprod Genet 1999;16:268–75.

[39] Reinhold C, Tafazoli F, Mehio A, et al. Uterine adenomyosis: endovaginal US and MR imaging features with histopathologic correlation. Radiographics 1999;19 Spec No:S147–60.

[40] McLucas B, Perrella R. Adenomyosis: MRI of the uterus treated with uterine artery embolization. AJR Am J Roentgenol 2004;182:1084–5.

[41] Siskin GP, Tublin ME, Stainken BF, et al. Uterine artery embolization for the treatment of adenomyosis: clinical response and evaluation with MR imaging. AJR Am J Roentgenol 2001; 177:297–302.

[42] Liu P, Chen C, Liu L, et al. [Investigation of the hemodynamic changes during uterine arterial embolization in the treatment of adenomyosis]. Zhonghua Fu Chan Ke Za Zhi 2002;37:536–8.

[43] Jha RC, Takahama J, Imaoka I, et al. Adenomyosis: MRI of the uterus treated with uterine artery embolization. AJR Am J Roentgenol 2003; 181:851–6.

[44] Kim MD, Won JW, Lee DY, et al. Uterine artery embolization for adenomyosis without fibroids. Clin Radiol 2004;59:520–6.

[45] Pelage JP, Jacob D, Fazel A, et al. Midterm results of uterine artery embolization for symptomatic adenomyosis: initial experience. Radiology 2005;234:948–53.

[46] McLucas B, Adler L, Perrella R. Uterine fibroid embolization: nonsurgical treatment for symptomatic fibroids. J Am Coll Surg 2001;192:95–105.

[47] Jakab A, Ovari L, Juhasz B, et al. Detection of feeding artery improves the ultrasound diagnosis of endometrial polyps in asymptomatic patients. Eur J Obstet Gynecol Reprod Biol 2005; 119:103–7.

[48] Fleischer AC, Shappell HW. Color Doppler sonohysterography of endometrial polyps and submucosal fibroids. J Ultrasound Med 2003; 22:601–4.

[49] Timmerman D, Verguts J, Konstantinovic ML, et al. The pedicle artery sign based on sonography with color Doppler imaging can replace second-stage tests in women with abnormal vaginal bleeding. Ultrasound Obstet Gynecol 2003;22:166–71.

[50] Alcazar JL, Galan MJ, Minguez JA, et al. Transvaginal color Doppler sonography versus sonohysterography in the diagnosis of endometrial polyps. J Ultrasound Med 2004;23:743–8.

[51] Reinhold C, Khalili I. Postmenopausal bleeding: value of imaging. Radiol Clin North Am 2002; 40:527–62.

[52] Salem S, Wilson SR. Gynecologic ultrasound. In: Rumack CM, Wilson SR, Charboneau JW, editors. 3rd edition. Diagnostic ultrasound, Vol 2. St. Louis (MO): Elsevier, Mosby; 2004. p. 527–87.

[53] Aleem F, Predanic M, Calame R, et al. Transvaginal color and pulsed Doppler sonography of the endometrium: a possible role in reducing the number of dilatation and curettage procedures. J Ultrasound Med 1995;14:139–45.

[54] Carter J, Saltzman A, Hartenbach E, et al. Flow characteristics in benign and malignant gynecologic tumors using transvaginal color flow Doppler. Obstet Gynecol 1994;83:125–30.

[55] Alcazar JL, Castillo G, Minguez JA, et al. Endometrial blood flow mapping using transvaginal power Doppler sonography in women with postmenopausal bleeding and thickened endometrium. Ultrasound Obstet Gynecol 2003; 21:583–8.

[56] Kurjak A, Kupesic S. Three dimensional ultrasound and power doppler in assessment of uterine and ovarian angiogenesis: a prospective study. Croat Med J 1999;40:413–20.

[57] Bonilla-Musoles F, Marti MC, Ballester MJ, et al. Normal uterine arterial blood flow in postmenopausal women assessed by transvaginal color Doppler ultrasonography. J Ultrasound Med 1995;14:491–4.

[58] Alcazar JL, Galan MJ, Jurado M, et al. Intratumoral blood flow analysis in endometrial carcinoma: correlation with tumor characteristics and risk for recurrence. Gynecol Oncol 2002; 84:258–62.

[59] Lee CN, Cheng WF, Chen CA, et al. Angiogenesis of endometrial carcinomas assessed by measurement of intratumoral blood flow, microvessel density, and vascular endothelial growth factor levels. Obstet Gynecol 2000;96: 615–21.

[60] Cheng WF, Chen CA, Lee CN, et al. Preoperative ultrasound study in predicting lymph node metastasis for endometrial cancer patients. Gynecol Oncol 1998;71:424–7.

[61] Cheng WF, Chen TM, Chen CA, et al. Clinical application of intratumoral blood flow study in patients with endometrial carcinoma. Cancer 1998;82:1881–6.

[62] Ghi T, Giunchi S, Rossi C, et al. Three-dimensional power Doppler sonography in the diagnosis of arteriovenous malformation of the uterus. J Ultrasound Med 2005;24: 727–31.

[63] Damani N, Wilson SR. Nongynecologic applications of transvaginal US. Radiographics 1999; 19 Spec No:S179–200.

[64] Polat P, Suma S, Kantarcy M, et al. Color Doppler US in the evaluation of uterine vascular abnormalities. Radiographics 2002;22:47–53.

[65] Kwon JH, Kim GS. Obstetric iatrogenic arterial injuries of the uterus: diagnosis with US and treatment with transcatheter arterial embolization. Radiographics 2002;22:35–46.

[66] Huang MW, Muradali D, Thurston WA, et al. Uterine arteriovenous malformations: gray-scale and Doppler US features with MR imaging correlation. Radiology 1998;206:115–23.

[67] Henrich W, Fuchs I, Luttkus A, et al. Pseudoaneurysm of the uterine artery after cesarean delivery: sonographic diagnosis and treatment. J Ultrasound Med 2002;21:1431–4.

[68] Langer JE, Cope C. Ultrasonographic diagnosis of uterine artery pseudoaneurysm after hysterectomy. J Ultrasound Med 1999;18:711–4.

[69] Laubach M, Delahaye T, Van Tussenbroek F, et al. Uterine artery pseudo-aneurysm: diagnosis

and therapy during pregnancy. J Perinat Med 2000;28:321–5.

[70] Lee WK, Roche CJ, Duddalwar VA, et al. Pseudoaneurysm of the uterine artery after abdominal hysterectomy: radiologic diagnosis and management. Am J Obstet Gynecol 2001;185: 1269–72.

[71] Zhou Q, Lei XY, Xie Q, et al. Sonographic and Doppler imaging in the diagnosis and treatment of gestational trophoblastic disease: a 12-year experience. J Ultrasound Med 2005; 24:15–24.

[72] Fraser-Hill F, Wilson SR. Gestational trophoblastic neoplasia. In: Rumack CM, Wilson SR, Charboneau JW, editors. 3rd edition. Diagnostic ultrasound, Vol 2. St. Louis (MO): Elsevier, Mosby; 2004. p. 589–601.

[73] Dogra V, Paspulati RM, Bhatt S. First trimester bleeding evaluation. Ultrasound Q 2005;21: 69–85.

[74] Fleischer AC, James Jr AE, Krause DA, et al. Sonographic patterns in trophoblastic diseases. Radiology 1978;126:215–20.

[75] Soper JT. Identification and management of high-risk gestational trophoblastic disease. Semin Oncol 1995;22:172–84.

[76] Mangili G, Spagnolo D, Valsecchi L, et al. Transvaginal ultrasonography in persistent trophoblastic tumor. Am J Obstet Gynecol 1993;169: 1218–23.

[77] Taylor KJ, Schwartz PE, Kohorn EI. Gestational trophoblastic neoplasia: diagnosis with Doppler US. Radiology 1987;165:445–8.

[78] Desai RK, Desberg AL. Diagnosis of gestational trophoblastic disease: value of endovaginal color flow Doppler sonography. AJR Am J Roentgenol 1991;157:787–8.

[79] Carter J, Fowler J, Carlson J, et al. Transvaginal color flow Doppler sonography in the assessment of gestational trophoblastic disease. J Ultrasound Med 1993;12:595–9.

[80] Paspulati RM, Bhatt S, Nour S. Sonographic evaluation of first-trimester bleeding. Radiol Clin North Am 2004;42:297–314.

[81] Avva R, Shah HR, Angtuaco TL. US case of the day. Placenta increta. Radiographics 1999;19: 1089–92.

[82] Lazebnik N, Lazebnik RS. The role of ultrasound in pregnancy-related emergencies. Radiol Clin North Am 2004;42:315–27.

[83] Taipale P, Orden MR, Berg M, et al. Prenatal diagnosis of placenta accreta and percreta with ultrasonography, color Doppler, and magnetic resonance imaging. Obstet Gynecol 2004;104: 537–40.

[84] Hoffman-Tretin JC, Koenigsberg M, Rabin A, et al. Placenta accreta. Additional sonographic observations. J Ultrasound Med 1992;11:29–34.

[85] Rosemond RL, Kepple DM. Transvaginal color Doppler sonography in the prenatal diagnosis of placenta accreta. Obstet Gynecol 1992;80: 508–10.

[86] Lerner JP, Deane S, Timor-Tritsch IE. Characterization of placenta accreta using transvaginal sonography and color Doppler imaging. Ultrasound Obstet Gynecol 1995;5:198–201.

[87] Levine D, Hulka CA, Ludmir J, et al. Placenta accreta: evaluation with color Doppler US, power Doppler US, and MR imaging. Radiology 1997;205:773–6.

[88] Miller DA, Chollet JA, Goodwin TM. Clinical risk factors for placenta previa-placenta accreta. Am J Obstet Gynecol 1997;177:210–4.

[89] Krapp M, Baschat AA, Hankeln M, et al. Gray scale and color Doppler sonography in the third stage of labor for early detection of failed placental separation. Ultrasound Obstet Gynecol 2000;15:138–42.

[90] Finberg HJ, Williams JW. Placenta accreta: prospective sonographic diagnosis in patients with placenta previa and prior cesarean section. J Ultrasound Med 1992;11:333–43.

[91] Megier P, Du Rouchet E, Desroches A, et al. [Prenatal diagnosis of a placenta praevia percreta with color Doppler. A case report. Review of the literature]. J Gynecol Obstet Biol Reprod (Paris) 1994;23:315–7.

[92] Passini Jr R, Knobel R, Barini R, et al. Placenta percreta with silent rupture of the uterus. Sao Paulo Med J 1996;114:1270–3.

[93] Mathieu E, Dufour P, Ernoult P, et al. [Uterine rupture after twenty-two weeks of amenorrhea due to placenta praevia percreta. A case report]. Rev Fr Gynecol Obstet 1995;90:228–32.

[94] Lee W, Lee VL, Kirk JS, et al. Vasa previa: prenatal diagnosis, natural evolution, and clinical outcome. Obstet Gynecol 2000;95:572–6.

[95] Stafford IP, Neumann DE, Jarrell H. Abnormal placental structure and vasa previa: confirmation of the relationship. J Ultrasound Med 2004; 23:1521–2.

[96] Oyelese KO, Turner M, Lees C, et al. Vasa previa: an avoidable obstetric tragedy. Obstet Gynecol Surv 1999;54:138–45.

[97] Oyelese Y, Spong C, Fernandez MA, et al. Second trimester low-lying placenta and in-vitro fertilization? Exclude vasa previa. J Matern Fetal Med 2000;9:370–2.

[98] Schachter M, Tovbin Y, Arieli S, et al. In vitro fertilization is a risk factor for vasa previa. Fertil Steril 2002;78:642–3.

[99] Sepulveda W, Rojas I, Robert JA, et al. Prenatal detection of velamentous insertion of the umbilical cord: a prospective color Doppler ultrasound study. Ultrasound Obstet Gynecol 2003; 21:564–9.

[100] Hertzberg BS, Kliewer MA. Vasa previa: prenatal diagnosis by transperineal sonography with Doppler evaluation. J Clin Ultrasound 1998;26: 405–8.

[101] Sadan O, Golan A, Girtler O, et al. Role of sonography in the diagnosis of retained products of conception. J Ultrasound Med 2004; 23:371–4.

[102] Achiron R, Goldenberg M, Lipitz S, et al. Trans-vaginal duplex Doppler ultrasonography in bleeding patients suspected of having residual trophoblastic tissue. Obstet Gynecol 1993;81: 507–11.

[103] Cetin A, Cetin M. Diagnostic and therapeutic decision-making with transvaginal sonography for first trimester spontaneous abortion, clinically thought to be incomplete or complete. Contraception 1998;57:393–7.

[104] Keogan MT, Hertzberg BS, Kliewer MA. Low resistance Doppler waveforms with retained products of conception: potential for diagnostic confusion with gestational trophoblastic disease. Eur J Radiol 1995;21:109–11.

[105] Dillon EH, Feyock AL, Taylor KJ. Pseudogestational sacs: Doppler US differentiation from normal or abnormal intrauterine pregnancies. Radiology 1990;176:359–64.

[106] Alcazar JL. Transvaginal ultrasonography combined with color velocity imaging and pulsed Doppler to detect residual trophoblastic tissue. Ultrasound Obstet Gynecol 1998;11:54–8.

[107] Dillon EH, Case CQ, Ramos IM, et al. Endovaginal US and Doppler findings after first-trimester abortion. Radiology 1993;186:87–91.

[108] Warner MA, Fleischer AC, Edell SL, et al. Uterine adnexal torsion: sonographic findings. Radiology 1985;154:773–5.

[109] Lee EJ, Kwon HC, Joo HJ, et al. Diagnosis of ovarian torsion with color Doppler sonography: depiction of twisted vascular pedicle. J Ultrasound Med 1998;17:83–9.

[110] Graif M, Itzchak Y. Sonographic evaluation of ovarian torsion in childhood and adolescence. AJR Am J Roentgenol 1988;150:647–9.

[111] Pellerito JS, Troiano RN, Quedens-Case C, et al. Common pitfalls of endovaginal color Doppler flow imaging. Radiographics 1995;15:37–47.

[112] Vijayaraghavan SB. Sonographic whirlpool sign in ovarian torsion. J Ultrasound Med 2004;23: 1643–9.

[113] Pracros JP, Sann L, Genin G, et al. Ultrasound diagnosis of midgut volvulus: the "whirlpool" sign. Pediatr Radiol 1992;22:18–20.

[114] Shimanuki Y, Aihara T, Takano H, et al. Clockwise whirlpool sign at color Doppler US: an objective and definite sign of midgut volvulus. Radiology 1996;199:261–4.

[115] Albayram F, Hamper UM. Ovarian and adnexal torsion: spectrum of sonographic findings with pathologic correlation. J Ultrasound Med 2001; 20:1083–9.

[116] Fleischer AC, Stein SM, Cullinan JA, et al. Color Doppler sonography of adnexal torsion. J Ultrasound Med 1995;14:523–8.

[117] Brown JM, Taylor KJ, Alderman JL, et al. Contrast-enhanced ultrasonographic visualization of gonadal torsion. J Ultrasound Med 1997; 16:309–16.

[118] Beyth Y, Bar-On E. Tuboovarian autoamputation and infertility. Fertil Steril 1984;42:932–4.

[119] Shalev J, Mashiach R, Bar-Hava I, et al. Sub-torsion of the ovary: sonographic features and clinical management. J Ultrasound Med 2001; 20:849–54.

[120] Chiang G, Levine D. Imaging of adnexal masses in pregnancy. J Ultrasound Med 2004;23:805–19.

[121] Cacciatore B, Stenman UH, Ylostalo P. Early screening for ectopic pregnancy in high-risk symptom-free women. Lancet 1994;343:517–8.

[122] Braffman BH, Coleman BG, Ramchandani P, et al. Emergency department screening for ectopic pregnancy: a prospective US study. Radiology 1994;190:797–802.

[123] Atri M, Leduc C, Gillett P, et al. Role of endovaginal sonography in the diagnosis and management of ectopic pregnancy [discussion 775]. Radiographics 1996;16:755–74.

[124] Stein MW, Ricci ZJ, Novak L, et al. Sonographic comparison of the tubal ring of ectopic pregnancy with the corpus luteum. J Ultrasound Med 2004;23:57–62.

[125] Atri M. Ectopic pregnancy versus corpus luteum cyst revisited: best Doppler predictors. J Ultrasound Med 2003;22:1181–4.

[126] Atri M, Chow CM, Kintzen G, et al. Expectant treatment of ectopic pregnancies: clinical and sonographic predictors. AJR Am J Roentgenol 2001;176:123–7.

[127] Parvey HR, Dubinsky TJ, Johnston DA, et al. The chorionic rim and low-impedance intrauterine arterial flow in the diagnosis of early intrauterine pregnancy: evaluation of efficacy. AJR Am J Roentgenol 1996;167:1479–85.

[128] Wherry KL, Dubinsky TJ, Waitches GM, et al. Low-resistance endometrial arterial flow in the exclusion of ectopic pregnancy revisited. J Ultrasound Med 2001;20:335–42.

[129] Prieto-Nieto MI, Perez-Robledo JP, Rodriguez-Montes JA, et al. Acute appendicitis-like symptoms as initial presentation of ovarian vein thrombosis. Ann Vasc Surg 2004;18:481–3.

[130] Grant TH, Schoettle BW, Buchsbaum MS. Postpartum ovarian vein thrombosis: diagnosis by clot protrusion into the inferior vena cava at sonography. AJR Am J Roentgenol 1993;160: 551–2.

[131] Kurjak A, Zalud I, Alfirevic Z. Evaluation of adnexal masses with transvaginal color ultrasound. J Ultrasound Med 1991;10:295–7.

[132] Weiner Z, Thaler I, Beck D, et al. Differentiating malignant from benign ovarian tumors with transvaginal color flow imaging. Obstet Gynecol 1992;79:159–62.

[133] Hamper UM, Sheth S, Abbas FM, et al. Transvaginal color Doppler sonography of adnexal masses: differences in blood flow impedance in benign and malignant lesions. AJR Am J Roentgenol 1993;160:1225–8.

[134] Brown DL, Frates MC, Laing FC, et al. Ovarian masses: can benign and malignant lesions be differentiated with color and pulsed Doppler US? Radiology 1994;190:333–6.

[135] Fleischer AC, Rodgers WH, Kepple DM, et al. Color Doppler sonography of ovarian masses: a multiparameter analysis. J Ultrasound Med 1993;12:41–8.

[136] Shaharabany Y, Akselrod S, Tepper R. A sensitive new indicator for diagnostics of ovarian malignancy, based on the Doppler velocity spectrum. Ultrasound Med Biol 2004;30:295–302.

[137] Fleischer AC, Cullinan JA, Kepple DM, et al. Conventional and color Doppler transvaginal sonography of pelvic masses: a comparison of relative histologic specificities. J Ultrasound Med 1993;12:705–12.

[138] Kinkel K, Hricak H, Lu Y, et al. US characterization of ovarian masses: a meta-analysis. Radiology 2000;217:803–11.

[139] Jain KA. Prospective evaluation of adnexal masses with endovaginal gray-scale and duplex and color Doppler US: correlation with pathologic findings. Radiology 1994;191:63–7.

[140] Reles A, Wein U, Lichtenegger W. Transvaginal color Doppler sonography and conventional sonography in the preoperative assessment of adnexal masses. J Clin Ultrasound 1997;25: 217–25.

[141] Marret H, Sauget S, Giraudeau B, et al. Contrast-enhanced sonography helps in discrimination of benign from malignant adnexal masses. J Ultrasound Med 2004;23:1629–39.

[142] Orden MR, Gudmundsson S, Kirkinen P. Contrast-enhanced sonography in the examination of benign and malignant adnexal masses. J Ultrasound Med 2000;19:783–8.

[143] Orden MR, Jurvelin JS, Kirkinen PP. Kinetics of a US contrast agent in benign and malignant adnexal tumors. Radiology 2003;226:405–10.

ULTRASOUND
CLINICS

Ultrasound Clin 1 (2006) 223–230

Index

Note: Page numbers of article titles are in **boldface** type.

doi:10.1016/S1556-858X(05)00038-1